A GUIDE TO
RADIOLOGICAL
PROCEDURES

For Elsevier:

Commissioning Editor: Timothy Horne
Development Editor: Lulu Stader
Project Manager: Kerrie-Anne McKinlay
Designer/Design Direction: Kirsteen Wright
Illustrator: David Gardner

CHAPMAN & NAKIELNY

A GUIDE TO RADIOLOGICAL PROCEDURES

FIFTH EDITION

Edited by

Frances Aitchison MB, ChB, FRCP, FRCR
Consultant Radiologist,
City Hospital, Birmingham,
Honorary Senior Clinical Lecturer,
University of Birmingham, Birmingham, UK

FOURTH EDITION

Edited by

Stephen Chapman MBBS, MRCS, FRCP, FRCPCH, FRCR
Consultant Paediatric Radiologist,
Diana, Princess of Wales Children's Hospital,
Birmingham Children's Hospital NHS Trust, Birmingham,
Honorary Senior Clinical Lecturer, University of Birmingham,
Birmingham, UK

Richard Nakielny MA, BM, BCh, FRCR
Consultant Radiologist (CT Scanning),
Royal Hallamshire Hospital, Sheffield,
Honorary Clinical Lecturer, University of Sheffield,
Sheffield, UK

Edinburgh • London • New York • Oxford • Philadelphia •
St Louis • Sydney • Toronto 2009

SAUNDERS

ELSEVIER

First published 2001

ISBN: 9780702029820

British Library Cataloguing in Publication Data
A catalogue record for this book is available from the British Library

Library of Congress Cataloging in Publication Data
A catalog record for this book is available from the Library of Congress

Notice
Knowledge and best practice in this field are constantly changing. As new research and experience broaden our knowledge, changes in practice, treatment and drug therapy may become necessary or appropriate. Readers are advised to check the most current information provided (i) on procedures featured or (ii) by the manufacturer of each product to be administered, to verify the recommended dose or formula, the method and duration of administration, and contraindications. It is the responsibility of the practitioner, relying on their own experience and knowledge of the patient, to make diagnoses, to determine dosages and the best treatment for each individual patient, and to take all appropriate safety precautions. To the fullest extent of the law, neither the Publisher nor the Editors assume any liability for any injury and/or damage to persons or property arising out or related to any use of the material contained in this book.

The Publisher

ELSEVIER your source for books, journals and multimedia in the health sciences

www.elsevierhealth.com

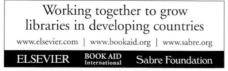

Working together to grow libraries in developing countries

www.elsevier.com | www.bookaid.org | www.sabre.org

ELSEVIER   BOOK AID International   Sabre Foundation

The Publisher's policy is to use **paper manufactured from sustainable forests**

Printed in China

Preface

During the 7 years since the previous edition of this book on radiological procedures was published, there have been considerable changes in technology and intravenous contrast media which have altered everyday radiological practice. These changes include increased use of magnetic resonance imaging (MRI) contrast, the introduction of iso-osmolar contrast media and increasing sophistication of cross-sectional imaging equipment, which has rendered obsolete some of the procedures previously included. Re-reading the preface to the second edition, which I used as a trainee, it is clear that similar changes occurred between the first and second editions of the book: low osmolar contrast media had just become widely available for clinical use at that time and the techniques which were becoming obsolete included air encephalography. It was, therefore, both an honour and a challenge to edit the fifth edition of the text.

The aim of the book is to build on the successful format established by Steve Chapman and Richard Nakielny in the first four editions and produce a current, practical and concise guide to radiological procedures. I was extremely fortunate that two of the contributors to the previous edition agreed to update or re-write sections of the book. Several new contributors have revised or re-written chapters about which they have subspecialty knowledge and three new chapters have been added: breast procedures, sedation and monitoring and medical emergencies in the radiology department.

In this project I was helped by other specialist colleagues who generously gave advice: Teri Millane and Alp Notghi with Chapter 8, Swarup Chavda with Chapters 15 and 16, Laura Wilkinson with Chapter 17 and Katharine Foster with the Paediatric text throughout the book.

Heartfelt thanks also go to Lulu Stader, the publishing editor, for her encouragement, patience and persistence.

F. Aitchison
Birmingham 2008

Dedication

For Rebecca and Emma

Contributors

The numbers in brackets refer to the chapters written or co-written by the contributor.

J.F.C. Olliff MRCP, FRCR, FBIR
[3, 4, 5, 6]
Consultant Radiologist
Queen Elizabeth Hospital
Birmingham
Senior Clinical Lecturer
University of Birmingham

F.M. Bryden FRCP, FRCR
[7, 8]
Consultant Radiologist
Stobhill Hospital
Glasgow
Senior Clinical Lecturer
University of Glasgow

M.S. Moss MRCP, FRCR
[9, 10]
Consultant Radiologist
City Hospital
Birmingham

P.J. Guest FRCP, FRCR
[11 and all nuclear medicine text]
Consultant Radiologist
Queen Elizabeth Hospital
Birmingham
Senior Clinical Lecturer
University of Birmingham

V. Cassar-Pullicino FRCR
[12, 14]
Consultant Radiologist
Robert Jones and Agnes Hunt Hospital
Oswestry
Senior Clinical Lecturer
University of Birmingham

A.C. Thomas DM, FRCR, MSc
[13]
Consultant Radiologist
Queens Medical Centre
Nottingham
Senior Clinical Lecturer
University of Nottingham

H.M. Dobson FRCP, FRCR
[17]
Consultant Radiologist
West Scotland Breast Screening Service
Glasgow
Senior Clinical Lecturer
University of Glasgow

Z.P. Khan DA, FRCA
[18, 19]
Consultant Anaesthetist
City Hospital
Birmingham
Senior Clinical Lecturer
University of Birmingham

Contents

Contents

Contents

Contents

General notes

RADIOLOGY

The procedures are laid out under a number of sub-headings, which follow a standard sequence. The general order is outlined below, together with certain points that have been omitted from the discussion of each procedure in order to avoid repetition. Minor deviations from this sequence will be found in the text where this is felt to be more appropriate.

Methods
A description of the technique for each procedure.

Indications
Appropriate clinical reasons for using each procedure.

Contraindications
All radiological procedures carry a risk. The risk incurred by undertaking the procedure must be balanced against the benefit to the patient as deduced from the information obtained. Contraindications may be relative (the majority) or absolute. Factors that increase the risk to the patient can be categorized under three headings: due to radiation; due to the contrast medium; due to the technique.

Risk due to radiation
Radiation effects on humans may be:

1. hereditary, i.e. revealed in the offspring of the exposed individual, or
2. somatic injuries, which fall into two groups: stochastic and deterministic. The latter, e.g. skin erythema and cataracts, occur when a critical threshold has been reached and are rarely relevant to diagnostic radiology. Stochastic effects, such as malignancy, are 'all or none'. The cancer produced by a small

dose is the same as the cancer produced by a large dose, but the frequency of its appearance is less with the smaller dose. The current consensus held by national and international radiological protection organizations is that, for comparatively low doses, the risk of both radiation-induced cancer and hereditary disease is assumed to increase linearly with increasing radiation dose, with no threshold (the so-called linear no threshold model).[1] It is impossible to totally avoid staff and patient exposure to radiation. The adverse effects of radiation, therefore, cannot be completely eliminated, but must be minimized. There is an excess of cancers following diagnostic levels of irradiation to the fetus[2] and the female breast,[3] and trends of increased rates of cancer are seen in workers in the nuclear power industry exposed to low doses.[4] In the United Kingdom about 0.6% of the overall cumulative risk of cancer by the age of 75 years could be attributable to diagnostic X-rays. This percentage is equivalent to about 700 new cases of cancer per year.[5]

There are legal regulations which guide the use of diagnostic radiation (see Appendix I). These are the basic principles:

1. *Justification* that a proposed examination is of net benefit to the patient.
2. *ALARP* – doses should be kept *As Low As Reasonably Practicable*; economic and social factors being taken into account.[6]

Justification is particularly important when considering the irradiation of women of reproductive age, because of the risks to the developing fetus. The mammalian embryo and fetus are highly radiosensitive. The potential effects of in-utero radiation exposure on a developing fetus include prenatal death, intrauterine growth restriction, small head size, mental retardation, organ malformation and childhood cancer. The risk of each effect depends on the gestational age at the time of the exposure and the absorbed radiation dose.[2] Most diagnostic radiation procedures will lead to a fetal absorbed dose of less than 1 mGy for imaging beyond the maternal abdomen/pelvis and less than 10 mGy for direct abdominal/pelvic or nuclear medicine imaging.[7] There are important exceptions which result in higher doses. Computed tomography (CT) scanning of the maternal pelvis may result in fetal doses below the level thought to induce neurologic detriment to the fetus, but, theoretically, may double the fetal risk for developing a childhood cancer.[8]

Almost always, if a diagnostic radiology examination is medically indicated, the risk to the mother of not doing the procedure is greater than the risk of potential harm to the fetus.[9] However, whenever possible, alternative investigation techniques not involving ionizing radiation should be considered before a decision is taken to use ionizing radiation in a female of reproductive age. It is extremely important to have a robust process in place that prevents inappropriate or unnecessary ionizing radiation exposure to the fetus. Previous guidelines recommended that all non-emergency examinations that would involve irradiation of the lower abdomen or pelvis in women of child-bearing age be restricted to the first 10 days (10-day rule) or 28 days (28-day rule) following the onset of a menstrual period.[10] This led to some potential practical difficulties, e.g. for women who denied recent sexual intercourse, for those with an irregular menstrual cycle or for those who had been taking the oral contraceptive pill. There are also concerns:

- about the safety of irradiation of the unfertilized ovum during the first part of the menstrual cycle, which may be as hazardous as irradiation of the conceptus
- that, although it had been thought that a damaging radiation dose to the fetus in the first few weeks of pregnancy would result in miscarriage, evidence exists that some carcinogenic mutations are compatible with continuing development of the fetus[10]
- that the most sensitive fetal gestational age might be the 4th to 8th week after conception when organogenesis takes place. Therefore, irradiation after conception but before the next expected menstrual cycle may be less damaging to organogenesis.

Joint guidance from the National Radiological Protection Board, the College of Radiographers and the Royal College of Radiologists recommends the following:[11]

When a female of reproductive age presents for an examination in which the primary beam irradiates the pelvic area, or for a procedure involving radioactive isotopes, she should be asked whether she is or might be pregnant. If the patient cannot exclude the possibility of pregnancy, she should be asked if her menstrual period is overdue. Her answer should be recorded and, depending on the answer, the patient assigned to one of the following four groups:

1. **No possibility of pregnancy** – proceed with the examination.
2. **Patient definitely, or probably, pregnant** – review the justification for the proposed examination and decide whether to defer until after delivery, bearing in mind that delaying an essential procedure until later in pregnancy may present a greater risk to the fetus.
3. **Low-dose examination, pregnancy cannot be excluded** – proceed with the examination provided that the period is not overdue. If the period is overdue, follow the advice in the section above.
4. **High-dose examination, pregnancy cannot be excluded** – either apply the 10-day rule or re-book patients who attend for such examinations and are identified to be in the second half of their menstrual cycle, of child-bearing age and in whom pregnancy cannot be excluded.

If the examination is necessary, a technique that minimizes the number of views and the absorbed dose per examination should be utilized. However, the quality of the examination should not be reduced to the level where its diagnostic value is impaired. The risk to the patient of an incorrect diagnosis may be greater than the risk of irradiating the fetus. Radiography of areas that are remote from the pelvis and abdomen may be safely performed at any time during pregnancy with good collimation and lead protection.

Risk due to the contrast medium

The risks associated with administration of iodinated contrast media and magnetic resonance imaging (MRI) contrast are discussed in detail in Chapter 2 and guidelines are given for prophylaxis of adverse reactions to intravascular contrast.

Contraindications to other contrast media, e.g. barium, water-soluble contrast media for the gastrointestinal tract and biliary contrast media, are given in the relevant sections.

Risks due to the technique

Skin sepsis can occur at the needle puncture site.

Specific contraindications to individual techniques are discussed with each procedure.

Contrast medium

Volumes given are for a 70 kg man.

Equipment

For many procedures this will also include a trolley with a sterile upper shelf and a non-sterile lower shelf. Emergency drugs and resuscitation equipment should be readily available (see Chapter 17).

See Chapter 9 for introductory notes on angiography catheters.

If only a simple radiography table and overcouch tube are required, then this information has been omitted from the text.

Patient preparation

1. Will admission to hospital be necessary?
2. If the patient is a woman of child-bearing age, the examination should be performed at a time when the risks to a possible fetus are minimal (see above). Any female presenting for radiography or a nuclear medicine examination at a time when her period is known to be overdue should be considered to be pregnant unless there is information indicating the absence of pregnancy. If her cycle is so irregular that it is difficult to know whether a period has been missed and it is not practicable to defer the examination until menstruation occurs, then a pregnancy test or pelvic ultrasound (US) examination may help to determine whether she is pregnant. The '10-day rule' should still apply for

hysterosalpingography, so that the risks of mechanical trauma to an early pregnancy are reduced.

3. Except in emergencies, in circumstances when consent cannot be obtained, patient consent to treatment is a legal requirement for medical care.[12] Consent should be obtained in a suitable environment and only after appropriate and relevant information has been given to the patient.[13] Patient consent may be:

   a. implied consent – for a very low-risk procedure, the patient's actions at the time of the examination will indicate whether they are content for the procedure to be performed

   b. express consent – for a procedure of intermediate risk, such as barium enema, express consent should be given by the patient, either verbally or in writing

   c. written consent – must be obtained for any procedure that involves significant risk and/or side-effects.

   The radiologist must assess a child's capacity to decide whether to give consent for or refuse an investigation. At age 16 years a young person can be treated as an adult and can be presumed to have the capacity to understand the nature, purpose and possible consequences of the proposed investigation, as well as the consequences of non-investigation. Following case law in the United Kingdom (Gillick v West Norfolk and Wisbech Area Health Authority) and the introduction of The Children Act 1989, in which the capacity of children to consent has been linked with the concept of individual ability to understand the implications of medical treatment, there has come into existence a standard known as 'Gillick competence'. Under the age of 16 years children may have the capacity to consent depending on their maturity and ability to understand what is involved. When a competent child refuses treatment, a person with parental responsibility or the court may authorize investigations or treatment which is in the child's best interests. In Scotland the situation is different: parents cannot authorize procedures a competent child has refused. Legal advice may be helpful in dealing with these cases.[14]

4. If an interventional procedure carries a risk of causing bleeding then the patient's blood clotting should be measured before proceeding. If a bleeding disorder is discovered, or if the patient is being treated with anticoagulant therapy, the appropriate steps should be taken to normalize clotting before performing the procedure.

5. Cleansing bowel preparation may be used prior to investigation of the gastrointestinal tract or when considerable faecal loading obscures other intra-abdominal organs. For other radiological investigations of abdominal organs, bowel preparation is not always necessary, and when given may result in excessive bowel

gas. Bowel gas may be reduced if the patient is kept ambulant prior to the examination and those who routinely take laxatives should continue to do so.

6. Previous films and notes should be obtained.
7. Premedication will be necessary for painful procedures or where the patient is unlikely to cooperate for any other reason. Suggested premedication for adults and children is described in Chapter 18.

Preliminary film

The purpose of these films is:

1. to make any final adjustments in exposure factors, centering, collimation and patient position, for which purpose the film should always be taken using the same equipment as will be used for the remainder of the procedure
2. to exclude prohibitive factors such as residual barium from a previous examination or excessive faecal loading
3. to demonstrate, identify and localize opacities which may be obscured by contrast medium
4. to elicit radiological physical signs.

Every radiographic view taken should have on it the patient's name, registration number, date and a side marker. The examination can only proceed if satisfactory preliminary films have been obtained.

Technique

1. For aseptic technique the skin is cleaned with chlorhexidine 0.5% in 70% industrial spirit or its equivalent.
2. The local anaesthetic used is lidocaine 1% without adrenaline (epinephrine).
3. Gonad protection is used whenever possible, unless it obscures the region of interest.

Films

When films are taken during the procedure rather than at the end of it, they have, for convenience, been described under 'Technique'.

Additional techniques *or* modifications of technique
Aftercare

May be considered as:

1. instructions to the patient
2. instructions to the ward.

Complications

Complications may be considered under the following three headings:

Due to the anaesthetic
1. General anaesthesia
2. Local anaesthesia:
   a. allergic – unusual
   b. toxic.

Anaesthetic lozenges contribute to the total dose. Symptoms are of paraesthesia and muscle twitching which may progress to convulsions, cardiac arrhythmias, respiratory depression and death due to cardiac arrest. Treatment is symptomatic and includes adequate oxygenation.

Due to the contrast medium
Intravascular contrast media (see Chapter 2)
Barium (see Chapter 3).

Due to the technique
Specific details are given with the individual procedures and may be conveniently classified as:
1. local
2. distant or generalized.

References
1. Wall, B.F., Kendall, G.M., Edwards, A.A., et al. (2006) What are the risks from medical X-rays and other low dose radiation? *Br. J. Radiol.* **79(940)**, 285–294.
2. McCollough, C.H., Scheuler, B.A., Atwell, T.D., et al. (2007) Radiation exposure and pregnancy: when should we be concerned? *Radiographics* **27(4)**, 909–917.
3. Einstein, A.J., Henzlova, M.J. & Rajagopalan, S. (2007) Estimating risk of cancer associated with radiation exposure from 64-slice computed tomography coronary angiography. *JAMA* **298(3)**, 317–323.
4. Cardis, E., Vrijheid, M., Blettner, M., et al. (2007) The 15-Country Collaborative Study of Cancer Risk among Radiation Workers in the Nuclear Industry: estimates of radiation-related cancer risks. *Radiat. Res.* **167(4)**, 396–416.
5. Berrington de González, A. & Darby, S. (2004) Risk of cancer from diagnostic X-rays: estimates from the UK and 14 other countries. *Lancet* **363 (9406)**, 345–351.
6. International Commission on Radiological Protection. (2006) The optimization of radiological protection: broadening the process. ICRP publication 101. *Ann. ICRP* **36(3)**.
7. Lowe, S.A. (2004) Diagnostic radiography in pregnancy: risks and reality. *Aust. N. Z. J. Obstet. Gynaecol.* **44(3)**, 191–196.
8. Hurwitz, L.M., Yoshizumi, T., Reiman, R.E., et al. (2006) Radiation dose to the fetus from body MDCT during early gestation. *Am. J. Roentgenol.* **186 (3)**, 871–876.
9. International Commission on Radiological Protection (2000) Pregnancy and medical radiation. IRCP publication 84. *Ann. ICRP* **30(1)**, 1–43.

10. Bury, B., Hufton, A. & Adams, J. (1995) Editorial. Radiation and women of childbearing potential. *BMJ* **310**, 1022–1023.
11. Sharp, C., Shrimpton, J.A. & Bury, R.F. (1998) *Diagnostic Medical Exposures: Advice on Exposure to Ionising Radiation during Pregnancy.* London: National Radiological Protection Board.
12. The Royal College of Radiologists (2005) *Standards for Patient Consent Particular to Radiology.* London: The Royal College of Radiologists.
13. General Medical Council (2008) *Consent: Patients and Doctors Making Decisions Together.* London: General Medical Council.
14. General Medical Council (2007) *0–18 years: Guidance for all Doctors.* London: General Medical Council.

RADIONUCLIDE IMAGING

RADIOPHARMACEUTICALS

Radionuclides are shown in symbolic notation, the most frequently used in nuclear medicine being ^{99m}Tc, a 140-keV gamma-emitting radioisotope of the element technetium with $T_{1/2} = 6.0$ hours.

Radioactive injections

In the UK, the Administration of Radioactive Substances Advisory Committee (ARSAC) advises the health ministers on the Medicines (Administration of Radioactive Substances) Regulations 1978 (MARS). These require that radioactive materials may only be administered to humans by a doctor or dentist holding a current ARSAC certificate or by a person acting under their direction. Administration of radioactive substances can only be carried out by an individual who has received appropriate theoretical and practical training, as specified in the Ionising Radiation (Medical Exposure) Regulations 2000[1] (see Appendix III). These will place responsibilities on the referrer to provide medical data to justify the exposure, the practitioner (ARSAC licence holder) to justify individual exposure, and operators (persons who carry out practical aspects relating to the exposure).

Activity administered

The maximum activity values quoted in the text are those currently recommended as diagnostic reference levels in the ARSAC Guidance Notes.[2] The unit used is the SI unit, the megabecquerel (MBq). Millicuries (mCi) are still used in some countries, notably the US; 1 mCi = 37 MBq.

Radiation doses are quoted as the adult effective dose (ED) in millisieverts (mSv) from the ARSAC Guidance Notes.

The regulations require that doses to patients are kept as low as reasonably practicable (the ALARP principle) and that exposure follows accepted practice. Centres will frequently be able to administer activities below the maximum, depending upon the capabilities of their equipment and local protocols. Typical figures are given in the text where they differ from the diagnostic reference levels. In certain circumstances, the person clinically directing (ARSAC licence holder) may use activity higher than the recommended maximum for a named patient, for example for an obese patient where attenuation would otherwise degrade image quality.

ARSAC recommends that activities administered for paediatric investigations should be reduced according to body weight, but no longer in a linear relationship. The guidance notes include a table of suggested scaling factors based on producing comparable quality images to those expected for adults, with a minimum activity of 10% of the adult value for most purposes. However, organs develop at different rates (e.g. the brain achieves 95% of its adult size by age 5 years) and some radiopharmaceuticals behave differently in children, so the administered activity may need to be adjusted accordingly. It should be noted that when scaling activity according to the suggested factors, the radiation dose for a child may be higher than that for an adult.

Equipment

Gamma cameras usually have one or two imaging heads. Double-headed systems have the advantage of being able to image two sites simultaneously, which in many cases can roughly halve the imaging time. This can be a great advantage for SPECT (single-photon emission computed tomography) scans where minimizing patient movement can be critical.

Recent developments on double-headed systems include transmission line sources for measured attenuation correction, and coincidence imaging systems for PET (positron emission tomography). Hybrid systems are now available where multislice CT forms part of an integrated system as a single machine with either a double-headed gamma camera (CT-SPECT) or a PET scanner (CT-PET). Amongst a number of advantages is the better anatomical localization of abnormal areas of activity on co-registered or fused images.

All gamma cameras are now supplied with imaging computer systems, and the text assumes that all images are acquired by the computer for appropriate processing.

Technique

Patient positioning

The resolution of gamma camera images is critically dependent upon the distance of the collimator surface from the patient, falling off approximately linearly with distance. Every effort should, there-fore, be made to position the camera as close to the patient as possi-ble. For example, in posterior imaging with the patient supine, the thickness of the bed separates the patient from the camera, as well as interposing an attenuating medium. In this case, imaging with the patient sitting or standing directly against the camera is preferable.

Patient immobilization for the duration of image acquisition is very important. If a patient is uncomfortable or awkwardly posi-tioned, they will have a tendency to move gradually and perhaps imperceptibly, which will have a blurring effect on the image. Point marker sources attached to the patient away from areas being exam-ined can help to monitor and possibly permit correction for move-ment artefact.

'Oldendorf' bolus injection[3]

For some investigations the Oldendorf technique is recommended to provide an abrupt bolus:

1. Place a butterfly needle (20 G or larger) in the antecubital vein.
2. Attach to a three-way tap connected to two syringes, one containing 10 ml of saline and the other the radiopharmaceutical in a small volume (<1 ml).
3. Place a blood-pressure cuff on the arm and inflate to below diastolic pressure for about 1 min to suffuse veins.
4. Inflate above systolic pressure for 1–2 min to provoke reactive hyperaemia when cuff is released.
5. Inject radionuclide.
6. Release cuff and flush with saline.

Images

The image acquisition times quoted in the text should only be con-sidered an approximate guide since the appropriate time will depend upon such factors as the sensitivity of the available equipment, the amount of activity injected and the size of the patient. An acceptable acquisition time will usually be a compromise between the time available, the counts required for a diagnostic image and the ability of the patient to remain motionless.

Aftercare

Radiation safety

Special instructions should be given to patients who are breast feed-ing regarding expression of milk and interruption of feeding.[2] Precautions may have to be taken with patients leaving hospital or returning to wards, depending upon the radionuclide and activity administered. These precautions were reviewed following the in-troduction of the Ionising Radiation Regulations 1999 and the adoption of lower dose limits to members of the public, and appropriate guidance has been published.[4]

Complications

With few exceptions (noted in the text), the amount of biologically active substance injected with radionuclide investigations is at trace levels and very rarely causes any systemic reactions. Those that may occasionally cause problems are labelled blood products, antibodies and substances of a particulate nature.

References

1. *The Ionising Radiation (Medical Exposure) Regulations* 2000. London: HMSO.
2. Administration of Radioactive Substances Advisory Committee (1998) *Notes for Guidance on the Clinical Administration of Radiopharmaceuticals and use of Sealed Radioactive Sources.* Didcot: NRPB.
3. Oldendorf, W.H., Kitano, M. & Shimizu, S. (1965) Evaluation of a simple technique for abrupt intravenous injection of radioisotope. *J. Nucl. Med.* **6**, 205–209.
4. Working Party of the Radiation Protection Committee of the British Institute of Radiology (1999) Patients leaving hospital after administration of radioactive substances. *Br. J. Radiol.* **72**, 121–125.

COMPUTED TOMOGRAPHY

Patient preparation

Many CT examinations require little physical preparation. An explanation of the procedure, the time it is likely to take, the necessity for immobility and the necessity for breath-holding whilst scanning chest and abdomen should be given. Waiting times should be kept to a minimum, as a long wait may increase anxiety. The patient should be as pain-free as is practical but too heavy sedation or analgesia may be counter-productive – patient cooperation is often required. Children under the age of 4 years will usually need sedation; please see Chapter 18. Children should also have an intravenous (i.v.) cannula inserted at the time sedation is administered or local anaesthetic cream applied to two sites if i.v. contrast medium is needed. If these simple steps are taken, the number of aborted scans will be reduced and the resultant image quality improved.

Intravenous contrast medium

Many CT examinations will require i.v. contrast medium. Essential information should be obtained from the patient and appropriate guidelines followed (see Chapter 2). An explanation of the need for contrast enhancement should be given to the patient.

The dose of contrast (using $300\,mg\,I\,ml^{-1}$) will depend on the area examined: e.g. head – 50 ml; chest or abdomen – 100 ml, usually given at $2\,ml\,s^{-1}$. The chest is usually scanned at 20 s after the start of the contrast injection. For arterial phase images of the abdomen or pelvis the acquisition of the scan is usually begun 30 s after the start of the contrast injection and for portal venous phase images 60 s after the start of the contrast injection. For CT angiography, a technique of bolus tracking may be used where the density of contrast in the vessel is monitored directly during the injection to allow optimum acquisition timing. In children a maximum total iodinated contrast dose of $2\,ml\,kg^{-1}$ body weight $(300\,mg\,I\,ml^{-1})$ should be observed.

Oral contrast medium

For examinations of the abdomen, opacifying the bowel satisfactorily can be problematic. Water-soluble contrast medium (e.g. 20 ml Urografin 150 diluted in 1 l of orange squash to disguise the taste, preflavoured contrast such as 20 ml Gastromiro diluted in 1 l of water) or low-density barium suspensions (2% w/v) can be used. Timing of administration is given in Table 1.1. Doses of contrast media in children depend upon age.

Pelvic scanning

Rarely, it may be necessary to opacify the rectum using direct instillation of contrast medium or air via catheter. The concentration of contrast medium should be the same as for oral administration; 150 ml is adequate. Vaginal tampons may also be used. The air trapped by the tampon produces good negative contrast.

CT colonography

This requires thorough cleansing preparation of the large bowel and insufflation of air via a rectal catheter to adequately distend the colon during the examination.

Table 1.1 Timing and volume for oral contrast medium in CT

	Volume (ml)	Time before scan (min)
Adult		
Full abdomen and pelvis	1000	Gradually over 1 h before scanning
Upper abdomen, e.g. pancreas	500	Gradually over 0.5 h before scanning
Child		
Newborn	60–90	Full dose 1 h before scanning and a further half dose immediately prior to the scan
1 month–1 year	120–240	
1–5 years	240–360	
5–10 years	360–480	
Over 10 years	As for adult	
If the large bowel needs to be opacified then give the contrast medium the night before or 3–4 h before scanning		

MAGNETIC RESONANCE IMAGING

Patient preparation

As for CT scanning, a full description of the purpose and nature of the examination should be given to the patient and waiting times kept to a minimum. Some patients find the interior of the scanner a very disconcerting environment, and report claustrophobic and even acute anxiety symptoms. This may occur in as many as 10% of patients. Most of these patients are able to complete their examination, but approximately 1% of investigations may have to be curtailed as a result. To decrease the number of scans aborted, the counselling, explanation to and reassurance of patients by well-trained staff should be routine. A small number of adult patients may require sedation before an MRI scan is undertaken. Sedation or general anaesthesia are often required for MRI scans in young children; details of suggested protocols are given in Chapter 18.

If i.v. contrast is required it is extremely helpful to insert the i.v. cannula before the examination begins. It is critically important that detailed preparation regarding patient safety is made for each MRI examination.

SAFETY IN MAGNETIC RESONANCE IMAGING

MRI has generally been a very safe process because of the care taken by equipment manufacturers and MRI staff. However, there are significant potential hazards[1] to patients and staff due to:

1. magnetic fields:
   a. static field
   b. gradient field
   c. radiofrequency field
2. the auditory effects of noise
3. inert gas quench
4. claustrophobia
5. i.v. contrast agents (see Chapter 2).

Effects due to magnetic fields

Static field

The strength of the static magnetic field used in MRI is measured in units of gauss or tesla (10000 gauss = 1 tesla (T)). The earth's magnetic field is approximately 0.6 gauss. Current guidelines on MRI field strength are given in Table 1.2.

Biological effects

Despite extensive research, no significant deleterious physiological effects have been proven. There have been reports of minor changes, such as alteration in electrocardiogram (T-wave elevation)[2] presumed to be due to electrodynamic forces on moving ions in blood vessels which might result in a reduction of blood-flow velocity. This change is purely temporary and disappears on removal from the field. Studies of volunteers exposed to 8 T static magnetic fields have shown no clinically significant effect on heart rate, respiratory rate, systolic and diastolic blood pressure, finger pulse oxygenation levels and core body temperature.[3] However, it was noted that movement within the 8 T field could cause vertigo. Teratogenesis in humans is thought unlikely at the field strengths used in clinical MRI.

Non-biological effects

There are two main areas of concern:

1. Ferromagnetic materials may undergo rotational or translational movement as a result of the field. Rotational movement occurs as a result of an elongated object trying to align with the field. This may result in displacement of the object, and applies to certain types of surgical clip. Not all materials implanted are ferromagnetic and many are only weakly so. Each type should be checked individually for any such risk. In many cases, post-operative fibrosis (greater than 6 weeks) is strong enough to anchor the material so that no danger of displacement exists. Translational movement occurs when loose ferromagnetic

Table 1.2 Guidelines on whole-body exposure to static magnetic fields[4]

Level	Magnetic field (T)
Normal operating mode	<2
First level operating mode (one or more outputs reach a value that may cause physiological stress and which requires medical supervision)	2–4
Second level operating mode (one or more outputs reach a value that may produce significant risk for patients, for which explicit ethical approval is required)	>4

objects are attracted to the field. Objects such as paperclips or hairgrips may reach considerable speeds and could potentially cause severe damage to patient or equipment. This is the so-called missile effect.

2. Electrical devices such as cardiac pacemakers may be affected by static field strengths as low as 5 gauss. Most modern pacemakers have a sensing mechanism that can be bypassed by a magnetically operated relay and this relay can be triggered by fields as low as 5 gauss. Relay closure can be expected in virtually all cardiac pacemakers placed in the bore of the magnet and these patients must not enter the controlled MRI area.

Gradient field
Biological effects
The rapidly switched magnetic gradients used in MRI can induce electric fields in a patient which may result in nerve or muscle stimulation, including cardiac muscle stimulation. The strength of these is dependent on the rate of change of the field and the size of the subject.[5] Studies have shown that the threshold for peripheral nerve stimulation is lower than that for cardiac or brain stimulation.[6] Although possible cardiac fibrillation or brain stimulation are major safety issues, peripheral nerve stimulation is a practical concern because, if sufficiently intense, it can be intolerable and result in termination of the examination. Recommendations for safety limits on gradient fields state that the system must not have a gradient output that exceeds the limit for peripheral nerve stimulation.[5] This will protect against cardiac fibrillation.

Non-biological effects
Rapidly varying fields can induce currents in conductors. Metal objects may heat up rapidly and cause tissue damage. Instances of

partial- and full-thickness burns, arising when conducting loops (e.g. ECG electrodes or surface imaging coils) have come into contact with skin, are well recorded.

Radiofrequency field

Radiofrequency energy at frequencies above 10 MHz, deposited in the body during an MRI examination, will be converted to heat, which will be distributed by connective heat transfer through blood flow. Energy deposited in this way is calculated as the average energy dissipated in the body per unit of mass and time, the specific absorption rate (SAR). Guidelines on radiofrequency exposure are designed to limit the rise in temperature of the skin, body core and local tissue to levels below those where systemic heat overload or thermal-induced local tissue damage occur. The extent to which local temperature rises depends on the SAR and on the blood flow and vascularity of the tissue. Areas of particular concern include those most sensitive to heat such as the hypothalamus and poorly perfused regions such as the lens of the eye.

For whole-body exposures, no adverse health effects are expected if the increase in body core temperature does not exceed 1°C. In the case of infants and those with circulatory impairment, the temperature increase should not exceed 0.5°C. With regard to localized heating temperatures, measured temperature in focal regions of the head should be less than 38°C, of the trunk less than 39°C, and in the limbs less than 40°C.[5]

Noise

During imaging, noise arises from vibration in the gradient coils and other parts of the scanner due to the varying magnetic fields. The amplitude of this noise depends on the strength of the magnetic fields, pulse sequence and scanner design.

Noise levels may reach as much as 95 dB for long periods of time. This level is greater than agreed noise limits in industry. Temporary or even permanent hearing loss has been reported.

Where noise levels are excessive the use of earplugs or headphones is advised.

Inert gas quench

Where superconducting magnets are used the coolant gases, liquid helium or nitrogen, could vaporize should the temperature inadvertently rise. This could potentially lead to asphyxiation or exposure to extreme cold resulting in frostbite. To prevent this, a well-ventilated room with some form of oxygen monitor to raise an alarm should be installed.

Intravenous contrast medium

See Chapter 2.

Recommendations for safety

Detailed MRI safety recommendations have been published by the American College of Radiology.[7] It is essential that all MRI units have clear MRI safety policies and protocols, including a detailed screening questionnaire for all patients and staff (Table 1.3).

Controlled and restricted access

Access to the scanning suite should be limited. Areas should be designated as restricted (5 gauss line) and, closer to the scanner, controlled (10 gauss line). No patient with a pacemaker should be allowed to enter the restricted area. Any person who enters this area should be made aware of the hazards; in particular the 'missile effect'. Any person entering the controlled area should remove all loose ferromagnetic materials, such as paperclips and pens, and it is advisable that wristwatches and any magnetic tape or credit cards do not come near the magnet. Other considerations include the use of specially adapted cleaning equipment, wheelchairs and

Table 1.3 Questions which should be included in a screening questionnaire for magnetic resonance imaging patients and staff

Question to patient or staff member	Action
Do you have a pacemaker or have you had a heart operation?	Pacemaker – if present patient must not enter controlled area. Heart operation – establish if any metal valve prosthesis, intravascular device or recent metallic surgical clip insertion and check MR compatibility.
Could you possibly be pregnant?	See text.
Have you ever had any penetrating injury, especially to the eyes, even if it was years ago?	Establish details. If necessary arrange X-ray of orbits or relevant area to determine if there is any metallic foreign body.
Have you ever had any operations to your head, chest or neck?	Find out details. If any metallic aneurysm or haemostatic clips or metallic prosthesis/implant then check MR compatibility.
Do you have any joint replacements or any other body implants?	Check details of surgery and MR compatibility of joint replacement or implant.
Have you removed all metal objects and credit cards from your clothing and possessions?	This must be done before entering the controlled area.

trolleys. Fire extinguishers and all anaesthetic or monitoring equipment must be constructed from non-ferromagnetic materials.

Implants

As mentioned above, persons with pacemakers must not enter the restricted area. All other persons must be screened to ensure there is no danger from implanted ferromagnetic objects, such as aneurysm clips, prosthetic heart valves, intravascular devices or orthopaedic implants. Where an object is not known to be 'magnet safe', then the person should not be scanned. Lists of safe and unsafe implants are available[8] and should be consulted for each individual object.

Specific questioning is also advisable to assess the risk of shrapnel and intraocular foreign body (Table 1.3).

Pregnancy

The developing fetus and embryo are susceptible to a variety of teratogens, including heat. Sensitivity varies during gestation and is usually greatest during organogenesis. Although no conclusive evidence of teratogenesis exists in humans, scanning should be avoided, particularly during the first trimester, unless alternative diagnostic procedures would involve the exposure of the fetus to ionizing radiation. Before a pregnant patient is accepted for an MRI examination, a risk–benefit analysis of the request should be made. Pregnant staff members are advised to remain outside the controlled area (10 gauss line) and to avoid exposure to gradient or RF fields.

MRI contrast agents should *not* be routinely administered to pregnant patients (see Chapter 2).

Occupational exposure

The safety of MRI workers is regulated by the EU Medical Devices Directive (amend. Direct 93/42/EEC) and established safety standards have been set by the International Electrotechnical Commission (IEC/EN 60601-2-33, 2nd amendment 2007).

MAGNETIC RESONANCE IMAGING SEQUENCES

During each MRI examination a series of radiofrequency events (pulses) and magnetic field gradient events (pulses) are applied to the patient that generate nuclear magnetic resonance signals. These signals are processed to produce the image. By varying the duration and timing of the radiofrequency and magnetic field gradient events, a huge range of possible pulse sequences is available which alters the form, speed and information content of the image. The appearance of tissues varies on each pulse sequence. By changing the technical factors, including pulse sequence repetition time (TR)

Water or CSF in ventricle	Fat	Muscle	Image type	Pulse sequence factors
			T1 weighted	Short TR Short TE
			T2 weighted	Long TR Long TE
			Proton density weighted	Long TR Short TE

Figure 1.1 Appearance of water, fat and muscle on basic MRI image types.

and echo time (TE), the following are some of the basic image types generated in MRI imaging:

- T1-weighted images
- T2-weighted images
- Proton density-weighted images.

The appearance of water, fat and muscle on each image type is illustrated in Figure 1.1.

References

1. ECRI Hazard Report. (2001) Patient death illustrates the importance of adhering to safety precautions in magnetic resonance enviroments. *Health Devices* **30(8)**, 311–314.
2. Jehenson, P., Duboc, D., Lavergne, T., et al. (1988) Change in human cardiac rhythm induced by a 2T static magnetic field. *Radiology* **166**, 227-230.
3. Chakeres, D.W., Kangarlu, A., Boudoulas, H., et al. (2003) Effect of static magnetic field exposure of up to 8T on sequential human vital sign measurements. *J. Mag. Res. Imaging* **18(3)**, 346–352.
4. International Electrotechnical Commission (1995 revised 2002) Medical electrical equipment – particular requirements for the safety of magnetic resonance equipment for medical diagnosis. *IEC* 60601–2–33.
5. The International Commission on Non-Ionizing Radiation Protection (2004) Medical magnetic resonance (MR) procedures: protection of patients. *Health Physics* **87(2)**, 197–216.
6. Nyenhuis, J.A., Bourland, J.D., Kildishev, A.V., et al. (2001) Health effects and safety of intense gradient fields. In: Shellock, F.G. (ed.) *Magnetic Resonance Procedures: Health Effects and Safety*. New York: CRC Press; 31–53.

7. Kanal, E., Barkovich, A.J., Bell, C., et al. (2007) ACR guidance document for safe MR practices. *Am. J. Roentgenol.* **188**, 1447–1474.
8. Shellock, F.G. *Reference Manual for Magnetic Resonance Safety, Implants, and devices.* 2007 edn. Los Angeles: Biomedical Research Publishing Company.

Further reading

Allisy-Roberts, P. & Williams, J. (eds) (2007) Magnetic resonance imaging. In: *Farr's Physics for Medical Imaging.* 2nd edn. Edinburgh: Saunders.

ULTRASONOGRAPHY

Patient preparation

For many US examinations no preparation is required. This includes examination of tissues such as thyroid, breast, testes, musculoskeletal, vascular and cardiac. In certain situations simple preparatory measures are required.

Abdomen

For optimal examination of the gallbladder it should be dilated. This requires fasting for 6–8 h before scanning. If detailed assessment of the pancreas is required it can be helpful to have clear fluid filling the stomach, which can then act as a transonic 'window'.

Pelvis

To optimally visualize the pelvic contents, bowel gas must be displaced. This is easily accomplished by filling the urinary bladder to capacity. This then acts as a transonic 'window'. The patient should be instructed to drink 1–2 pints of water during the hour prior to scanning and not to empty their bladder. In practice, both abdominal and pelvic scanning are often performed at the same attendance. Oral intake of clear fluids will not provoke gallbladder emptying and so the two examinations can be combined. However, it should be noted that in normal subjects who drink a large volume of oral fluid prior to the scan to fill their bladder, the renal collecting systems may appear slightly dilated. If this is the case, the patient should be asked to empty their bladder and the kidneys rescanned. If the renal collecting system dilatation is significant it will persist after the bladder is emptied.

Endoscopic

Endoscopic examination of rectum or vagina requires no physical preparation but an explanation of the procedure in a sympathetic manner is needed.

Examination of the oesophagus or transoesophageal echocardiography requires preparation similar to upper gastrointestinal endoscopy. The patient should be starved for 4 h prior to the procedure to minimize the risk of vomiting, reflux and aspiration. Anaesthesia and sedation are partly a matter of personal preference of the operator. Local anaesthesia of the pharynx can be obtained using 10% lidocaine spray. Care to avoid overdose is essential as lidocaine is rapidly absorbed via this route. The maximum dose of lidocaine should not exceed 200 mg; the Xylocaine spray metered dose applicator delivers 10 mg per dose. Sedation using i.v. benzodiazepines such as Diazemuls 10 mg or midazolam 2–5 mg may also be necessary. If local anaesthetic has been used then the patient must be instructed to avoid hot food and drink until the effect has worn off (1–2 h).

Children

US examination in children can, in most cases, be performed with no preparation apart from explanation and reassurance to both child and parent. In some cases where the child is excessively frightened or where immobility is required then sedation may be necessary. With echocardiography in infants, sedation is essential to obtain optimal recordings. The sedation regimes described in Chapter 18 may be used.

2

Intravascular contrast media

HISTORICAL DEVELOPMENT OF RADIOGRAPHIC AGENTS

The first report of opacification of the urinary tract after intravenous (i.v.) injection of a contrast agent appeared in 1923, when Osborne et al. took advantage of the fact that i.v.-injected, 10% sodium iodide solution, which was then used in the treatment of syphilis, was excreted in the urine. In 1928 German researchers synthesized a compound with a number of pyridine rings containing iodine in an effort to detoxify the iodine. This mono-iodinated compound was developed further into di-iodinated compounds and subsequently in 1952 the first tri-iodinated compound, sodium acetrizoate (Urokon), was introduced into clinical radiology. Sodium acetrizoate was based on a 6-carbon ring structure, tri-iodo benzoic acid, and was the precursor of all modern water-soluble contrast media.

Until the early 1970s all contrast media were ionic compounds and were hypertonic with osmolalities of 1200–2000 mosmol kg^{-1} water, 4–7 × the osmolarity of blood. These are referred to as high osmolar contrast media (HOCM) and are distinguished by differences at position 5 of the anion and by the cations sodium and/or meglumine. In 1969 Almén first postulated that many of the adverse effects of contrast media were the result of high osmolality and that by eliminating the cation, which does not contribute to diagnostic information but is responsible for up to 50% of the osmotic effect, it would be possible to reduce the toxicity of contrast media.[1]

Conventional ionic contrast media had a ratio of three iodine atoms per molecule to two particles in solution, i.e. a ratio of 3:2 or 1.5 (Table 2.1). In order to decrease the osmolality without changing the iodine concentration, the ratio between the number

Table 2.1 Schematic illustration of the development of contrast media

Description	Name	Chemical structure	Ratio of no. of iodine atoms/ions: no. of particles in solution	Osmolarity of a 280mg I ml⁻¹ solution	Osmolarity group
	Sodium Iodide	Na⁺ I⁻	0.5		
	Diodone	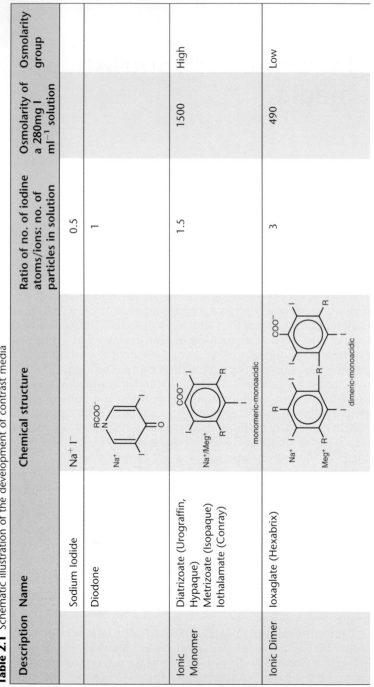	1		
Ionic Monomer	Diatrizoate (Urograffin, Hypaque) Metrizoate (Isopaque) Iothalamate (Conray)	monomeric-monoacidic	1.5	1500	High
Ionic Dimer	Ioxaglate (Hexabrix)	dimeric-monoacidic	3	490	Low

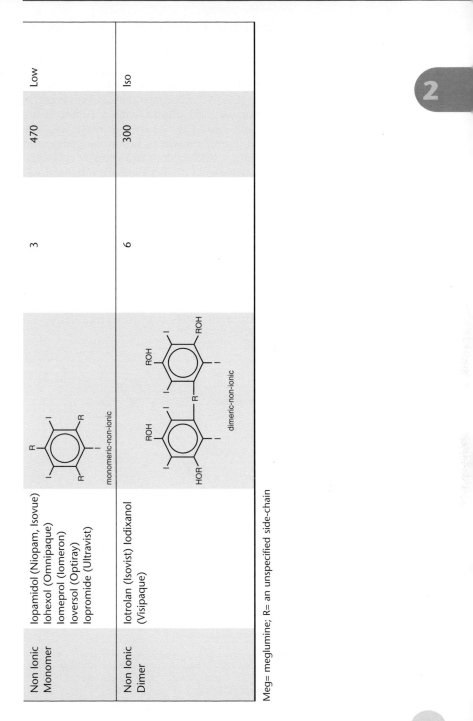

Non Ionic Monomer	Iopamidol (Niopam, Isovue) Iohexol (Omnipaque) Iomeprol (Iomeron) Ioversol (Optiray) Iopromide (Ultravist)	monomeric-non-ionic	3	470 Low
Non Ionic Dimer	Iotrolan (Isovist) Iodixanol (Visipaque)	dimeric-non-ionic	6	300 Iso

Meg= meglumine; R= an unspecified side-chain

of iodine atoms and the number of dissolved particles must be increased.

Further development proceeded along two separate paths (Table 2.1). The first was to combine two tri-iodinated benzene rings to produce an ionic dimer with six iodine atoms per anion, the low osmolar contrast medium (LOCM) ioxaglate (Hexabrix). Replacement of one of the carboxylic acid groups with a non-ionizing radical means that only one cation is needed per molecule. The alternative, more successful, approach was to produce a compound that does not ionize in solution and so does not provide radiologically useless cations. Contrast media of this type are referred to as non-ionic and are also LOCM. These include the non-ionic monomers iopamidol (Niopam, Iopamiron, Isovue, and Solutrast), iohexol (Omnipaque), iopromide (Ultravist), iomeprol (Iomeron) and ioversol (Optiray).

For both types of LOCM the ratio of iodine atoms in the molecule to the number of particles in solution is 3:1 and osmolality is decreased. Compared with high osmolar contrast material (HOCM), the LOCM show a theoretical halving of osmolality for equi-iodine solutions. However, because of aggregation of molecules in solution the measured reduction is approximately one-third (Fig. 2.1).

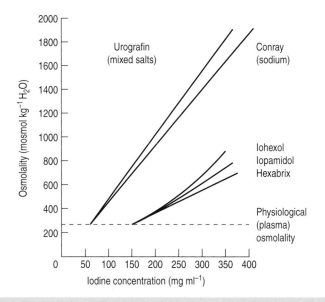

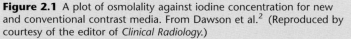

Figure 2.1 A plot of osmolality against iodine concentration for new and conventional contrast media. From Dawson et al.[2] (Reproduced by courtesy of the editor of *Clinical Radiology*.)

A further development in the search for the ideal contrast agent has been the introduction of non-ionic dimers – iotrolan (Isovist) and iodixanol (Visipaque). These have a ratio of six iodine atoms for each molecule in solution with satisfactory iodine concentrations at iso-osmolality; they are, therefore, called iso-osmolar contrast media. The safety profile of the iso-osmolar contrast agents is at least equivalent to LOCM, but any significant advantage of iso-osmolar contrast remains controversial.

The low- and iso-osmolar contrast media are 5–10 times safer than the HOCM.[3] Previously, HOCM were much less expensive than LOCM so were widely used despite the higher risk of adverse reaction and nephrotoxicity. LOCM were reserved for use in patients considered to be at increased risk of contrast reaction. Over the past few years, the relative cost of the non-ionic contrast media has fallen and the use of ionic contrast medium for i.v. injection has now ceased almost entirely. Ionic contrast media must *never* be used in the subarachnoid space.

With development having reached the stage of iso-osmolality, further research is now targeted on decreasing the chemotoxicity of the contrast molecule.

ADVERSE EFFECTS OF INTRAVENOUS WATER-SOLUBLE CONTRAST MEDIA

The toxicity of contrast media is a function of osmolarity, ionic charge (ionic contrast agents only), chemical structure (chemotoxicity) or lipophilicity.

Adverse reactions after administration of non-ionic iodinated contrast media are rare, occuring in less than 1% of all patients.[4] Of these reactions, the majority are mild and self-limiting. The incidence of severe or very severe non-ionic contrast reaction is 0.044%.[5]

TOXIC EFFECTS ON SPECIFIC ORGANS

Vascular toxicity

Venous

1. Pain at the injection site – usually the result of a perivenous injection
2. Pain extending up the arm – due to stasis of contrast medium in the vein. May be relieved by abducting the arm
3. Delayed limb pain – due to thrombophlebitis as a result of the toxic effect on endothelium.

Arterial

Arterial endothelial damage and vasodilatation are mostly related to hyperosmolality. Contrast medium injected during peripheral arteriography may cause a sensation of heat or pain.

Soft-tissue toxicity

Pain, swelling, erythema and even sloughing of skin may occur from extravasated contrast medium. The risk is increased when pumps are used to inject large volumes of contrast medium during computed tomography (CT) examinations. Treatment should consist of the application of cold packs and elevation of the limb. Systemic steroids, non-steroidal anti-inflammatory drugs and antibiotics have all been shown to be useful.

Cardiovascular toxicity

1. Intracoronary injection of contrast media may cause significant disturbance of cardiac rhythm.
2. Increased vagal activity may result in depression of the sino-atrial and atrio-ventricular nodes, causing bradycardia or asystole.
3. The injection of a hypertonic contrast medium causes significant fluid and ion shifts. Immediately after injection there is a significant increase in serum osmolality. This causes an influx of water from the interstitial space into the vascular compartment, an increase in blood volume, an increase in cardiac output and a brief increase of systemic blood pressure. Peripheral dilatation causes a more prolonged fall of blood pressure. Injection into the right heart or pulmonary artery causes transitory pulmonary hypertension and systemic hypotension; injection into the left ventricle or aorta causes brief systemic hypertension followed by a more prolonged fall.

Haematological changes

1. In the presence of a high concentration of contrast medium, such as withdrawal of blood into a syringe of contrast medium, damage to red cell walls occurs and haemolysis follows. Haemolysis and haemoglobinuria have been reported following angiocardiography. It is advisable not to re-inject blood that has been mixed with contrast medium.
2. Red cell aggregation and coagulation may occur in the presence of a high concentration of contrast medium, e.g. 350 mg I ml^{-1}. However, disaggregation occurs easily and this is not likely to be of any clinical significance.[6]
3. Contrast media impair blood clotting and platelet aggregation. Low- and iso-osmolar contrast media have a minimal effect compared to HOCM.[7]

4. Contrast media have a potentiating effect on the action of heparin.
5. Thrombus formation also occurs and is more common when blood is mixed with LOCM. However, the role of the syringe is also significant and thrombus formation is maximal when blood is slowly withdrawn into a syringe so that it layers on top of the contrast medium, against the wall of the syringe. Activation of coagulation by the tube material probably plays a significant role.
6. Contrast media have been shown to cause HbSS blood to sickle in vitro and sickle cell crisis has been provoked by contrast medium. Iso-osmolar contrast agents have a lesser effect and their use is indicated in this disease.[8]
7. When red blood cells are placed in a hypertonic contrast medium, water leaves the interior of the cells by osmosis and they become more rigid and less deformable. Isosmolar solutions may also have an effect on red cell deformability, indicating that there may also be a chemical effect. Red cells that deform less easily are less able to pass through capillaries and may occlude them. This is the explanation for the transient rise in pulmonary arterial pressure during pulmonary arteriography and may also be a factor in contrast-induced nephropathy.
8. Transient eosinophilia may occur 24–72 h after administration of contrast medium.

Nephrotoxicity

Reviews on the incidence of contrast-induced nephrotoxicity (CIN) suggest an incidence of approximately 1–6%. In those affected, the serum creatinine concentration starts to rise within the first 24 h, reaches a peak by 2–3 days and usually returns to baseline by 3–7 days. In rare cases patients may need temporary or permanent dialysis. There are a number of predisposing factors:

1. The most important risk factor is pre-existing impairment of renal function. This is present in 90% of reported cases of CIN. Patients with normal renal function are at very low risk and those with GFR of <30 ml/min are most at risk.[9] However, most patients have not had a recent GFR measurement and guidelines recommend the use of serum creatinine level of >130 μmol l[-1] as an imperfect, but readily available, indicator of patients at increased risk of CIN.[3]
2. Diabetes mellitus is present in 50% of cases of CIN.
3. Dehydration is a risk factor.
4. Age is also a factor because of the greater incidence of cardiovascular disease in the elderly.
5. Very large doses of contrast medium increase the risks.

6. Multiple myeloma increases the risks.
7. The presence of other nephrotoxic drugs is also a risk factor.

The mechanisms of CIN are summarized below:[10]

1. Impaired renal perfusion:
   a. adverse cardiotoxic effects
   b. increased peripheral vasodilatation
   c. renal vascular bed changes (increased blood flow followed by a more prolonged decrease)
   d. increased rigidity of red cells
   e. pre-dehydration
   f. osmotic diuresis.
2. Glomerular injury:
   a. impaired perfusion
   b. hyperosmolar effects
   c. chemotoxic effects.
3. Tubular injury:
   a. impaired perfusion
   b. hyperosmolar effects
   c. chemotoxic effects
   (all manifest histologically as cytoplasmic vacuolation).
4. Obstructive nephropathy:
   a. cytoplasmic vacuolation in tubules
   b. precipitation of Tamm-Horsfall protein
   c. precipitation of Bence Jones protein in multiple myeloma.

It was hoped that the iso-osmolar contrast agents might be less nephrotoxic than LOCM and HOCM. However, clinical trials have so far yielded conflicting results.[9,11] CIN has a complex aetiology and the positive benefit of reduction in osmolarity achieved with iso-osmolar contrast medium may be negated by the accompanying increase in viscosity.[12]

A further hazard for patients who suffer impairment of renal function as a result of intravenous iodinated contrast is reduced clearance of drugs excreted by the kidneys. This is well recognized as a clinical problem with metformin, an oral hypoglycaemic drug which is exclusively excreted via the kidneys. The resultant accumulation of metformin may result in the development of the potentially fatal complication lactic acidosis.

See Table 2.3 for guidelines on prophylaxis of renal adverse reaction to iodinated contrast.

Neurotoxicity

Contrast medium delivered to the brain via the arterial route may cross the blood–brain barrier. Neurotoxicity is caused by both osmolality and chemotoxic effects and i.v. contrast medium may rarely provoke convulsions in patients with epilepsy or cerebral tumours.

Convulsions may also occur secondary to the cerebral hypoxia caused by hypotension ± cardiac arrest after severe contrast reaction.

Thyroid function

1. Thyrotoxicosis may occur in patients with non-toxic goitres or be exacerbated in those with pre-existing thyrotoxic symptoms.[13]
2. Contrast media may interfere with thyroid function tests.

IDIOSYNCRATIC REACTIONS

Excluding death, adverse reactions can be classified in terms of severity as:

1. Major reactions, i.e. those that interfere with the examination and require treatment.
2. Intermediate reactions, i.e. those that interfere with the examination but do not require treatment.
3. Minor reactions, i.e. those that do not interfere with the examination but require patient reassurance.

Minor and intermediate reactions are not uncommon; major adverse reactions are rare (Table 2.2).

Fatal reactions

Deaths caused by iodinated contrast agents are very rare, occuring at a rate of 1.1–1.2 per million contrast media packages distributed. Most are attributed to renal failure, anaphylaxis or allergic reaction.[18]

Table 2.2 Adverse reaction rates for intravenous ionic* and non-ionic# contrast media

Study	Number of examinations	Minor	Intermediate	Severe	Fatal
Dillman et al. [USA–Paediatric only][14]	11 306#	1:706	1:11 300	1:3766	–
Palmer [Australasia][15]	79 000*	1:30	1:284	1:1117	1:40 000
	30 000#	1:96	1:1010	1:6056	–
Katayama et al. [Japan][16]	169 284*			1:394	1:169 000
	168 363#			1:2215	1:168 000
Wolf et al. [USA][17]	6006*	1:35	1:86	1:316	–
	8857#	1:227	1:738	1:8857	–

Almost all fatal reactions occur in the minutes following injection and patients must be under close observation during this time. The fatal event may be preceded by trivial events, such as nausea and vomiting, or may occur without warning. The majority of deaths occur in those over 50 years of age. Causes of death include cardiac arrest, pulmonary oedema, respiratory arrest, consumption coagulopathy, bronchospasm, laryngeal oedema and angioneurotic oedema.

Non-fatal reactions

1. *Flushing, metallic taste in the mouth, nausea, sneezing, cough and tingling* are common and related to dose and speed of injection.
2. *Perineal burning*, a desire to empty the bladder or rectum and an erroneous feeling of having been incontinent of urine are more common in women.
3. *Urticaria.*
4. *Angioneurotic oedema.* Most commonly affects the face. May persist for up to 3 days and its onset may be delayed.
5. *Rigors.*
6. *Necrotizing skin lesions.* Rare and mostly in patients with pre-existing renal failure (particularly those with systemic lupus erythematosus).
7. *Bronchospasm.* Predisposed to by a history of asthma and by therapy with ß-blockers. In most patients the bronchospasm is subclinical. Mechanisms include:
   a. direct histamine release from mast cells and platelets
   b. cholinesterase inhibition
   c. vagal overtone
   d. complement activation
   e. direct effect of contrast media on bronchi.
8. *Non-cardiogenic pulmonary oedema.* During acute anaphylaxis or hypotensive collapse and possibly due to increased capillary permeability.
9. *Arrhythmias.*
10. *Hypotension.* Usually accompanied by tachycardia but in some patients there is vagal over-reaction with bradycardia. The latter is rapidly reversed by atropine 0.6–2 mg i.v. Hypotension is usually mild and is treatable by a change of posture. Rarely, it is severe and may be accompanied by pulmonary oedema.
11. *Abdominal pain.* May be a symptom in anaphylactic reactions or vagal overactivity. Should be differentiated from the loin pain that may be precipitated in patients with upper urinary tract obstruction.
12. *Delayed-onset reactions* – (1 h–1 week after injection) include rashes, headaches, itching and parotid gland swelling. Risk factors for delayed reaction are previous contrast medium reaction and therapy with interleukin-2.[19]

MECHANISMS OF IDIOSYNCRATIC CONTRAST-MEDIUM REACTIONS

Idiosyncratic contrast medium reactions are usually labelled anaphylactoid since they have all the features of anaphylaxis but are IgE negative in most cases.[20] Possible mechanisms include those outlined below.

Histamine release

Histamine is the primary mediator of anaphylaxis/anaphylactoid reaction and contrast media cause the release of histamine from mast cells and basophils. This could provide a mechanism for the phenomena of flushing, urticaria, metallic taste, hypotension, collapse and angioneurotic oedema. While hyperosmolality is a factor, isosmolar concentrations of contrast media will also stimulate histamine release. Bronchospasm may be due to the effect of contrast medium on pulmonary-bed mast cells and dysrrhythmias from the effect on cardiac mast cells.

Complement activation

Contrast medium may activate the complement system leading to the formation of anaphylatoxins which induce the release of histamine and other biological mediators from basophils and mast cells.[20] However, there is uncertainty as some studies have failed to show an increase in complement fraction levels in patients after reaction to i.v. iodinated contrast.

Protein binding, enzyme inhibition and immune receptors

Contrast media are weakly protein bound and the degree of protein binding correlates well with their ability to inhibit the enzyme acetylcholinesterase. Contrast medium side-effects such as vasodilatation, bradycardia, hypotension, bronchospasm and urticaria are all recognized cholinergic effects. It was previously thought that they might be related more to cholinesterase inhibition than osmolality; however, this has not been conclusively proven. More recently, it has been postulated that weakly protein bound drugs, such as iodinated contrast, may directly activate T cells which bear immune receptors. It is thought that these may interact with the drug and that contrast medium may have an effect on cytokine production by helper T cells[21] to mediate the acute reaction.

Chemotoxicity

In addition to the toxicity of both ionic and non-ionic contrast media, because of their intrinsic structure, the ionic contrast agents had an electrical charge on the particles. This was almost certainly the cause of the high incidence of severe adverse reactions during intracoronary and intrathecal use of these agents.

Although the major adverse effect on erythrocytes is due to hyperosmolality, even contrast medium which is iso-osmolar with plasma produces changes in red-blood-cell morphology that reveal the intrinsic chemotoxicity of contrast medium molecules.

Anxiety

Many years ago, Lalli[22] postulated that most, if not all, contrast medium reactions are the result of the patient's fear and apprehension. The high autonomic nervous system activity in an anxious patient will be stimulated further when the patient experiences the administration of contrast medium. Furthermore, contrast medium crossing the blood–brain barrier can stimulate the limbic area and hypothalamus to produce further autonomic activity. This autonomic activity is responsible for contrast medium reactions by the sequence of events illustrated in Figure 2.2.

PROPHYLAXIS OF ADVERSE CONTRAST MEDIUM EFFECTS

Guidelines for prophylaxis of renal and non-renal adverse contrast media reaction are given in Tables 2.3 and 2.4. Sources used in these tables include documents of the Royal College of Radiologists[3] and

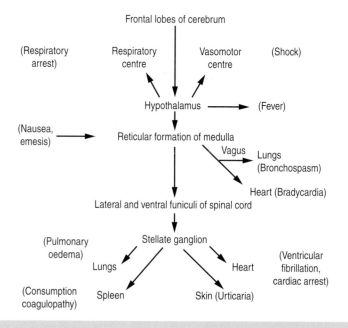

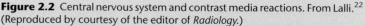

Figure 2.2 Central nervous system and contrast media reactions. From Lalli.[22] (Reproduced by courtesy of the editor of *Radiology*.)

Table 2.3 Guidelines for prophylaxis of renal adverse reactions to iodinated contrast medium

Renal adverse reactions
Identification of patients at increased risk:

1. The referring clinician should identify patients with pre-existing renal impairment and inform the radiology department.
2. Serum creatinine should be measured within 1 week before the administration of contrast in patients:
  a. **with previously raised serum creatinine**
  b. **who are diabetic and taking metformin**
  c. **who will undergo intra-arterial contrast injection**
  d. **with clinical history suggesting increased risk of renal impairment** (e.g. diabetes, renal surgery or administration of nephrotoxic drugs).

Precautions for patients with significant renal impairment (any patient with serum creatinine $>130\ \mu mol\ l^{-1}$):
1. Consider an alternative imaging method, not using iodinated contrast media. 2. 48 h before the procedure stop any treatment with metformin. This should be withheld for a further 48 h after the procedure and renal function re-assessed before restarting metformin treatment. 3. 24 h before the procedure stop all nephrotoxic drugs, mannitol and loop diuretics. 4. 6 h before the procedure start hydrating the patient either orally, or in the case of high dose or intra-arterial administration, intravenously. 5. Use the smallest possible dose of contrast medium. 6. Use low- or iso-osmolar contrast medium. There is insufficient evidence to support the use of prophylactic administration of N-acetyl cysteine for patients at high risk of contrast nephropathy.
There is no definite evidence that haemodialysis or peritoneal dialysis protect patients with impaired renal function from contrast medium induced nephrotoxicity.
Patients with normal renal function on treatment with metformin:
1. If <100 ml of contrast agent is to be used intravenously then no special precaution is required. 2. If >100 ml of contrast is to be used intravenously or the intra-arterial route is to be used, the metformin should be withheld for 48 h after the procedure.

Table 2.4 Guidelines for prophylaxis of non-renal adverse reactions to iodinated contrast medium

Non-renal adverse reactions
Identification of patients at increased risk of anaphylactoid contrast reaction:
It is essential that before administration of iodinated contrast *every* patient must be specifically asked whether they have a history of: 1. **previous contrast reaction** – associated with a sixfold increase in reactions to contrast medium.[20] Determine exact nature and specific agent used.   2. **asthma** – history of asthma associated with a six to tenfold increase in risk of severe reaction.[24] Determine whether patient has true asthma or COPD and whether asthma is currently well controlled. If asthma not currently well controlled and examination is non-emergency, the patient should be referred back for appropriate medical therapy.   3. **previous allergic reaction requiring medical treatment** – determine the nature of the allergies and their sensitivity (there is no specific cross reactivity with shellfish or topical iodine in acute reactions).
Precautions for patients at increased risk of anaphylactoid contrast reaction:

1. Consider an alternative test not requiring iodinated contrast.
 2. If the injection is considered necessary:
   a. Use a non-ionic low or iso-osmolar contrast agent
   b. For previous reactors to iodinated contrast use a different non-ionic low- or iso-osmolar contrast to that used previously
   c. Maintain close supervision
   d. Leave the cannula in place and observe for 30 min
   e. Be ready to treat promptly any adverse reaction and ensure that emergency drugs and equipment are ready.
 There are no conclusive data supporting the use of premedication in the prevention of severe reactions to contrast media in patients at increased risk and clinical opinion remains divided.[25,26]
 	
 If it is decided to use premedication for patients at increased risk, a suitable regime is prednisolone 30 mg orally given 12 h and 2 h before contrast medium.
 	
 Pre-treatment with antihistamines is of no benefit and is associated with an increased incidence of flushing. Pre-testing by applying contrast medium to the cornea or injecting a 1 ml test dose intravenously a few minutes prior to the full injection has also been abandoned.

Other situations:
Pregnancy – In exceptional circumstances, iodinated contrast may be given. Thyroid function of the neonate should be checked during the first week of life.[27]

Treatment with ß-blockers – ß-blockers may impair the response to treatment of bronchospasm induced by contrast medium.

Lactation – No special precaution required. Breast feeding can continue normally.

Thyrotoxicosis – Intravascular contrast should not be given if the patient is hyperthyroid. Avoid thyroid radio-isotope tests and treatment for 2 months after iodinated contrast medium administration.

Phaeochromocytoma – When detected biochemically it is advised that α and ß-adrenergic blockade with orally administered drugs is arranged before administration of iodinated contrast.

Sickle cell anaemia – There is risk of precipitating a sickle cell crisis. Iso-osmolar contrast should be used.

Myelomatosis – Bence Jones protein may be precipitated in renal tubules. Risk diminished by ensuring good hydration.

the European Society of Urogenital Radiology[23] on contrast medium administration; the full text of these documents can be downloaded from the internet at *www.rcr.ac.uk* and *www.esur.org* respectively. General safety issues are:

- a doctor should be immediately available in the department to deal with any severe reaction
- facilities for treatment of acute adverse reaction should be readily available and regularly checked
- a patient must not be left alone or unsupervised for the first 5 min following injection of the contrast agent
- the patient should remain in the department for at least 15 min after the contrast injection. In patients at increased risk of reaction this should be increased to 30 min.

References

1. Almén, T. (1969) Contrast agent design. Some aspects of synthesis of water-soluble contrast agents of low osmolality. *J. Theor. Biol.* **24**, 216–226.
2. Dawson, P., Grainger, R.G. & Pitfield, J. (1983) The new low-osmolar contrast media: a simple guide. *Clin. Radiol.* **34**, 221–226.
3. The Royal College of Radiologists (2005) *Standards for Intravenous Iodinated Contrast Administration to Adult Patients*. London: The Royal College of Radiologists.
4. Mortelé, K.J., Oliva, M.R., Ondategui, S., et al. (2005) Universal use of nonionic iodinated contrast medium for CT: evaluation of safety in a large urban teaching hospital. *Am. J. Roentgenol.* **184(1)**, 31–34.
5. Katayama, H., Yamaguchi, K., Kozuka, T., et al. (1990) Adverse reactions to ionic and non-ionic contrast media. *Radiology* **175(3)**, 621–628.

6. Dawson, P., McCarthy, P., Allison, D.J., et al. (1988) Non-ionic contrast agents, red cell aggregation and coagulation. *Br. J. Radiol.* **61**, 963–965.

7. Aspelin, P., Stacul, F., Thomsen, H.S., et al. (2006) Effects of iodinated contrast media on blood and endothelium. *Eur. Radiol.* **16(5)**, 1041–1049.

8. Losco, P., Nash, G., Stone, P., et al. (2001) Comparison of the effects of radiographic contrast media on dehydration and filterability of red blood cells from donors homozygous for hemoglobin A or hemoglobin S. *Am. J. Hematol.* **68(3)**, 149–158.

9. Benko, A., Fraser-Hill, M., Magner, P., et al. (2007) Canadian Association of Radiologists: consensus guidelines for the prevention of contrast induced nephropathy. *Can. Assoc. Radiol. J.* **58(2)**, 79–87.

10. Persson, P.B., Hansell, P. & Liss, P. (2005) Pathophysiology of contrast medium-induced nephropathy. *Kidney Int.* **68(1)**: 14–22.

11. Liss, P., Persson, P.B., Hansell P., et al. (2006) Renal failure in 57 925 patients undergoing coronary procedures using iso-osmolar or low-osmolar contrast media. *Kidney Int.* **70(10)**, 1811–1817.

12. Brunette, J., Mongrain, R., Rodés-Cabau, J., et al. (2008) Comparative rheology of low- and iso-osmolarity contrast agents at different temperatures. *Catheter Cardiovasc. Interv.* **71(1)**:78–83.

13. van der Molen, A.J., Thomsen, H.S., Morcos, S.K., et al. (2004) Effect of iodinated contrast media on thyroid function in adults. *Eur. Radiol.* **14(5)**, 902–907.

14. Dillman, J.R., Strouse, P.J., Ellis, J.H., et al. (2007) Incidence and severity of acute allergic-like reactions to i.v. non-ionic iodinated contrast material in children. *Am. J. Roentogenol.* **188(6)**, 1643–1647.

15. Palmer, F.J. (1988) The R.A.C.R. survey of intravenous contrast media reactions: final report. *Australas. Radiol.* **32**, 426–428.

16. Katayama, H., Yamaguchi, K., Kozuka, T., et al. (1990) Adverse reactions to ionic and non-ionic contrast media. A report from the Japanese Committee on the Safety of Contrast Media. *Radiology* **175**, 621–628.

17. Wolf, G.L., Mishkin, M.M., Roux, S.G., et al. (1991) Comparison of the rates of adverse drug reactions. Ionic contrast agents, ionic agents combined with steroids and nonionic agents. *Invest. Radiol.* **26**, 404–410.

18. Wysowski, D.K. & Nourjah, P. (2006) Deaths attributed to X-ray contrast media on U.S. death certificates. *Am. J. Roentgenol.* **186**, 613–615.

19. Webb, J.A., Stacul, F., Thomsen, H.S., et al. (2003) Late adverse reactions to intravascular iodinated contrast media. *Eur. Radiol.* **13(1)**, 181–184.

20. Morcos, S.K. (2005) Acute serious and fatal reactions to contrast media: our current understanding. *Br. J. Radiol.* **78(932)**, 686–693.

21. Böhm, I., Speck, U. & Schild, H. (2003) Cytokine profiles after nonionic dimeric contrast medium injection. *Invest. Radiol.* **38(12)**, 776–783.

22. Lalli, A.F. (1974) Urographic contrast media reactions and anxiety. *Radiology* **112(2)**, 267–271.

23. European Society of Urogenital Radiology Contrast Media Safety Committee (2007) ESUR guidelines on contrast media Version 6.0, ***www.esur.org***

24. Morcos, S.K. & Thomsen H.S. (2001) Adverse reactions to iodinated contrast media. *Eur. Radiol.* **11(7)**, 1267–1275.

25. Tramèr, M.R., von Elm, E., Loubeyre, P., et al. (2006) Pharmacological prevention of serious anaphylactic reactions due to iodinated contrast media: systematic review. *BMJ* **333(7570)**, 675.

26. Thomsen, H.S. (2003) Guidelines for contrast media from the European Society of Urogenital Radiology. *Am. J. Roentgenol.* **181**, 1463–1471.
27. Webb, J.A., Thomsen, H.S., Morcos, S.K., et al. (2005) The use of iodinated and gadolinium contrast media during pregnancy and lactation. *Eur. Radiol.* **15(6)**, 1234–1240.

CONTRAST AGENTS IN MAGNETIC RESONANCE IMAGING

HISTORICAL DEVELOPMENT

Shortly after the introduction of clinical MRI, the first contrast-enhanced human MRI studies were reported in 1981 using ferric chloride as a contrast agent in the gastrointestinal tract. In 1984, Carr et al. first demonstrated the use of a gadolinium compound as a diagnostic intravascular MRI contrast agent.[1] Currently, around one-quarter of all MRI examinations are performed with contrast agents.

MECHANISM OF ACTION

Whilst radiographic contrast agents use a direct alteration in tissue density to allow the visualization of structures, the MRI contrast agents act indirectly by altering the magnetic properties of hydrogen ions (protons) in water and lipid which form the basis of the image in MRI. To enhance the inherent contrast between tissues, MRI contrast agents must alter the rate of relaxation of protons within the tissues. The changes in relaxation vary and, therefore, different tissues produce differential enhancement of the signal (see Figs 2.3 and 2.4). These figures show that, for a given time t, if the T1 relaxation is more rapid then a larger signal is obtained (brighter images), but the opposite is true for T2 relaxation, where more rapid relaxation produces reduced signal intensity (darker images). There are different means by which these effects on protons can be produced using a range of MRI contrast agents.

MRI contrast agents must exert a large magnetic field density (a property imparted by their unpaired electrons) to interact with the magnetic moments of the protons in the tissues and so shorten their T1 relaxation time which will produce an increase in signal intensity (see Fig. 2.3). The electron magnetic moments also cause local changes in the magnetic field, which promotes more rapid proton dephasing and so shortens the T2 relaxation time. All contrast

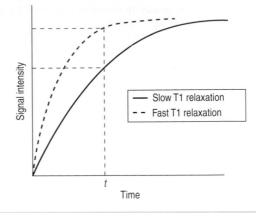

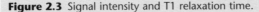

Figure 2.3 Signal intensity and T1 relaxation time.

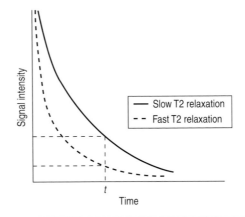

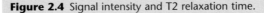

Figure 2.4 Signal intensity and T2 relaxation time.

agents shorten both T1 and T2 relaxation times but some will predominantly affect T1 (longitudinal relaxation rate) and other predominantly T2 (transverse relaxation rate).

Agents with unpaired electron spins are potential contrast agents in MRI. These may be classified under three headings:

1. *Ferromagnetic*. These retain magnetism even when the applied field is removed. This may cause particle aggregation and interfere with cell function, making them unsafe for clinical use as MRI contrast agents.

2. *Paramagnetic* – e.g. gadolinium. These contrast agents have magnetic moments which align to the applied field, but once the gradient field is turned off, thermal energy within the tissue is enough to overcome the alignment. Gadolinium compounds may be made soluble by chelation and can, therefore, either be injected intravenously or used as an oral preparation. Their maximum effect is on protons in the water molecule, shortening the T1 relaxation time and hence producing increased signal intensity (white) on T1 images (Fig. 2.3).

3. *Superparamagnetic* – e.g. particles of iron oxide (Fe_3O_4). These cause abrupt changes in the local magnetic field which results in rapid proton dephasing and reduction in the T2 relaxation time, and hence producing decreased signal intensity (black) on T2 images (Fig. 2.4). Superparamagnetic compounds were initially produced only as large particles in a colloid suspension for gastrointestinal contrast. However, more recently they have become available as small particles of iron oxide (SPIO) agents and ultrasmall particles of iron oxide (USPIO) agents. Both SPIO and USPIO agents have submicron global particle diameters and are small enough to form a stable solution which can be injected intravenously.

GADOLINIUM

The gadolinium (GD) chelates represent the largest group of MRI contrast media and are available in three forms:

1. Extracellular fluid (ECF) agents: by far the most commonly used form of gadolinium. Includes (i) Gd-diethylenetriaminepenta-acetic acid (DTPA), dimeglumine gadopentetate (Magnevist, Schering), (ii) Gadodiamide (Gd-DTPA-bismethylamide) (Omniscan, Nycomed Amersham) and (iii) Gd-DO3A, Gadoteridol (ProHance, Bracco, Merck, Squibb). They all contain gadolinium, an 8-coordinate ligand binding to gadolinium and a single water molecule coordination site to gadolinium and all have a molecular weight similar to iodinated contrast agents. After intravenous injection they circulate within the vascular system and are excreted unchanged by the kidneys. The ECF agents do not cross the normal blood–brain barrier but do cross the abnormal blood–brain barrier. ECF agents are used for angiography but rapidly leak out of the vascular space into the interstitial space so are used only for dynamic arterial studies. There is a wide range of indications for these contrast media including improved detection rates and more accurate delineation and characterization of tumours.

2. Liver agents: the excretion pathway of the gadolinium chelates can be altered to produce compounds such as Gd-BOPTA (gadobenate, Multihance) and Gd-DTPA (Primovist), which are

taken up by hepatocytes and cleared intact via the hepato-biliary system. Another paramagnetic liver specific contrast agent is the manganese chelate Mn-DPDP (Telescan). These agents are used to improve detection of liver lesions which do not contain hepatocytes (therefore do not take up the contrast), such as liver metastases, and to characterize lesions which do take up the contrast, such as hepatocellular carcinoma. They can also be used to provide positive contrast (T1 weighted) of the hepato-biliary system.

3. Blood pool agents: the blood pool agents remain longer in the vascular space than ECF agents and allow a wider range of vascular imaging. The first of these contrast agents approved for clinical use in Europe, gadofosveset trisodium (Vasovist, Bayer Schering),[2] has recently been introduced.

Dose

For ECF gadolinium agents, usually $0.1 \, \text{mmol kg}^{-1}$ body weight (e.g. 0.2 ml of Magnevist kg^{-1}); up to $0.2 \, \text{mmol kg}^{-1}$ when used in low-field magnets.

Adverse reactions

Gadolinium contrast agents are very safe and well tolerated; they have a much lower incidence of adverse reactions than iodinated contrast agents. Adverse reactions to gadolinium are mostly mild and self-limiting and can be divided into acute and delayed reactions. The incidence is shown in Table 2.5.

Acute adverse reactions
These are rare, but the following have been described:

1. Urticaria and rash
2. Nausea/vomiting
3. Dizziness and confusion
4. Dyspnoea, chest discomfort and palpitation
5. Anaphylactoid shock.

Table 2.5 Acute adverse reaction rates for gadolinium contrast agents

Study	Number of examinations	Mild	Moderate	Severe	Fatal
Li et al. [Hong Kong][3]	9528	1:212	1:9528	1:9528	None
Dillman et al. [USA][4]	78353	1:1958	1:7835	1:19588	None
Cochran et al. [USA][5]	28340	1:1574	None	1:28340	None

Patients with a history of previous adverse reaction to gadolinium contrast agents have up to an eightfold increase in likelihood of experiencing adverse reactions,[6] and those with asthma, documented allergies or previous adverse reaction to iodinated contrast are also at increased risk of adverse reaction.[7]

Delayed adverse reactions

1. Renal impairment – when used at the standard doses given above, gadolinium contrast agents do not cause significant impairment of renal function. It was initially thought that gadolinium agents might be used as a replacement for iodinated contrast for those at increased risk of contrast nephrotoxicity. However, when used at the high doses required to give equivalent X-ray attenuation, gadolinium-based contrast media have more nephrotoxic potential than iodinated contrast.[8]

2. Nephrogenic systemic fibrosis (NSF) – this systemic disorder, first described in 2000, is characterized by increased deposition of collagen with thickening and hardening of the skin, contractures and, in some patients, clinical involvement of other tissues.[9] NSF only occurs in patients with renal disease and almost all patients with NSF have been exposed to gadolinium-based contrast agents within 2–3 months prior to the onset of the disease. The mechanism by which renal failure and gadolinium-based contrast agents trigger NSF is not known. The overwhelming majority of reported cases of NSF represent patients who had previously been given gadodiamide (Omniscan, GE Healthcare),[10] but there are some reports of NSF associated with other gadolinium contrast agents. Reported figures from Denmark show that 5% of all patients with severe renal impairment who had been given Omniscan developed NSF.[7]

Precautions for prevention of adverse reactions

Detailed guidelines are available from the American College of Radiology[7] and the European Society of Urogenital Radiology.[11] These form the basis for the following advice.

Acute adverse reactions

1. Identify patients at increased risk of reaction because of previous gadolinium reaction, asthma, allergies or previous adverse reaction to iodinated contrast.

2. For those at increased risk consider an alternative test not requiring a gadolinium agent.

3. If proceeding with i.v. gadolinium contrast:
   a. patients who have previously reacted to one gadolinium-based contrast agent should be injected with a different agent if they are re-studied
   b. although there is no clinical evidence of the effectiveness of premedication, it is suggested that consideration be given to

the use of premedication such as oral prednisolone 30 mg orally 12 and 2 hours before contrast medium

c. those with at increased risk of adverse reaction should be monitored more closely after injection.

Delayed adverse reaction:

1. Identify patients at risk of NSF because of impaired renal function (GFR <30 ml/min or any patient having renal dialysis). Patients with mild renal impairment do not require special precautions except to note that patients with any level of renal impairment should not receive Omniscan.

2. For patients at increased risk consider an alternative test not requiring a gadolinium agent.

3. If proceeding with gadolinium contrast, after a risk–benefit analysis for that particular patient:
   a. use the lowest possible dose of gadolinium-based contrast agent
   b. some authorities recommend routine haemodialysis after gadolinium contrast agents in patients with significant renal impairment.

IRON-OXIDE MAGNETIC RESONANCE IMAGING CONTRAST AGENTS (SPIO AND USPIO)

After i.v. injection, the superparamagnetic SPIO contrast agents are taken up via the reticulo-endothelial system into the liver and spleen resulting in decreased signal intensity in normal liver and spleen on T2-weighted images. Malignant tumour tissue or other lesions which do not contain reticulo-endothelial cells will not take up the contrast and, therefore, retain their high MRI signal. Iron-oxide contrast agents are useful for detection of liver tumour, particularly hepatocellular carcinoma.[12]

The USPIO contrast agents have greater T1 shortening effects and a longer plasma circulation time than the SPIO agents. In addition, they have greater uptake in bone marrow and lymph nodes and their use for imaging bone marrow and lymph nodes is being developed.[13]

GASTROINTESTINAL CONTRAST AGENTS

These are used to distinguish bowel from adjacent soft-tissue masses. As with CT, all bowel contrast agents need to mix readily with the bowel contents to ensure even distribution. They must also be palatable. They can be divided into two groups:

Positive agents

These include fatty oils and gadolinium. They act by T1 shortening effects and appear white on T1 images.

Disadvantages
1. The high signal increases the effect of bowel-motion artifact.
2. The effect varies with the pulse sequence and the contrast concentration within the bowel. This can produce non-uniformity in the signal which may cause confusion.

Negative agents

These include ferrite and barium sulphate (60–70% w/w). These act by T2 shortening effects and appear black on T2 images.

Disadvantages
1. High concentrations result in image distortion and blurring of adjacent structures.
2. The required dose of ferrite is a potentially lethal dose and so enteric preparations need to be chelated to reduce the absorption of iron.

MRI Contrast agents in Pregnancy and Lactation

MRI contrast agents should not be routinely given to pregnant patients.[7] Although there are no reports of teratogenic or mutagenic effects in humans, there are no case controlled prospective studies in large numbers of patients and the precise risk to the fetus is not known. The decision to administer an MRI contrast agent to a pregnant patient should be made on a case by case basis and accompanied by a thoughtful and well documented risk–benefit analysis.

Only tiny amounts of gadolinium based contrast medium given intravenously to a lactating mother reach the milk and a minute proportion entering the baby's gut is absorbed. The very small risk associated with absorption of contrast medium may be considered insufficient to warrant stopping breast feeding for 24 h following gadolinium contrast agents.[14]

References
1. Carr, D.H., Brown, J., Bydder G.M., et al. (1984) Intravenous chelated gadolinium as a contrast agent in NMR imaging of cerebral tumours. *Lancet* **1(8375)**, 484–486.
2. Fink, C., Goyen, M. & Lotz, J. (2007) Magnetic resonance angiography with blood-pool contrast agents: future applications. *Eur. Radiol.* **17 Sup 2**, B38–44.
3. Li, A., Wong, C.S., Wong, M.K., et al. (2006) Acute adverse reactions to magnetic resonance contrast media- gadolinium chelates. *Br. J. Radiol.* **79**, 368–371.
4. Dillman, J.R., Ellis, J.H., Ellis, J.H., et al. (2007) Frequency and severity of acute allergic-like reactions to gadolinium-containing i.v. contrast media in children and adults. *Am. J. Roentgenol.* **189(6)**, 1533–1538.
5. Cochran, S.T., Bomyea, K. & Sayre, J.W. (2001) Trends in adverse events after iv administration of contrast media. *Am. J. Roentgenol.* **176(6)**, 1385–1388.
6. Nelson, K.L., Gifford, L.M., Lauber-Huber, C., et al. (1995) Clinical safety of gadopentetate dimeglumine. *Radiology* **196(2)**, 439–443.
7. Kanal, E., Barkovich, A.J., Bell, C., et al. (2007) ACR guidance document for safe MR practices. *Am. J. Roentgenol.* **188(6)**, 1447–1474.

8. Thomsen, H.S., Almèn, T. & Morcos, S.K. (2002) Gadolinium-containing contrast media for radiographic examinations: a position paper. *Eur. Radiol.* **12(10)**, 2600–2605.
9. Cowper, S.E., Robin, H.S., Steinberg, S.M., et al. (2000) Scleromyxoedema-like cutaneous diseases in renal dialysis patients. *Lancet* **356(9234)**, 1000–1001.
10. Kuo, P.H., Kanal, E., Abu-Alfa, A.K., et al. (2007) Gadolinium-based MR contrast agents and nephrogenic systemic fibrosis. *Radiology* **242(3)**, 647–649.
11. www.esur.org/fileadmin/Guidelines/ESUR_2007_Guideline_6_Kern_Ubersicht_pdf
12. Gandhi, S.N., Brown, M.A., Wong, J.G., et al. (2006) MR contrast agents for liver imaging: what, when, how. *Radiographics* **26(6)**, 1621–1636.
13. Misselwitz, B. (2006) MR contrast agents in lymph node imaging. *Eur. J. Radiol.* **58(3)**, 375–382.
14. Webb, J.A., Thomsen, H.S., Morcos, S.K., et al. (2005) The use of iodinated and gadolinium contrast media during pregnancy and lactation. *Eur. Radiol.* **15(6)**, 1234–1240.

Further reading

Edelman, R.R., Hesselink, J.R., Zlatkin, M.B., et al. (2006) *Clinical Magnetic Resonance Imaging.* 3rd edn. Philadelphia: Saunders Elsevier.
Symposium on Nephrogenic Systemic Fibrosis. Special Issue. (2008) *J. Am. Coll. Radiol.* **5(1)**, 21–56.

CONTRAST AGENTS IN ULTRASONOGRAPHY

During the late 1960s, studies were published describing the intracardiac injection of agents during echocardiography, which were the first reported use of ultrasound (US) contrast. Considerable progress has now been made in the development and clinical application of US contrast agents. These agents contain microbubbles of air, nitrogen or fluorocarbon gas coated with a thin shell of material such as albumin, galactose or lipid. The contrast is often injected intravenously, but in order to cross the pulmonary filter and reach the arterial circulation the microbubbles must be smaller than 7 μm, approximately the size of a red blood cell. Bubbles of this size only remain intact for a very short time in blood. All US contrast media are echo-enhancers and their effect is based on the marked difference in acoustic impedance between microbubbles and surrounding blood or tissue.[1]

Clinical applications of US contrast agents include the following:[2]

1. Assessment of the macrovasculature and microvasculature in different tissues.
2. Identification and characterization of lesions, particularly in the liver, but also in the spleen, pancreas, kidney, prostate, ovary and breast.

3. Voiding urosonography can be used to detect vesico-ureteric reflux in children; here US contrast is administered directly into the bladder.
4. Assessment of fallopian tubal patency at hysterosonosalpinography.
5. Echocardiography applications.

There are a number of different microbubble contrast agents available. Levovist (Schering) is one of the most widely used; it consists of microbubbles of air enclosed by a thin layer of palmitic acid in a galactose solution and is stable in blood for 1–4 min. SonoVue (Bracco), another microbubble contrast agent, is an aqueous suspension of stabilized sulphur hexafluoride microbubbles; after reconstitution of the lyophilisate with saline the suspension is stable and can be used for up to 4 h.

The US agents in clinical use are well tolerated and serious adverse reactions are rarely observed. Allergy-like reactions occur rarely and adverse events are usually mild and self-resolving.[3]

References

1. Calliada, F., Campani, R., Bottinelli, O., et al. (1998) Ultrasound contrast agents: basic principles. *Eur. J. Radiol.* **27**, S157–S160.
2. Quaia, E. (2007) Microbubble ultrasound contrast agents: an update. *Eur. Radiol.* **17(8)**, 1995–2008.
3. Jakobsen, J.A, Oyen, R., Thomsen, H.S., et al (2005) Safety of ultrasound contrast agents. *Eur. Radiol.* **15(5)**, 941–945.

Further reading

Burns, P.N. & Wilson, S.R. (2006) Microbubble contrast for radiological imaging 1. Principles. *Ultrasound Q.* **22(1)**, 5–13.
Wilson, S.R. & Burns, P.N. (2006) Microbubble contrast for radiological imaging 2. Applications. *Ultrasound Q.* **22(1)**, 15–18.

3

Gastrointestinal tract

Methods of imaging the gastrointestinal tract

1. Plain film
2. Barium swallow
3. Barium meal
4. Barium follow-through
5. Small bowel enema
6. Barium enema
7. Ultrasound (US):
   a. Transcutaneous
   b. Endosonography
8. Computed tomography (CT)
9. Magnetic resonance imaging (MRI)
10. Angiography
11. Radionuclide imaging:
    a. Inflammatory bowel disease
    b. Gastro-oesophageal reflux
    c. Gastric emptying
    d. Bile reflux study
    e. Meckel's scan
    f. Gastrointestinal bleeding.

Further reading

Ambrosini, R., Barchiesi, A., Di Mizio, V., et al. (2007) Inflammatory chronic disease of the colon: how to image. *Eur. J. Radiol.* **61(3)**, 442–448.

Brochwicz-Lewinski, M.J., Paterson-Brown, S. & Murchison, J.T. (2003) Small bowel obstruction – the water soluble follow-through revisited. *Clin. Radiol.* **58(5)**, 393–397.

Gasparaitis, A.E. & MacEneaney, P. (2002) Enteroclysis and computed tomography enteroclysis. *Gastroenterol. Clin. North Am.* **31(3)**, 715–730.

INTRODUCTION TO CONTRAST MEDIA

BARIUM

Barium suspension is made up from pure barium sulphate. (Barium carbonate is poisonous.) The particles of barium must be small (0.1–3 m), since this makes them more stable in suspension. A non-ionic suspension medium is used, for otherwise the barium particles would aggregate into clumps. The resulting solution has a pH of 5.3, which makes it stable in gastric acid.

There are many varieties of barium suspensions in use. Exact formulations are secret. In most situations the preparation will be diluted with water to give a lower density (Table 3.1).

Examinations of different parts of the gastrointestinal tract require barium preparations with differing properties:

1. *Barium swallow*, e.g. E-Z HD 200–250% 100 ml (or more, as required).
2. *Barium meal*, e.g. E-Z HD 250% w/v. A high-density, low-viscosity barium is required for a double-contrast barium meal to give a good thin coating that is still sufficiently dense to give satisfactory opacification. E-Z HD fulfils these requirements. It also contains simethicone (an anti-foaming and coating agent) and sorbitol (a coating agent).

Table 3.1 Barium suspensions and dilutions with water to give a lower density

Proprietary name	Density (w/v) – use
Baritop 100	100% – all parts gastrointestinal tract
EPI-C	150% – large bowel
E-Z-Cat	1–2% – computed tomography of gastrointestinal tract
E-Z HD	250% – oesophagus, stomach and duodenum
E-Z Paque	100% – small intestine
Micropaque DC	100% – oesophagus, stomach and duodenum
Micropaque liquid	100% – small and large bowel
Micropaque powder	76% – small and large bowel
Polibar	115% – large bowel
Polibar rapid	100% – large bowel

3. *Barium follow-through*, e.g. E-Z Paque 60–100% w/v 300 ml (150 ml if performed after a barium meal). This preparation contains sorbitol, which produces an osmotic hurrying and is partially resistant to flocculation.
4. *Small bowel enema*, e.g. two tubs of E-Z Paque made up to 1500 ml (60% w/v). N.B. As the transit time through the small bowel is relatively short in this investigation, there is a reduced chance of flocculation. This enables the use of barium preparations which are not flocculation-resistant. Some advocate the addition of Gastrografin to the mixture as this may help reduce the transit time still further.
5. *Barium enema*, e.g. Polibar 115% w/v 500 ml (or more, as required).

Advantages

1. The main advantage when compared to water-soluble contrast agents is the excellent coating which can be achieved with barium, allowing the demonstration of normal and abnormal mucosal patterns.
2. Cost.

Disadvantages

1. Subsequent abdominal CT and US are rendered difficult (if not impossible) to interpret. Patients may be asked to wait for up to 2 weeks to allow satisfactory clearance of the barium. If also required, it is advised that the CT and/or US be performed before the barium study.
2. High morbidity associated with barium in the peritoneal cavity.

Complications

1. *Perforation*. The escape of barium into the peritoneal cavity is rare. If large amounts enter the peritoneal spaces it is extremely serious, and will produce pain and severe hypovolaemic shock. Despite treatment, which should consist of intravenous (i.v.) fluids, steroids and antibiotics, there is still a 50% mortality rate. Of those that survive, 30% will develop peritoneal adhesions and granulomata. Intramediastinal barium also has a significant mortality rate. It is, therefore, imperative that a water-soluble contrast medium is used for any investigation in which there is a risk of perforation, or in which perforation is already suspected.
2. *Aspiration*. Barium if aspirated is relatively harmless. Sequelae include pneumonitis and granuloma formation. Physiotherapy is the only treatment required (for both aspirated barium and low osmolar contrast material (LOCM)), and should be arranged before the patient leaves hospital.

3. *Intravasation.* This may result in a barium pulmonary embolus, which carries a mortality of 80%.

For further complications (e.g. constipation and impaction), see the specific procedure involved.

Further reading

Karanikas, I.D., Kakoulidis, D.D., Gouvas, Z.T., et al. (1997) Barium peritonitis: a rare complication of upper gastrointestinal contrast investigation. *Postgrad. Med. J.* **73**, 297–298.

WATER-SOLUBLE CONTRAST AGENTS

Indications

1. Suspected perforation.
2. Meconium ileus.
3. To distinguish bowel from other structures on CT. A dilute solution of water-soluble contrast medium (e.g. 15 ml of Gastrografin in 1 l of flavoured drink) is used so that minimal artifact 'shadow' is produced.
4. LOCM is used if aspiration is a possibility.

Complications

1. Pulmonary oedema if aspirated (not LOCM).
2. Hypovolaemia in children – due to the hyperosmolality of the contrast media drawing fluid into the bowel (not with LOCM).
3. May precipitate in hyperchlorhydric gastric acid (i.e. 0.1 M HCl) – not non-ionics.

GASES

1. Oesophagus, stomach and duodenum – Carbon dioxide and, less often, air are used in conjunction with barium to achieve a 'double contrast' effect. For the upper gastrointestinal tract, CO_2 is administered orally in the form of gas producing granules/ powder.

   The requirements of these agents are as follows:
   a. Production of an adequate volume of gas – 200–400 ml
   b. Non-interference with barium coating
   c. No bubble production
   d. Rapid dissolution, leaving no residue
   e. Easily swallowed
   f. Low cost.

   Carbex granules and fluid satisfy most of these requirements, but have the disadvantage of being relatively costly.

2. Large bowel – For the large bowel, room air is administered per rectum via a hand pump attached to the enema tube. Carbon dioxide is said to cause less abdominal pain, but inferior bowel distension when compared to air.[1]

Reference
1. Holemans, J.A., Matson, M.B., Hughes, J.A., et al. (1998) A comparison of air, carbon dioxide and air/carbon dioxide mixture as insufflation agents for double contrast barium enema. *Eur. Radiol.* **8**, 274–276.

Further reading
Gellett, L.R., Farrow, R., Bloor, C., et al. (1999) Pain after small bowel meal and pneumocolon: a randomized controlled trial of carbon dioxide versus air insufflation. *Clin. Radiol.* **54**, 381–383.

PHARMACOLOGICAL AGENTS
Hyoscine-N-butyl bromide (Buscopan)
This is an antimuscarinic agent and, therefore, inhibits both intestinal motility and gastric secretion. It is not recommended in children.

Adult dose
20 mg i.v.

Advantages
1. Immediate onset of action
2. Short duration of action (approx. 5–10 min)
3. Cost.

Disadvantages
Antimuscarinic side-effects (uncommon and short-lived) include:
1. blurring of vision
2. dry mouth
3. transient bradycardia followed by tachycardia
4. urinary retention
5. acute gastric dilatation.

Contraindications[1]
1. Closed angle glaucoma
2. Myasthenia gravis
3. Paralytic ileus
4. Pyloric stenosis
5. Prostatic enlargement.
   Glucagon may be used in these circumstances.

Glucagon

This polypeptide hormone produced by the alpha cells of the islets of Langerhans in the pancreas has a predominantly hyperglycaemic effect but also causes smooth muscle relaxation.

Adult dose

0.3 mg i.v. for barium meal
1.0 mg i.v. for barium enema.

Advantages

1. It is a more potent smooth muscle relaxant than Buscopan
2. Short duration of action (approx. 15 min)
3. It does not interfere with the small-bowel transit time.

Disadvantages

1. Hypersensitivity reactions are possible, as it is a protein molecule
2. Relatively long onset of action (1 min)
3. Cost.

Contraindications

1. Phaeochromocytoma. Glucagon can cause the tumour to release catecholamines, resulting in sudden and marked hypertension; 5–10 mg phentolamine mesilate may be administered i.v. in an attempt to control the blood pressure.
2. Caution is advised in the following conditions:[1]
   a. Insulinoma: an initial increase in blood glucose may be followed by severe hypoglycaemia
   b. Glucagonoma.

Side-effects

1. Nausea and vomiting
2. Abdominal pain
3. Hypokalaemia
4. Hypotension
5. Rarely hypersensitivity reactions.

Metoclopramide (Maxolon)

This dopamine antagonist stimulates gastric emptying and small-intestinal transit.

Adult dose

20 mg oral or i.v.

Advantages

1. Produces rapid gastric emptying and, therefore, increased jejunal peristalsis
2. Anti-emetic.

Disadvantages
Extrapyramidal side-effects may occur if the dose exceeds 0.5 mg kg^{-1}.
This is more likely to occur in children/young adults.

Reference
1. British National Formulary (2007) **54**.

General points
In all barium work a high-kV technique is used (90–110 kV).

As in all radiological procedures, the ALARP (*As Low As Reasonably Practicable*) principle should be adhered to.

As regards women of child-bearing age, the '10-day rule' is generally applied for both upper and lower gastrointestinal investigations.

Barium has superior contrast qualities and, unless there are specific contraindications, its use (rather than water-soluble agents) is preferred. The barium swallow is often done in conjunction with a barium meal.

CONTRAST SWALLOW

Indications – suspected oesophageal pathology
1. Dysphagia
2. Anaemia
3. Pain
4. Assessment of tracheo-oesophageal fistulae
5. Assessment of the site of perforation.

Contraindications
None.

Contrast medium
1. E-Z HD 200–250% 100 ml (or more, as required)
2. Iodide-based contrast agent if perforation is suspected (e.g. Conray, Gastrografin)
3. LOCM (approx. 300 mg I ml^{-1}).

N.B.
1. Gastrografin should **NOT** be used for the investigation of a tracheo-oesophageal fistula or when aspiration is a possibility.
2. Barium should **NOT** be used if perforation is suspected.

Equipment

Rapid serial radiography (6 frames per s) or video recording may be required for assessment of the laryngopharynx and upper oesophagus during deglutition.

Patient preparation

None (but as for barium meal if the stomach is also to be examined – see p. 57).

Preliminary film

A control film is advised prior to a water-soluble study if perforation is suspected.

Technique

1. The patient is in the erect, right anterior oblique (RAO) position to throw the oesophagus clear of the spine. An ample mouthful of barium is swallowed, and spot films of the upper and lower oesophagus are taken. Oesophageal varices are better seen in the prone, right posterior oblique (RPO) position, as they will be more distended.
2. If rapid serial radiography is required, it may be performed in the right anterior oblique (RAO) and posterior anterior (PA) positions.

Modification of technique

To demonstrate a tracheo-oesophageal fistula in infants, a 'pull back' nasogastric tube oeosophogram may be performed. A nasogastric tube is introduced to the level of the mid-oesophagus, and the contrast agent (barium or LOCM) is syringed in to distend the oesophagus. This will force the contrast medium through any small fistula which may be present. It is important to take radiographs in the lateral projection during simultaneous injection of the contrast medium and withdrawal of the tube. Although some authors recommend that the infant be examined in the prone position whilst lying on the footstep of a vertical tilting table, satisfactory results are possible with children on their side on a horizontal table. It is important to watch for any possibility of aspiration into the airway from overspill. Overspill may lead to the incorrect diagnosis of tracheo-oesophageal fistula if it is not possible to determine whether contrast medium in the bronchi is due to a small fistula which is difficult to see or to aspiration.

Recently, it has been proposed that pull-back studies are not necessary in the majority of children, as tracheo-oesophageal fistulas can usually be demonstrated on standard contrast swallow examination, providing the oesophagus is distended well with contrast media.[1] Pull-back studies are still necessary for intubated patients, or those who are at high risk of aspiration. It is important to remember that fistulas are usually quite high, and the orifice can be occluded by an endotracheal tube. This can prevent the fistula being opacified. This can be rectified by altering the patients position, or slightly withdrawing the ET tube.

Aftercare

None.

Complications

1. Leakage of barium from an unsuspected perforation
2. Aspiration.

Reference

1. Laffan, E.E., Daneman, A., Ein, S.H., et al. (2006) Tracheoesophageal fistula without esophageal atresia: are pull-back tube esophagograms needed for diagnosis? *Pediatr. Radiol.* **36**, 1141–1147.

BARIUM MEAL

Methods

1. *Double contrast* – the method of choice to demonstrate mucosal pattern.
2. *Single contrast* – uses:
   a. children – since it usually is not necessary to demonstrate mucosal pattern
   b. to demonstrate gross pathology only.

Indications

1. Failed upper gastrointestinal endosocpy
2. Dyspepsia
3. Weight loss
4. Upper abdominal mass
5. Gastrointestinal haemorrhage (or unexplained iron-deficiency anaemia)
6. Partial obstruction
7. Assessment of site of perforation – it is essential that a water-soluble contrast medium, e.g. Gastrografin or LOCM, is used.

Contraindications

Complete large-bowel obstruction.

Contrast medium

1. E-Z HD 250% w/v 135 ml
2. Carbex granules (double contrast technique).

Patient preparation

1. Nil orally for 6 h prior to the examination
2. It should be ensured that there are no contraindications to the pharmacological agents used.

Preliminary film

None.

Technique

The double contrast method (Fig. 3.1):

1. A gas-producing agent is swallowed.
2. The patient then drinks the barium while lying on the left side, supported by the elbow. This position prevents the barium from reaching the duodenum too quickly and so obscuring the greater curve of the stomach.
3. The patient then lies supine and slightly on the right side, to bring the barium up against the gastro-oesophageal junction. This manoeuvre is screened to check for reflux, which may be revealed by asking the patient to cough or to swallow water while in this position. The significance of reflux produced by tipping the patient's head down is debatable, as this is an unphysiological position. If reflux is observed, spot films are taken to record the level to which it ascends.
4. An i.v. injection of a smooth muscle relaxant (Buscopan 20 mg or glucagon 0.3 mg) is given. The administration of Buscopan has been shown not to affect the detection of gastro-oesophageal reflux or hiatus hernia.
5. The patient is asked to roll onto the right side and then quickly over in a complete circle, to finish in an RAO position. This roll is performed to coat the gastric mucosa with barium. Good coating has been achieved if the areae gastricae in the antrum are visible.

Films

There is a great variation in views recommended, and the following is only the scheme used in our departments. In some departments fewer films are taken to reduce the cost and radiation dose:

1. Spot films of the stomach (lying):
   a. RAO – to demonstrate the antrum and greater curve
   b. Supine – to demonstrate the antrum and body
   c. LAO – to demonstrate the lesser curve *en face*
   d. Left lateral tilted, head up 45° – to demonstrate the fundus.

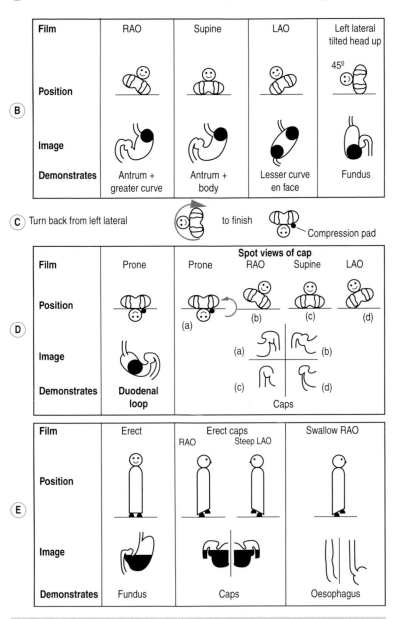

Figure 3.1 Barium meal sequence. Please note in a, b, c and d, the patient position is depicted as if the operator were standing at the end of the screening table looking towards the patient's head. ■ = Barium

From the left lateral position the patient returns to a supine position and then rolls onto the left side and over into a prone position. This sequence of movements is required to avoid barium flooding into the duodenal loop, which would occur if the patient were to roll onto the right side to achieve a prone position.

2. Spot film of the duodenal loop (lying):
   a. Prone – the patient lies on a compression pad to prevent barium from flooding into the duodenum.

   An additional view to demonstrate the anterior wall of the duodenal loop may be taken in an RAO position.

3. Spot films of the duodenal cap (lying):
   a. Prone
   b. RAO – the patient attains this position from the prone position by rolling first onto the left side, for the reasons mentioned above
   c. Supine
   d. LAO.

4. Additional views of the fundus in an erect position may be taken at this stage, if there is suspicion of a fundal lesion.

5. Spot films of the oesophagus are taken, while barium is being swallowed, to complete the examination.

Modification of technique for young children

The main indication will be to identify a cause for vomiting. The examination is modified to identify the three major causes of vomiting – gastro-oesophageal reflux, pyloric obstruction and mal-rotation, and it is essential that the position of the duodeno-jejunal flexure is demonstrated:

1. Single contrast technique using 30% w/v barium sulphate and no paralytic agent.

2. A relatively small volume of barium – enough to just fill the fundus – is given to the infant in the supine position. A film of the distended oesophagus is exposed.

3. The child is turned semi-prone into a LPO or RAO position. A film is exposed as barium passes through the pylorus. The pylorus is shown to even better advantage if 20–40° caudocranial angulation can be employed with an overhead screening unit. Gastric emptying is prolonged if the child is upset. A dummy coated with glycerine is a useful pacifier.

4. Once barium enters the duodenum, the infant is returned to the supine position, and with the child perfectly straight a second film is exposed as barium passes around the duodenojejunal flexure.

5. Once malrotation has been diagnosed or excluded, a further volume of barium is administered until the stomach is reasonably full and barium lies against the gastro-oesophageal junction. The child is gently rotated through 180° in an attempt to elicit gastro-oesophageal reflux.

In newborn infants with upper intestinal obstruction, e.g. duodenal atresia, the diagnosis may be confirmed if 20 ml of air is injected down the nasogastric tube (which will almost certainly have already been introduced by the medical staff). If the diagnosis remains in doubt, it can be replaced by a positive contrast agent (dilute barium or LOCM if the risk of aspiration is high).

Aftercare

1. The patient should be warned that his bowel motions will be white for a few days after the examination and may be difficult to flush away.
2. The patient should be advised to eat and drink normally to avoid barium impaction. Laxatives may be taken if required.
3. The patient must not leave the department until any blurring of vision produced by the Buscopan has resolved.

Complications

1. Leakage of barium from an unsuspected perforation
2. Aspiration of stomach contents due to the Buscopan
3. Conversion of a partial large bowel obstruction into a complete obstruction by the impaction of barium
4. Barium appendicitis, if barium impacts in the appendix (exceedingly rare)
5. Side-effects of the pharmacological agents used.

N.B. It must be emphasized that there are many variations in technique, according to individual preference, and that the best way of becoming familiar with the sequence of positioning is actually to perform the procedure oneself.

BARIUM FOLLOW-THROUGH

Methods

1. Single contrast
2. With the addition of an effervescent agent
3. With the addition of a pneumocolon technique.

Indications

1. Pain
2. Diarrhoea
3. Anaemia/gastrointestinal bleeding
4. Partial obstruction
5. Malabsorption
6. Abdominal mass.

Contraindications

1. Complete obstruction. This may not be an absolute contraindication if the surgical team are aware of this.
2. Suspected perforation (unless a water-soluble contrast medium is used).

Contrast medium

E-Z Paque 100% w/v 300 ml usually given in 10–15-min increments, although some radiologists give the full 300 ml at once. The transit time through the small bowel has been shown to be reduced by the addition of 10 ml of Gastrografin to the barium. In children, 3–4 ml kg^{-1} is a suitable volume.

In situations where barium is contraindicated, non-ionic water-soluble solutions have been shown to be a satisfactory alternative.[1]

Patient preparation

Metoclopramide 20 mg orally may be given before or during the examination.

Preliminary film

Plain abdominal film is used if small bowel obstruction is thought possible.

Technique

The aim is to deliver a single column of barium into the small bowel. This is achieved by laying the patient on his right side after the barium has been ingested. Metoclopramide enhances the rate of gastric emptying. If the transit time through the small bowel is found to be slow, the addition of an osmotic water-soluble contrast agent may help to speed it up. If a follow-through examination is combined with a barium meal, glucagon is used for the duodenal cap views rather than Buscopan because it has a short length of action and does not interfere with the small-bowel transit time.

Films

1. Prone PA films of the abdomen are taken every 15–20 min during the first hour, and subsequently every 20–30 min until the colon is reached. The prone position is used because the pressure on the abdomen helps to separate the loops of small bowel.
2. Spot films of the terminal ileum are taken supine, using a compression pad.

Additional films

1. To separate loops of small bowel:
   a. compression with fluoroscopy
   b. obliques

    c. with X-ray tube angled into the pelvis

    d. with the patient tilted head down.

2. To demonstrate diverticula: erect film – this position will reveal any fluid levels caused by contrast medium retained within the diverticula.

Aftercare

As for barium meal.

Complications

As for barium meal.

References
1. Jobling, C., Halligan, S. & Bartram, C. (1999) The use of water-soluble contrast agents for small bowel follow-through examinations. *Eur. Radiol.* **9**, 706–710.

Further reading
Ha, H.K., Shin, J.H., Rha, S.E., et al. (1999) Modified small bowel follow through: use of methylcellulose to improve bowel transradiance and prepare barium suspension. *Radiology* **211**, 197-201.

Summers, D.S., Roger, M.D., Allan, P.L., et al. (2007) Accelerating the transit time of barium sulphate suspensions in small bowel examinations. *Eur. J. Radiol.* **62(1)**, 122–125.

SMALL-BOWEL ENEMA

Advantage

This procedure gives better visualization of the proximal small bowel than that achieved by a barium follow-through because rapid infusion of a large, continuous column of contrast medium directly into the jejunum provides better distension of the proximal small bowel. This is less effective in the ileum.

Disadvantages

1. Intubation may be unpleasant for the patient, and may occasionally prove difficult.
2. It is more time-consuming for the radiologist.
3. There is a higher radiation dose to the patient (screening the tube into position).

Indications and Contraindications

These are the same as for a barium follow-through. In some departments it is only performed in the case of an equivocal follow-through.

Contrast medium

1. E-Z Paque 70% w/v diluted
2. Dilute Baritop
3. 600 ml of 0.5% methylcellulose after 500 ml of 70% w/v barium.[1]

It may be difficult to obtain good distension and double-contrast effect of the distal small bowel and terminal ileum.

Equipment

A choice of tubes is available:
1. Bilbao-Dotter tube with a guidewire (the tube is longer than the wire so that there is reduced risk of perforation when introducing the wire).
2. Silk tube (E. Merck Ltd). This is a 10-F, 140-cm long tube. It is made of polyurethane and the stylet and the internal lumen of the tube are coated with a water-activated lubricant to facilitate the smooth removal of the stylet after insertion.

Patient preparation

1. NBM after midnight
2. If the patient is taking any antispasmodic drugs, they must be stopped 1 day prior to the examination
3. Tetracaine lozenge 30 mg, 30 min before the examination.

Immediately before the examination the pharynx is anaesthetized with lidocaine spray.

Preliminary film

Plain abdominal film is used if a small bowel obstruction is suspected.

Technique

1. The patient sits on the edge of the X-ray table. The pharynx is thoroughly anaesthetized with lidocaine spray. If a per nasal approach is planned, the patency of the nasal passages is checked by asking the patient to sniff with one nostril occluded. The silk tube should be passed with the guidewire pre-lubricated and fully within the tube, whereas for the Bilbao-Dotter tube it may be more comfortable to introduce the guidewire after the tube tip is in the stomach.

2. The tube is then passed through the nose or the mouth, and brief lateral screening of the neck may be helpful in negotiating the epiglottic region. The patient is asked to swallow with the neck flexed, as the tube is passed through the pharynx. The tube is then advanced into the gastric antrum.

3. The patient then lies down and the tube is passed into the duodenum. Various manoeuvres may be used alone or in combination, to help this part of the procedure, which may be difficult:

   a. Lay the patient on his left side so that the gastric air bubble rises to the antrum, thus straightening out the stomach.

   b. Advance the tube whilst applying clockwise rotational motion (as viewed from the head of the patient looking towards the feet).

   c. In the case of the Bilbao-Dotter tube, introduce the guidewire.

   d. Get the patient to sit up, to try to overcome the tendency of the tube to coil in the fundus of the stomach.

   e. Metoclopramide (20 mg i.v.) may help.

4. When the tip of the tube has been passed through the pylorus, the guidewire tip is maintained at the pylorus as the tube is passed over it along the duodenum to the level of the ligament of Treitz. Clockwise torque applied to the tube may again help in getting past the junction of the first and second parts of the duodenum. The tube is passed beyond the duodenojejunal flexure to diminish the risk of aspiration due to reflux of barium into the stomach.

5. Barium is then run in quickly, and spot films are taken of the barium column and its leading edge at the regions of interest, until the colon is reached. If methylcellulose is used, it is infused continuously, after an initial bolus of 500 ml of barium, until the barium has reached the colon.

6. The tube is then withdrawn, aspirating any residual fluid in the stomach. Again, this is to decrease the risk of aspiration.

7. Finally, prone and supine abdominal films are taken.

Modification of technique

In patients with malabsorption, especially if an excess of fluid has been shown on the preliminary film, the volume of barium should be increased (240–260 ml). Compression views of bowel loops should be obtained before obtaining double contrast. Flocculation is likely to occur early. If it is important to obtain images of the duodenum, the catheter tip should be sited proximal to the ligament of Trietz.

Aftercare

The patient should be warned that diarrhoea may occur as a result of the large volume of fluid given.

Complications

1. Aspiration
2. Perforation of the bowel owing to manipulation of the guidewire (very rare).

Reference

1. Ha, H.K., Park, K.B., Kim, P.N., et al. (1998) Use of methylcellulose in small bowel follow through examination: comparison with conventional series in normal subjects. *Abdom. Imaging* **23**, 281–285.

Further reading

Cirillo, L.C., Camera, L., Della Noce, M., et al. (2000) Accuracy of enteroclysis in Crohn's disease of the small bowel: a retrospective study. *Eur. Radiol.* **10(12)**, 1894–1898.

Minordi, L.M., Vecchioli, A., Guidi, L., et al. (2006) Multidetector CT enteroclysis versus barium enteroclysis with methylcellulose in patients with suspected small bowel disease. *Eur. Radiol.* **16(7)**, 1527–1536.

Nolan, D.J. (1997) The true yield of the small intestinal barium study. *Endoscopy* **29**, 447–453.

BARIUM ENEMA

Methods

1. *Double contrast* – the method of choice to demonstrate mucosal pattern.
2. *Single contrast* – uses:
   a. children – since it is usually not necessary to demonstrate mucosal pattern
   b. reduction of an intussusception (see p. 71)
   c. localization of an obstructing colonic lesion.

Indication

Suspected large bowel pathology.

N.B. If a tight stricture is demonstrated, only run a small volume of barium proximally to define the upper margin, as otherwise the barium may impact.

Contraindications

Absolute
1. Toxic megacolon (double-contrast barium enema is said to be no better than clinical judgement in this situation, and is clearly more dangerous[1])
2. Pseudomembranous colitis
3. Recent rectal biopsy[2] via:
   a. rigid endoscope within previous 5 days
   b. flexible endoscope within previous 24 h.

Relative
1. Incomplete bowel preparation
2. Recent barium meal – it is advised to wait for 7–10 days
3. Patient frailty.

Contrast medium
1. Polibar 115% w/v 500 ml (or more, as required)
2. Air.

Equipment
Miller disposable enema tube.

Patient preparation
Many regimes for bowel preparation exist. A suggested regime is as follows:

For 3 days prior to examination
Low residue diet.

On the day prior to examination
1. Fluids only
2. Picolax – at 08.00 h and 18:00 h.
   Consider admitting the elderly and those with social problems.

On the day of the examination
It is advisable to place diabetics first on the list.

Technique
The double-contrast method (Fig. 3.2):
1. The patient lies on their left side, and the catheter is inserted gently into the rectum. It is taped firmly in position. Connections are made to the barium reservoir and the hand pump for injecting air.
2. An i.v. injection of Buscopan (20 mg) or glucagon (1 mg) is given. Some radiologists choose to give the muscle relaxant half way through the procedure.

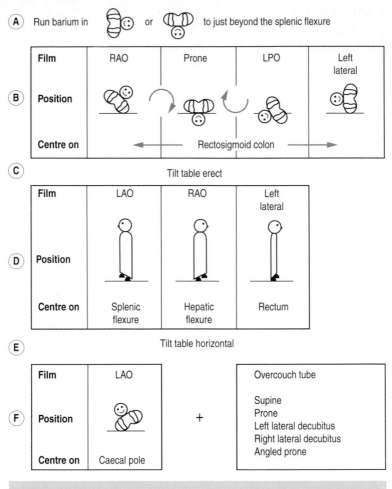

Figure 3.2 Barium enema sequence. Please note in a, b and f the patient position is depicted as if the operator were standing at the end of the screening table looking towards the patient's head.

3. The infusion of barium is commenced. Intermittent screening is required to check the progress of the barium. The infusion is terminated when the barium reaches the hepatic flexure. The column of barium within the sigmoid colon is run back out by either lowering the infusion bag to the floor or tilting the table to the erect position.

4. Air is gently pumped into the bowel, forcing the column of barium round towards the caecum, and producing the double-

contrast effect. Some centres use CO_2 as the negative contrast agent as it has been shown to reduce the incidence of severe, post-double-contrast enema pain.[3]

Films

There is a great variation in views recommended. Fewer films may be taken to reduce the radiation dose and cost.

The sequence of positioning enables the barium to flow proximally to reach the caecal pole. Air is pumped in as required to distend the colon:

1. Spot films of all areas of the large bowel are taken including oblique views. Particular emphasis should be taken with the rectosigmoid and caecum/proximal right colon.
2. Overcouch films (usually with a ceiling tube) to demonstrate the entire large bowel (lying):
   a. Supine
   b. Prone
   c. Left lateral decubitus
   d. Right lateral decubitus
   e. Prone, with the tube angled 45° caudad and centred 5 cm above the posterior superior iliac spines. This view separates overlying loops of sigmoid colon.
3. Extra spot films of any regions of abnormality are taken as required.

Aftercare

1. Patients should be warned that their bowel motions will be white for a few days after the examination, and to eat and drink normally to avoid barium impaction.
2. The patient must not leave the department until any blurring of vision produced by the Buscopan has resolved.

Complications (all are rare)

1. Perforation of the bowel. There is an increased risk of this in:
   a. Infants and the elderly
   b. Obstructing neoplasm
   c. Ulceration of the bowel wall
   d. Inflation of a Foley catheter balloon in a colostomy, or the rectum
   e. Patients on steroid therapy
   f. Hypothyroidism.
2. Transient bacteraemia
3. Side-effects of the pharmacological agents used (see p. 53)
4. Cardiac arrhythmia due to rectal distension
5. Intramural barium
6. Venous intravasation. This may result in a barium pulmonary embolus, which carries 80% mortality.

References
1. Marion, J.F. & Present, D.H. (1997) The modern medical management of acute severe ulcerative colitis. *Eur. J. Gastroenterol. Hepatol.* **9**, 831–835.
2. Low, V.H. (1998) What is the current recommended waiting time for performance of a gastrointestinal barium study after endoscopic biopsy of the upper or lower gastrointestinal tract? *Am. J. Roentgenol.* **170**, 1104–1105.
3. Taylor, P.N. & Beckly, D.E. (1991) Use of air in double contrast barium enema: is it still acceptable? *Clin. Radiol.* **44**, 183–184.

Further reading
Cittadini, G., Sardanelli, F., De Cicco, E., et al. (1999) Bowel preparation for the double contrast barium enema: how to maintain coating with cleansing? *Clin. Radiol.* **54**, 216–220.
Ferrucci, J.T. (2006) Double-contrast barium enema: use in practice and implications for CT colonography. *Am. J. Roentgenol.* **187(1)**, 170–173.
Martin, C.J. (2004) A review of factors affecting patient doses for barium enemas and meals. *Br. J. Radiol.* **77(922)**, 864–868.
Rollandi, G.A., Biscaldi, E. & DeCicco, E. (2007) Double contrast barium enema: technique, indications, results and limitations of a conventional imaging methodology in the MDCT virtual endoscopy era. *Eur. J. Radiol.* **61(3)**, 382–327.

THE 'INSTANT' ENEMA

Indications

1. To identify the level of suspected large bowel obstruction.
2. To show the extent and severity of mucosal lesions in active ulcerative colitis.

Contraindications

1. Toxic megacolon
2. Rectal biopsy (as for barium enema)
3. Chronic ulcerative colitis – a formal barium enema should be performed to exclude a carcinoma
4. Crohn's colitis – assessment in this situation is unreliable.

Contrast medium

Water-soluble contrast.

Preliminary film

Plain abdominal film – to exclude:
1. toxic megacolon
2. perforation.

Technique

1. The contrast medium is run until it flows into:
   a. an obstructing lesion
   b. dilated bowel loops
   c. the caecum.
2. Air insufflation is not required – i.e. single contrast technique.

Films

These are obtained as required, e.g.:

1. prone
2. left lateral decubitus
3. erect.

AIR ENEMA

Indications

Demonstrate extent of ulcerative colitis.

Technique

1. Insert 14–16-F Foley catheter into rectum and inflate balloon (10–20 ml)
2. Take preliminary overcouch anterior posterior (AP) film of abdomen
3. View film and without the patient moving give relaxant, e.g. Buscopan and then inflate air (gentle puffs) into catheter lumen
4. Take AP film of abdomen.

REDUCTION OF AN INTUSSUSCEPTION

This procedure should only be attempted in full consultation with the surgeon in charge of the case and when an anaesthetist with adequate paediatric training and experience, and with paediatric anaesthetic equipment, is available.[1,2]

Methods

1. Using air and fluoroscopy[3] – barium is no longer used in the majority of centres as air reduction has the following advantages:
   a. more rapid reduction, because the low viscosity of air permits rapid filling of the colon

    b. reduced radiation dose because of the above

    c. more effective reduction

    d. in the presence of a perforation, air in the peritoneal cavity is preferable to barium, and gut organisms are not washed into the peritoneal cavity

    e. there is more accurate control of intraluminal pressure

    f. less mess, and a dry infant will not lose heat

    g. less expensive.

2. Using a water-soluble contrast medium and US.

Contraindications

1. Peritonitis or perforation
2. The pneumatic method should probably not be used in children over 4 years of age as there is a higher incidence of significant lead points which may be missed[4]
3. Successful reduction is less likely in patients with prolonged symptoms or radiographic signs of obstruction, but this does not preclude an attempt at reduction if the patient is well hydrated and stable.[5]

Patient preparation

1. Sedation is of questionable value, but analgesia is important (e.g. morphine $50\,\mu g\,kg^{-1}$ if <1 year or $50–100\,\mu g\,kg^{-1}$ if >1 year).
2. Some institutions perform the examination under general anaesthesia. This has the advantages of greater muscle relaxation, which may increase the likelihood of successful reduction, and also enables the child to go to surgery quickly in the event of a failed radiological reduction.
3. Correction of fluid and electrolyte imbalance. The child has an i.v. line in-situ.
4. Antibiotic cover is not routine.

Preliminary investigations

1. Plain abdominal film – to assess bowel distension and to exclude perforation. A right-side-up decubitus film is often helpful in confirming the diagnosis by showing a failure of caecal filling with bowel gas because of the presence of the soft-tissue mass of the intussusception. Normal plain films do not exclude the diagnosis, and the clinical findings and/or history should be sufficient indications.
2. US – should confirm or exclude the diagnosis. Absence of blood flow within the intussusceptum on colour-flow Doppler should lead to cautious reduction.[6] US may identify a lead point; if so, even attempted reduction (to facilitate surgery) should be followed by surgery. If US identifies fluid trapped between the intussusceptum and intussuscipiens, the success rate is significantly reduced.[7]

Contrast medium

1. Air
2. Barium sulphate 100% w/v (now rarely used)
3. Water-soluble contrast, e.g. LOCM 150 or dilute Gastrografin (1 part Gastrografin to 4 or 5 parts water).

Technique

A 16–22-F balloon catheter is inserted into the rectum and the buttocks taped tightly together to provide a seal. It may be necessary to inflate the balloon but if this is done it should be performed under fluoroscopic control so that the rectum is not over distended.

Pneumatic reduction

1. The child is placed in the prone position so that it is easier to maintain the catheter in the rectum and the child is disturbed as little as possible during the procedure.
2. Air is instilled by a hand or mechanical pump and the intussusception is pushed back by a sustained pressure of up to 80 mmHg. If this fails, the pressure may be increased to 120 mmHg. Pressure should be monitored at all times and there should be a pressure release valve in the system to ensure that excessive pressures are not delivered.
3. Reduction is successful when there is free flow of air into the distal ileum.
4. If the intussusception does not move after 3 min of sustained pressure, the pressure is reduced and the child rested for 3 min. If, after three similar attempts, the intussusception is still immovable it is considered irreducible and arrangements are made for surgery.
5. The intussusception is only considered completely reduced when the terminal ileum is filled with air. However, it is not uncommon for there to be a persisting filling defect in the caecum at the end of the procedure, with or without reflux of air into the terminal ileum. This is often due to an oedematous ileocaecal valve. In the presence of a soft-tissue caecal mass, a clinically well and stable child should be returned to the ward to await a further attempt at reduction after a period of 2–8 h rather than proceed to surgery. A second enema is often successful at complete reduction or showing resolution of the oedematous ileocaecal valve.[8]
6. When air (or barium) dissects between the two layers of the intussusception – the dissection sign – reduction is less likely.[9]

Barium reduction: now rarely used

1. Patient positioning is as for the pneumatic method.
2. The bag containing barium is raised 100 cm above the table top and barium run in under hydrostatic pressure. Progress of the column of barium is monitored by intermittent fluoroscopy.

3. If the intussusception does not move after 3 min of sustained pressure, the bag of barium is lowered to table-top height and the child rested for 3 min. If, after three similar attempts, the intussusception is still immovable it is considered irreducible and arrangements are made for surgery.
4. The points regarding failed or incomplete reduction discussed above also apply to hydrostatic reduction.

Ultrasound reduction
1. To facilitate scanning the child must be supine.
2. The intussusception can be identified with US. The contrast medium is run as far as the obstruction and its passage around the colon and the reducing head of the intussusception monitored by US.
3. The points regarding failed or incomplete reduction discussed above also apply to this technique.

Films
1. Spot films as required
2. Post-reduction film.

Aftercare
Observation in hospital for 24 h.

Complications
Perforation. For the pneumatic method, if a pump is used without a pressure-monitoring valve, perforation may result in a tension pneumoperitoneum, resulting in respiratory embarrassment. Puncture of the peritoneal cavity with a 'green' 23-G needle may be life-saving.

References
1. The Royal College of Anaesthetists (1999) *Guidelines for the Provision of Anaesthetic Services*. Guidance on the Provision of Paediatric Anaesthesia, pp 24–26. London: Royal College of Anaesthetists.
2. The British Association of Paediatric Surgeons (1994, revised 1995) *A Guide for Purchasers and Providers of Paediatric Surgeons*. London: British Association of Paediatric Surgeons.
3. Kirks, D.R. (1995) Air intussusception reduction: 'The winds of change'. *Pediatr. Radiol.* **25**, 89–91.
4. Stringer, D.A. & Ein, S.H. (1990) Pneumatic reduction: advantages, risks and indications. *Pediatr. Radiol.* **20**, 475–477.
5. Daneman, A. & Navarro, O. (2004) Intussusception Part 2: An update on the evolution of management. *Paediatr. Radiol.* **34**, 97–108.
6. Lim, H.K., Bae, S.H., Lee, K.H., et al. (1994) Assessment of reducibility of ileocolic intussusception in children: usefulness of color Doppler sonography. *Radiology* **191**, 781–785.
7. Britton, I. & Wilkinson, A.G. (1999) Ultrasound features of intussusception predicting outcome of air enema. *Pediatr. Radiol.* **29**, 705–710.

8. Gorenstein, A., Raucher, A., Serour, F., et al. (1998) Intussusception in children: reduction with repeated, delayed air enema. *Radiology* **206**, 721–724.

9. Barr, L.L., Stansberry, S.D., & Swischuk, L.E. (1990) Significance of age, duration, obstruction and the dissection sign in intussusception. *Pediatr. Radiol.* **20**, 454–456.

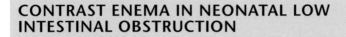

CONTRAST ENEMA IN NEONATAL LOW INTESTINAL OBSTRUCTION

The differential diagnosis of low intestinal obstruction in the new-born consists of five conditions which comprise nearly all causes. Three involve the colon: Hirschsprung's disease, functional immaturity of the colon (small left colon syndrome, meconium plug syndrome) and colonic atresia. Two involve the distal ileum: meconium ileus and ileal atresia. All infants with low intestinal obstruction require a contrast enema.

Contraindications

Perforation.

Patient preparation

The baby should already have i.v. access and be well hydrated prior to the procedure.

Contrast medium

Dilute ionic contrast medium as is used for cystography, e.g. Urografin 150. This has the advantage of not provoking large fluid shifts and being dense enough to provide satisfactory images. Non-ionic contrast media and barium offer no advantages and the latter is contraindicated with perforation as a possibility. Infants with meconium ileus or functional immaturity will benefit from a water-soluble contrast enema and so their therapeutic enema commences with the diagnostic study. The non-operative treatment of meconium ileus was first described using the hypertonic agent Gastrografin, which dislodged the sticky meconium by drawing water into the bowel lumen. However, most paediatric radiologists now believe that a hypertonic agent is not necessary for successful treatment.[1]

Technique

If the enema demonstrates that the entire colon is small (a microcolon; <1 cm in diameter) then the diagnosis is likely to be meconium ileus or ileal atresia. (The microcolon of prematurity and total colonic Hirschsprung's disease are alternative rare diagnoses.) For the treatment of meconium ileus, the aim is to run the water-soluble contrast medium into the small bowel to surround the meconium. An attempt should be made to get the contrast medium back into dilated small bowel. If successful, meconium should be passed in the next hour. If no result is seen and the infant's condition deteriorates then surgical intervention will be necessary. If the passage of meconium is incomplete and the clinical condition remains stable, multiple enemas over the succeeding few days will be necessary to ensure complete resolution of the obstruction.

Overall success rate is approximately 50–60%, with a perforation rate of 2%.[1]

Reference
1. Kao, S.C.S. & Franken, E.A. Jr. (1995) Nonoperative treatment of simple meconium ileus: a survey of the Society for Pediatric Radiology. *Pediatr. Radiol.* **25**, 97–100.

SINOGRAM

1. A water-soluble contrast medium should be used.
2. A preliminary film is taken to exclude the presence of a radio-opaque foreign body.
3. An appropriate-size Foley catheter is then inserted into the orifice of the sinus and the balloon inflated to prevent retrograde flow.
4. The contrast medium is injected carefully under fluoroscopic control.
5. Spot films are taken as required, including tangential views.

RETROGRADE ILEOGRAM

Indications
To demonstrate anatomy of small bowel in patients with an ileostomy.

Technique
1. Cannulate the ileostomy with an appropriate (16–22-F) Foley catheter. Carefully inflate the balloon.

2. Inject contrast. Dilute barium (Baritop) can be used as a single contrast or as double contrast with either air or water/methyl cellulose (see small bowel enema). Water-soluble contrast media may be used.

COLOSTOMY ENEMA

Indications

To demonstrate proximal colon following resection of the rectum.

Technique

1. Cannulate colostomy with a 22–26-F Foley catheter and gently inflate balloon.
2. Infuse barium as for a barium enema.

LOOPOGRAM

Indications

Appropriate in patients following bladder resection to demonstrate anatomy of ileal conduit, ureters, and renal pelvicalyceal systems.

Contrast

Low concentration water-soluble contrast agent (150 mg/ml^{-1}).

Technique

Cannulate ileal conduit with 14–18-F Foley catheter and gently inflate balloon. Inject contrast into ileal conduit.

HERNIOGRAM

Indications

1. History suggestive of a hernia with a normal/inconclusive physical examination.
2. Undiagnosed groin pain.

Contraindications

1. Infancy
2. Pregnancy
3. Intestinal obstruction
4. Allergy to contrast medium.

Patient preparation

The patient is asked to empty their bladder just prior to the examination.

Contrast medium

50–100 ml water-soluble medium (e.g. Omnipaque 300).

Technique

1. The patient lies supine on the X-ray table.
2. An aseptic technique is employed.
3. 5–10 ml of 1% lidocaine is injected into the skin, subcutaneous tissues and peritoneum. The injection site varies between operators; the midline just below the umbilicus is most common, the midpoint of the left lateral rectus muscle is one variation.
4. A 18G spinal needle is introduced into the peritoneal cavity and used to inject contrast into the peritoneal cavity.

Films

1. Prone
2. Erect films: frontal, obliques, lateral.

The patient is asked to cough and perform the Valsalva manoeuvre while these are taken. The tube may be angled 25° caudally.

Complications

These are uncommon, and patient admission for observation is all that is usually required:

1. Pain
2. Visceral puncture
3. Vascular puncture
4. Injection into the abdominal wall
5. Haematoma at the injection site
6. Allergy to contrast medium.

Further reading

Ekberg, O. (1981) Inguinal herniography in adults: technique, normal anatomy, and diagnostic criteria for hernias. *Radiology* **138**, 31–36.
Ekberg, O. (1983) Complications after herniography in adults. *Am. J. Roentgenol.* **140**, 490–495.

Garner, J.P., Patel, S., Glaves, J., et al. (2006) Is herniography useful? *Hernia* **10(1)**, 66–69.

Gwanmesia, I.I., Walsh, S., Bury, R., et al. (2001) Unexplained groin pain: safety and reliability of herniography for the diagnosis of occult hernias. *Postgrad. Med. J.* **77(906)**, 250–251.

3

EVACUATING PROCTOGRAM

Indications

1. Constipation
2. Suspected pelvic floor weakness – posterior (rectocoele/enterocoele/rectal intussuception)
3. Anorectal incontinence – anal manometry and anal US preferred.

Contraindications

Pregnancy.

Contrast medium

Thick barium paste (although commercial pastes are available, this may be satisfactorily prepared with barium powder and cereal, e.g. Readibrek).

Technique

1. One can of Baritop or equivalent given orally 1 hour prior to examination to opacify small bowel
2. For female patients, approximately 20–30 ml of water-soluble contrast mixed with US gel are introduced into the vagina through a Foley catheter
3. Approximately 120 ml of barium paste (or enough to fill the rectum) are instilled via a bladder syringe.

Films

1. These are taken in a lateral projection with the patient sitting on a commode
2. Video-recording at rest and during the Valsalva manoeuvre and during pelvic floor contractions
3. Video-recording during defecation using a maximum of 1- min screening time to minimize patient dose.

Further reading

Dobben, A.C., Wiersma, T.G., Janssen, L.W., et al. (2005) Prospective assessment of interobserver agreement for defecography in fecal incontinence. *Am. J. Roentgenol.* **185(5)**, 1166–1172.

Jones, H.J., Swift, R.I. & Blake, H. (1998) A prospective audit of the usefulness of evacuating proctography. *Ann. R. Coll. Surg. Engl.* **80(1)**, 40–45.

Kelvin, F.M., Maglinte, D.D., Hornback, J.A., et al. (1992) Pelvic prolapse: assessment with evacuation proctography (defecography). *Radiology* **184**, 547–551.

COELIAC AXIS, SUPERIOR MESENTERIC AND INFERIOR MESENTERIC ARTERIOGRAPHY

Indications

1. Gastrointestinal haemorrhage
2. Staging tumours prior to intervention (surgical or radiological)
3. Gastrointestinal ischaemia
4. Portal venography. (This is rarely needed except prior to intervention as CT/MR shows PV system well.)

Contrast medium

LOCM 280 to 370.

Equipment

1. Digital fluoroscopy with angiography facility
2. Pump injector
3. Catheter – selective femorovisceral, sidewinder or cobra catheter.

Technique

1. Femoral artery puncture – Seldinger technique
2. Bowel movement causing subtraction artifact can be reduced by using a smooth-muscle relaxant (e.g. Buscopan 10–20 mg) and abdominal compression
3. When performed for gastrointestinal bleeding, provided that the patient is actively bleeding at the time, a blood loss of $0.5–0.6\,\mathrm{ml\,min^{-1}}$ can be demonstrated. The site of active bleeding is revealed by extravasated contrast medium remaining in the bowel on the late films, when intravascular contrast has cleared. Vascular malformations, tumours and varices may be demonstrated.

Coeliac axis
Patient supine; 25–36 ml contrast medium at 5–6 ml s^{-1}.

(Angiography of the pancreas is best achieved by selective injection into the splenic, dorsal pancreatic and gastroduodenal arteries.)

Superior mesenteric artery
Patient supine; 25–42 ml contrast medium at 5–7 ml s^{-1}.

Late-phase visceral arteriography
Patient slightly RPO.

When selective catheterization of the coeliac or SMA has been achieved, delayed venous-phase films will show the portal vein.

N.B. If splenic vein opacification is required, then a late-phase splenic arteriogram is necessary.

Inferior mesenteric artery
If the inferior mesenteric artery is to be examined as part of a procedure which will examine the superior mesenteric artery or coeliac axis as well, e.g. to find the source of gastrointestinal bleeding, then the inferior mesenteric artery should be examined first so that contrast medium in the bladder will not obscure its terminal branches.

Patient 30° LPO (to open the sigmoid loop); 10–20 ml at 4 ml s^{-1}.

ULTRASOUND OF THE GASTROINTESTINAL TRACT

ENDOLUMINAL EXAMINATION OF THE OESOPHAGUS AND STOMACH

Indications

1. Staging of primary malignant disease of the upper gastrointestinal tract or mediastinal pathology, such as suspected lymphadenopathy or mass
2. US-guided biopsy of primary tumours or suspected nodal disease.

Equipment

Echoendoscope with 5.0–10-MHz 360° rotary transducer.

Patient preparation

Conscious sedation is usually required.

Technique

Monitoring with a pulse oximeter is recommended. If the stomach is to be examined, this may be filled with de-aerated water through the working channel before the patient is examined in a left lateral decubitus position. The echo-endoscope is passed during endoscopy, either combined with direct vision or blind by an experienced endoscopist. A 360° rotary transducer will provide transverse scans with respect to the long axis of the tube.

Aftercare

The patient should be observed by experienced nursing staff until the effects of any sedation have worn off, in the same manner as for other endoscopic procedures.

Further reading

Botet, J.F. & Lightdale, C. (1992) Endoscopic ultrasonography of the upper gastrointestinal tract. *Radiol. Clin. North Am.* **30**, 1067–1083.

Weber, W.A. & Ott, K. (2004) Imaging of esophageal and gastric cancer. *Semin. Oncol.* **31(4)**, 530–541.

TRANSABDOMINAL EXAMINATION OF THE LOWER OESOPHAGUS AND STOMACH

Indications

Not routinely indicated in adults.

HYPERTROPHIC PYLORIC STENOSIS

The typical patient is a 6-week-old male infant with non-bilious projectile vomiting.

Equipment

5–7.5-MHz linear or sector transducer.

Technique

1. The right upper quadrant is scanned with the patient supine. If the stomach is very distended, the pylorus will be displaced posteriorly and the stomach should be decompressed with a nasogastric tube. If the stomach is collapsed, the introduction of some dextrose, by mouth or via a nasogastric tube, will distend the antrum and differentiate it from the pylorus.
2. The pylorus is scanned in its longitudinal and transverse planes and images will resemble an olive and a doughnut, respectively. The poorly echogenic muscle is easily differentiated from the bright mucosa. Antral peristalsis can be seen and the volume of fluid passing through the pylorus with each antral wave can be assessed.

3. A number of measurements can be made. These include muscle thickness, canal length, pyloric volume and muscle thickness/wall diameter ratio, but there is no universal agreement as to which is the most discriminating parameter.

Further reading

King, S.J. (1997) Ultrasound of the hollow gastrointestinal tract in children. *Eur. Radiol.* **7**, 559–565.

Misra, D., Akhter, A., Potts, S.R., et al. (1997) Pyloric stenosis. Is over reliance on ultrasound scans leading to negative explorations? *Eur. J. Ped. Surg.* **7**, 328–330.

SMALL BOWEL

Indications

1. It is infrequent that US is used as a primary investigation for patients with suspected small-bowel disease, but the small bowel can be included in an examination of the abdomen, especially if the patient has right-iliac-fossa pain, inflammatory bowel disease or suspected small-bowel obstruction.
2. Midgut malrotation.

Technique

1. Dilated small-bowel loops and bowel wall thickening may be readily recognized. Doppler examination of the mesenteric vessels may be included to assess activity of inflammatory bowel disease.
2. Malrotation of the small bowel may be diagnosed by alteration of the normal relationship between the superior mesenteric artery and vein. The vein should lie anterior and to the right of the artery.

APPENDIX

Indications

Diagnosis of appendicitis and its complications.

Equipment

5–7.5-MHz linear array transducer.

Patient preparation

None.

Technique

The US transducer is used to apply graded compression to the right lower quadrant of the abdomen. This displaces bowel loops and compresses the caecum. The normal appendix should be compressible and have a maximum diameter of 6 mm. It should also exhibit peristalsis.

Further reading
Brown, J.J. (1991) Acute appendicitis – the radiologist's role. *Radiology* **180**, 13–14.
Simonovský, V. (1999) Sonographic detection of normal and abnormal appendix. *Clin. Radiol.* **54**, 533–539.

LARGE BOWEL

Indications
At present, colonoscopy, CT or barium examinations are first-line imaging investigations, but large-bowel masses can be visualized by US during a routine abdominal scan.

ENDOLUMINAL EXAMINATION OF THE RECTUM AND ANUS

Indications
1. Incontinence and suspected anal sphincter defects
2. Intersphincteric fistula.

Patient preparation
Simple bowel preparation using a small self-administered disposable enema.

Equipment
5–7-MHz radially scanning transducer. A linear transducer can be used but is less satisfactory.

Technique
1. The patient is placed in the left lateral position.
2. A careful digital rectal examination is carried out.
3. The probe is covered with a latex sheath containing contact jelly, and all air bubbles are expelled.
4. More jelly is placed over the latex sheath and the probe is introduced into the rectum.

Aftercare
None.

Further reading
Beynon, J., Feifel, G.A., Hildebrandt, U., et al. (1991) *An Atlas of Rectal Endosonography.* Berlin: Springer-Verlag.

CT OF THE GASTROINTESTINAL TRACT

Indications

1. Abdominal mass
2. Tumour staging
3. Appendicitis – focused appendiceal CT (FACT)
4. Large and small bowel obstruction
5. Altered bowel habit in the elderly and infirm.

Oral and i.v. contrast media are usually employed. Oral contrast should be given at least 24 and perhaps 48 h before the examination to opacify the large bowel. Iodinated or barium-based oral contrast may not be necessary with multi-slice CT scanners.

Oral contrast is not necessary and may be contraindicated in patients with suspected intestinal obstruction. Fluid within dilated bowel will act as a negative contrast agent and allow definition of the transition point. Scans are usually obtained in portal venous phase following i.v. contrast. Slice thickness will depend upon the specification of the CT scanner. Viewing images in coronal and sagittal as well as axial planes may be helpful.

N.B. CT gives a high radiation dose (see Appendix II).

Further reading

Boudiaf, M., Soyer, P., Terem, C., et al. (2001) CT evaluation of small bowel obstruction. *Radiographics* **21(3)**, 613–624.

Domjan, J., Blaquiere, R. & Odurny, A. (1998) Is minimal preparation CT comparable with barium enema in elderly patients with colonic symptoms? *Clin. Radiol.* **53**, 894–898.

Peck, J.J., Milleson, T. & Phelan, J. (1999) The role of computed tomography with contrast and small bowel follow-through in the management of small bowel obstruction. *Am. J. Surg.* **177**, 375–378.

Rao, P.M. & Boland, G.W. (1998) Imaging of acute right lower abdominal quadrant pain. *Clin. Radiol.* **53**, 639–649.

Wittenberg, J., Harisinghani, M.G., Jhaveri, K., et al. (2002) Algorithmic approach to CT diagnosis of the abnormal bowel wall. *Radiographics* **22(5)**, 1093–1107.

COMPUTED TOMOGRAPHIC COLONOGRAPHY

Indications

1. Incomplete colonoscopy – can be performed the same day with no further preparation
2. Patients at risk or who have aversion to colonoscopy
3. Patients with an obstructing lesion preventing full colonoscopy who require full evaluation of the colon

4. Other indications are controversial and include screening for colorectal cancer, and evaluation of colorectal cancer and colonic polyps.

Technique

1. Large-bowel preparation as for barium enema (see above). Diabetic patients may need to be admitted onto the ward for the duration of the bowel preparation
2. Patient to go to toilet immediately before procedure
3. Intravenous access obtained
4. Patient positioned on their side and Foley catheter placed in rectum and air insufflated. Alternatively an empty enema bag is filled with air. The rectal catheter is inserted into the rectum and gentle pressure on the enema bag is used to introduce air via the rectal tube to distend the large bowel. A CO_2 machine may be used to insufflate the colon, 20–25 psi to be maintained throughout the examination (4 l CO_2 initially maintained at 20–25 psi)
5. Patient turned into supine or prone position during gas insufflation
6. 20 mg i.v. Buscopan or 1 mg i.v. glucagon given during insufflation
7. CT scout performed to check satisfactory gaseous distension of large bowel
8. CT parameters will depend upon the type of CT scanner available. CT scans may be performed using a low-dose technique (e.g. 80 mA) without i.v. contrast, or i.v. iodinated contrast may be given and scans performed in portal phase (70 s delay) using usual diagnostic CT parameters
9. Patients may be scanned initially in a supine position using low dose and then turned prone; further insufflation may be needed (e.g. 2 l CO_2) and a further low-dose scan performed.

Further reading

Aschoff, A.J., Ernst, A.S., Brambs, H.J., et al. (2008) CT colonography: an update. *Eur. Radiol.* **18(3)**, 429–437.

Blachar, A. & Sosna, J. (2007) CT colonography (virtual colonoscopy): technique, indications and performance. *Digestion* **76(1)**, 34–41.

Geenen, R.W., Hussain, S.M., Cademartiri, F., et al. (2004) CT and MR colonography: scanning techniques, post processing, and emphasis on polyp detection. *Radiographics* **24(1)**, e18.

Mang, T., Maier, A., Plank, C., et al. (2007) Pitfalls in multi-detector row CT colonography: a systematic approach. *Radiographics* **27(2)**, 431–454.

Tolan, D.J., Armstrong, E.M. & Chapman, A.H. (2007) Replacing barium enema with CT colonography in patients older than 70 years: the importance of detecting extracolonic abnormalities. *Am. J. Roentgenol.* **189(5)**, 1104–1111.

MAGNETIC RESONANCE IMAGING OF THE GASTROINTESTINAL TRACT

Indications

1. Suspected perianal fistula
2. Local staging of rectal cancer
3. Evaluation of inflammatory bowel disease.

Contraindications

1. Standard MRI contraindications – see Chapter 1
2. Some gadolinium-based contrast agents are contraindicated in patients with known or suspected renal dysfunction – see Chapter 2.

Contrast agents

Contrast agents that can be used to alter the signal intensity within the bowel can be classified as positive contrast agents (high signal on T1-weighting) or negative agents (low signal on T2-weighting) or biphasic (e.g. Klean-Prep). However, air itself (within bowel) is a natural contrast agent and the addition of expensive contrast agents is not often necessary.

Motion artifacts

The time taken to obtain a scan can be in the order of several minutes if spin echo sequences are used. Consequently, it is important to minimize peristalsis and respiration artifacts. Glucagon or buscopan should be used to try and minimize peristalsis. A prone position or a compression band can be used to help reduce respiratory motion of the anterior abdominal wall. The artifact, which is propagated from the anterior abdominal wall during respiration, is also due to the high signal from fat. Consequently, fat suppression sequences can help to minimize this.

Pulse sequences

The sequences used for imaging the abdomen and gastrointestinal tract will depend on the nature of the clinical problem. Very fast sequences such as breath-hold gradient echo (GE) and single-shot fast-spin echo (SE) sequences may be used to minimize any movement artifact. However, they do suffer from relatively poor contrast resolution. Standard fast-spin echo T1-weighted and T2-weighted sequences (with gadolinium and fat suppression added as necessary) are often used as baseline sequences, but on occasion suffer from movement artifact. The plane of the sequences will depend on the clinical problem but axial scans are frequently used in the first instance with orthogonal planes (coronal or sagittal) as required.

Techniques
Suspected peri-anal fistula

1. No patient preparation required
2. Patient supine in MRI scanner
3. Axial and coronal high-resolution scans using T1W SE, T2W SE (with fat saturation) or short tau inversion recovery (STIR). Scans following intravenous gadolinium using T1W with fat saturation may be obtained to demonstrate active inflammatory change.

Local staging of colorectal cancer

1. Patient supine
2. Sagittal T2 -weighted SE sequence of central pelvic structures. Use this scan to plan orthogonal, high-resolution axial and coronal T2 W, e.g. (TR 6270 TE122) voxel size $0.9 \times 0.9 \times 3$ mm. SE 3 mm contiguous slices FOV 240 phase FOV 100%, phase resolution 256.

Small-bowel magnetic resonance enteroclysis

1. Obtain venous access
2. Pass Bilbao Dotter tube to DJ flexure using fluoroscopy
3. Transfer patient to MR scanner
4. Supine coronal fast imaging steady state precession (FISP)
5. Turn patient prone and connect Bilbao Dotter tube to enteroclysis pump (situated in control room if not MR compatible). Infuse (80–100 mL min^{-1}) Klean-Prep under MR fluoroscopy (thick slab single shot sequence, e.g. half Fourier acquisition single shot turbo spin echo (HASTE)) to monitor filling of small bowel to ileocaecal valve. Check for reflux to stomach
6. Give Buscopan 20 mg intravenously
7. Obtain sequences in coronal and axial planes using HASTE, FISP
8. 3D T1W fat suppressed, e.g. volumetric interpolated breathold examination (VIBE) sequences following intravenous gadolinium.

Small-bowel magnetic resonance enterography

1. Drink oral MR contrast (1.5 l)
2. Obtain venous access
3. Give Buscopan 20 mg i.v.
4. Obtain sequences in coronal and axial planes using HASTE, FISP sequences or other manufacturer's equivalent
5. Give gadolinium-based contrast agent i.v.
6. Obtain fast 3D T1W fat suppressed (e.g. VIBE) sequences.

Further reading

Berman, L., Israel, G.M., McCarthy, S.M., et al. (2007) Utility of magnetic resonance imaging in anorectal disease. *World J. Gastroenterol.* **13(23)**, 3153–3158.

Buchanan, G.N., Halligan, S., Bartram, C.I., et al. (2004) Clinical examination, endosonography, and MR imaging in preoperative assessment of fistula in ano: comparison with outcome-based reference standard. *Radiology* **233**, 674–681.

Fidler, J. (2007) MR imaging of the small bowel. *Radiol. Clin. North Am.* **45(2)**, 317–331.

Halligan, S. & Stoker, J. (2006) Imaging of fistula in ano. *Radiology* **239**, 18–33.

Schreyer, A.G., Geissler, A., Albrich, H., et al. (2004) Abdominal MRI after enteroclysis or with oral contrast in patients with suspected or proven Crohn's disease. *Clin. Gastroenterol. Hepatol.* **2(6)**, 491–497.

RADIONUCLIDE GASTRO-OESOPHAGEAL REFLUX STUDY

Indications

Diagnosis and quantification of suspected gastro-oesophageal reflux.

Contraindications

None.

Radiopharmaceuticals

^{99m}Tc-colloid or ^{99m}Tc-DTPA mixed with:

1. *Adults and older children*: 150–300 ml orange juice acidified with an equal volume of 0.1 M hydrochloric acid.
2. *Infants and young children*: normal milk feed.
   Typical adult dose is 10–20 MBq, max. 40 MBq (0.9 mSv ED).

Equipment

1. Gamma-camera
2. Low-energy general purpose collimator
3. Abdominal binder for compression test.

Patient preparation

Nil by mouth for 4–6 h. Infants may be studied at normal feed times.

Technique

Physiological test[1] – adults and older children

1. The liquid containing the tracer is given and washed down with unlabelled liquid to clear residual activity from the oesophagus.
2. The patient lies semi-recumbent with the camera centred over the stomach and lower oesophagus.
3. Dynamic imaging is commenced with 5-s 64×64 frames for 30–60 min.

Milk scan[1] – infants and younger children

1. The milk feed is divided into two parts and one mixed with the tracer.
2. The radiolabelled milk is given and washed down with the remaining unlabelled milk.
3. After eructation, the child is placed either supine or prone, according to natural behaviour (although reflux appears to occur more readily in the supine position), with the camera anterior over stomach and oesophagus.
4. Dynamic imaging is commenced with 5-s 64×64 frames for 30–60 min.
5. If pulmonary aspiration of feed is suspected, later imaging at 4 h may be performed. The test is specific but not very sensitive for this purpose.

Provocation with abdominal compression[2] – adults and older children

1. The abdominal binder is placed around the upper abdomen.
2. The radiolabelled liquid is given as above.
3. The patient lies supine with the camera centred over the stomach and lower oesophagus.
4. A 30-s image is taken.
5. The pressure in the binder is increased in steps of 20 mmHg up to 100 mmHg, being maintained at each step for 30 s while an image is taken.
6. The test is terminated as soon as significant reflux is seen.

Analysis

1. For dynamic studies, regions are drawn round the stomach and lower, middle and upper oesophagus.
2. Time–activity curves of these regions are produced, from which may be calculated the size, extent, frequency and duration of any reflux episodes.

Additional techniques

Oesophageal transit

The reflux study may be combined with a bolus transport investigation by fast-frame (0.2–0.5 s) dynamic imaging during swallowing and the generation of a functional compressed image incorporating information from each frame.

Aftercare

None.

Complications

None.

References

1. Guillet, J., Basse-Cathalinat, B., Christophe, E., et al. (1984) Routine studies of swallowed radionuclide transit in paediatrics: experience with 400 patients. *Eur. J. Nucl. Med.* **9**, 86–90.
2. Martins, J.C., Isaacs, P.E., Sladen, G.E., et al. (1984) Gastro-oesophageal reflux scintigraphy compared with pH probe monitoring. *Nucl. Med. Commun.* **5**, 201–204.

Further reading

Heyman, S. (1995) Paediatric gastrointestinal motility studies. *Semin. Nucl. Med.* **25**, 339–347.

Kjellén, G., Brudin, L. & Håkansson, H.O. (1991) Is scintigraphy of value in the diagnosis of gastro-oesophageal reflux disease? *Scand. J. Gastroenterol.* **26**, 425–430.

RADIONUCLIDE GASTRIC-EMPTYING STUDY

Indications

1. Investigation of symptoms suggestive of gastroparesis
2. Before or after gastric surgery
3. Investigation of the effects of gastric motility-altering drugs.

Contraindications

High probability of vomiting.

Radiopharmaceuticals

Many radiolabelled meals have been designed for gastric-emptying studies, but as yet no standard has emerged. Emptying rate measured by radiolabelling is influenced by many factors, for example meal bulk, fat content, calorie content, patient position during imaging and labelling stability in vivo. For this reason, so-called 'normal' emptying times need to be taken in the context of the particular meal and protocol used to generate them. It is important that the meal used is physiological and reproducible. For centres new to the technique it is better to use a meal for which published data exist, rather than create yet another formulation with inherently different behaviour.

Both liquid and solid studies may be performed, separately or simultaneously, as a dual isotope study. Liquids have generally shorter emptying times than solids, and tend to follow an exponential emptying pattern. Solids tend to empty linearly after a lag phase. Prolonged solid emptying is highly correlated with prolonged liquid emptying, and there is debate, therefore, as to whether both studies are routinely necessary.[1] Examples of meals used are:

1. *Liquid meal*: Max. 12 MBq ^{99m}Tc-tin colloid (0.3 mSv ED) mixed with 200 ml orange juice, or with milk or formula feed for infants.
2. *Solid meal*: Scrambled egg prepared with max. 12 MBq ^{99m}Tc-colloid (0.3 mSv ED) or ^{99m}Tc-DTPA. Bulk is made up with other non-labelled foods such as bread and milk.
3. *Dual isotope combined liquid and solid meal:*
   a. *Liquid*: 12 MBq ^{99m}Tc-colloid (0.3 mSv ED) mixed with 200 ml orange juice.
   b. *Solid*: 2 MBq ^{111}In-labelled resin beads (0.7 mSv ED) incorporated into a pancake containing 27 g fat, 18 g protein, 625 calories. Bulk is made up with other non-labelled foods. Only 2 MBq of ^{111}In is suggested (ARSAC max. is 12 MBq, 4 mSv ED) in order to minimize the downscatter into the ^{99m}Tc energy window.

Equipment

1. Gamma-camera, preferably dual-headed
2. Low-energy general purpose collimator for ^{99m}Tc, medium energy for ^{111}In/^{99m}Tc.

Patient preparation

1. Nil by mouth for 8 h
2. No smoking or alcohol from midnight before test
3. Where practical, stop medications affecting gastric motility such as dopaminergic agonists (e.g. metoclopramide, domperidone), cholinergic agonists (e.g. bethanechol), tricyclic antidepressants and anticholinergics for 24 h or more prior to the study, depending upon their biological half-life.

Technique

Imaging from a single projection can cause significant errors due to movement of the meal anteriorly as it transfers to the antrum, thereby altering the amount of tissue attenuation of gamma-photons. The problem is likely to be exacerbated in obese patients. This can largely be overcome by taking pairs of opposing views and calculating the geometric, mean stomach activity in each pair:

1. The patient ingests the meal as quickly as they comfortably can. (If dumping syndrome is suspected, the meal should be eaten in front of the camera with a fast-frame dynamic acquisition running, or the dumping episode may be missed.)
2. The patient is positioned standing.
3. Every 5 min a pair of 1-min anterior and posterior 128×128 images is obtained.
4. The patient sits and relaxes between images.
5. A liquid study should be continued for up to 60 min and a solid study for up to 90 min. If it can be seen that the majority of the meal has emptied inside this time, the study may be terminated.
6. If emptying is very slow, later pairs of images may be acquired at intervals of 30–60 min.

Analysis

1. Stomach region of interest is drawn.
2. Stomach time-activity curve is produced, using geometric mean if anterior and posterior imaging performed.
3. Half-emptying time is calculated.
4. Other parameters may be calculated, e.g. lag-phase duration for solid studies, or percentage left in the stomach at various time points.

Additional techniques

1. The small-bowel transit time (SBTT) can be ascertained by continuing imaging at intervals until the caecum is seen. Since the position of the caecum is often not obvious and may be overlain by small bowel, a 12–24 h image can be useful to determine the position of the large bowel.
2. Frequency analysis of fast dynamic scans (1-s frame time) can be used to characterize antral contraction patterns.[2]

Aftercare

None.

Complications

None.

References

1. Siegel, J.A., Krevsky, B., Maurer, A.H., et al. (1989) Scintigraphic evaluation of gastric emptying: are radiolabelled solids necessary? *Clin. Nucl. Med.* **14**, 40–46.

2. Urbain, J-L. & Charkes, N.D. (1995) Recent advances in gastric emptying scintigraphy. *Semin. Nucl. Med.* **25**, 318–325.

Further reading
Maughan, R.J. & Leiper, J.B. (1996) Methods for the assessment of gastric emptying in humans: an overview. *Diabet. Med.* **13(suppl 5)**, S6–10.

RADIONUCLIDE MECKEL'S DIVERTICULUM SCAN

Indications

Detection of a Meckel's diverticulum as a cause for gastrointestinal bleeding, obstruction or abdominal pain.

Contraindications

1. Barium study in previous 2–3 days (barium causes significant attenuation of gamma photons and may mask a diverticulum).
2. In-vivo, labelled red blood cell study in previous few days (due to likelihood of pertechnetate adhering to red cells).
3. Precautions and contraindications to any pre-administered drugs should be observed.

Radiopharmaceuticals

^{99m}Tc-pertechnetate, 200 MBq typical (2.5 mSv ED), 400 MBq max (5 mSv ED). Injected ^{99m}Tc-pertechnetate localizes in ectopic gastric mucosa within a diverticulum.

Equipment

1. Gamma-camera
2. Low-energy general purpose collimator.

Patient preparation

1. Nil by mouth for 6 h, unless emergency
2. It may be possible to enhance detection by prior administration of drugs, e.g. pentagastrin, cimetidine or ranitidine aimed at increasing the uptake of ^{99m}Tc-pertechnetate into gastric mucosa and inhibiting its release into the lumen of the stomach and progression into the bowel.

Technique

1. The bladder is emptied – a full bladder may obscure the diverticulum
2. The patient lies supine with the camera over the abdomen and pelvis. The stomach must be included in the field of view because diagnosis is dependent on demonstrating uptake of radionuclide in the diverticulum concurrent with uptake by gastric mucosa
3. Pertechnetate is administered i.v.
4. Dynamic imaging
5. Posterior and lateral images as required.

Aftercare

None.

Complications

Pre-administered drug sensitivity and side-effects.

Further reading

Elsayes, K.M., Menias, C.O., Harvin, H.J., et al. (2007) Imaging manifestations of Meckel's diverticulum. *Am. J. Roentgenol.* **189**, 81–88.

Ford, P.V., Bartold, S.P., Fink-Bennett, D.M., et al. (1999) Procedure guidelines for gastrointestinal bleeding and Meckel's diverticulum scintigraphy. *J. Nucl. Med.* **40**, 1226–1232.

RADIONUCLIDE IMAGING OF GASTROINTESTINAL BLEEDING

Indications

Gastrointestinal bleeding of unknown origin.

Contraindications

1. No active bleeding at time scheduled for study
2. Slow bleeding of less than approx. $0.5\,\mathrm{ml\,min^{-1}}$
3. Barium study in previous 2–3 days (barium causes significant attenuation of gamma photons and may mask a bleeding site).

Radiopharmaceuticals

1. ^{99m}Tc-labelled red blood cells, 400 MBq max (4 mSv ED). Red cells are pre-treated with a stannous agent. ^{99m}Tc-pertechnetate is added and is reduced by the stannous ions,

causing it to be retained intracellularly. Labelling efficiency is important, as false-positive scans can result from accumulations of free pertechnetate. In-vitro preparation gives the best labelling efficiency, but is most complex and time-consuming. However, commercial kits are available which can reduce the preparation time to around 30 min. In-vivo labelling is least efficient, and there is also a compromise in-vivo/vitro method where the labelling occurs in the syringe as blood is withdrawn from the patient.[1]

2. ^{99m}Tc-colloid, 400 MBq max (4 mSv ED).

This used to be a commonly used alternative to labelled red cells, but studies showed it to be a less sensitive tracer for detecting bleeding sites,[2] hence it is not recommended. Colloids are rapidly extracted from the circulation, so bleeding occurring only within 10 min or so of injection can be detected. It also localizes intensely in liver and spleen, masking upper gastrointestinal bleeding sites.

Equipment

1. Gamma-camera
2. Low-energy general purpose collimator.

Patient preparation

1. In-vivo or in-vivo/vitro methods: 'Cold' stannous agent (15 g kg^{-1} tin) is administered directly into a vein 20–30 min before the ^{99m}Tc-pertechnetate injection. (Injection via a plastic cannula will result in a poor label.)
2. The patient is asked to empty their bladder before each image is taken. Catheterization is ideal if appropriate.

Technique

1. The patient lies supine.
2. The camera is positioned over the anterior abdomen with the symphysis pubis at the bottom of the field of view.
3. ^{99m}Tc-pertechnetate (in-vivo method) or ^{99m}Tc-labelled red cells (in vitro or in vivo/vitro methods) are injected i.v.
4. A 128×128 dynamic acquisition is begun immediately with 2-s images for 1 min to help to demonstrate vascular blood pool anatomy, followed by 1-min images up to 45 min. Dynamic imaging permits cinematic viewing of images to detect bleed sites and movement through bowel.[3]
5. Further 15×1-min dynamic image sets are acquired at 1, 2, 4, 6, 8 and 24 h or until bleeding site is detected (imaging much beyond 24 h is limited by radioactive decay).
6. Oblique and lateral views may help to localize any abnormal collections of activity.

Aftercare

None.

Complications

None.

Alternative investigative imaging modalities

Catheter angiography
Multidetector CT [4]

References

1. Chaudhuri, T.K. (1991) Radionuclide methods of detecting acute gastrointestinal bleeding. *Int. J. Rad. Appl. Instrum.* Part B **18**, 655–661.
2. Bunker, S.R., Lull, R.J., Tanasescu, D.E., et al. (1984) Scintigraphy of gastrointestinal hemorrhage: superiority of ^{99m}Tc red blood cells over ^{99m}Tc sulfur colloid. *Am. J. Roentgenol.* **143**, 543–548.
3. Maurer, A.H. (1996) Gastrointestinal bleeding and cine-scintigraphy. *Semin. Nucl. Med.* **26**, 43–50.
4. Laing, C.J., Tobias, T., Rosenblum, D.I., et al. (2007) Acute gastrointestinal bleeding: emerging role of multidetector CT angiography and review of current imaging techniques. *Radiographics* **27**, 1055–1070.

LABELLED WHITE CELL SCANNING IN INFLAMMATORY BOWEL DISEASE

Described in Chapter 11

Liver, biliary tract and pancreas

Methods of imaging the hepatobiliary system
1. Plain film
2. Ultrasound (US):
   a. Transcutaneous
   b. Intraoperative
   c. Endoscopic.
3. CT including:
   a. Routine 'staging' (portal venous phase) CT
   b. Triple phase 'characterization' CT
   c. CT cholangiography.
4. MRI
5. Endoscopic retrograde cholangiopancreatography (ERCP)
6. Percutaneous transhepatic cholangiography (PTC)
7. Operative cholangiography
8. Post-operative (T-tube) cholangiography
9. Angiography – diagnostic and interventional
10. Radionuclide imaging:
    a. Static, with colloid
    b. Dynamic, with iminodiacetic acid derivatives.

Methods of imaging the pancreas
1. Plain abdominal films
2. US:
   a. Transcutaneous
   b. Intraoperative
   c. Endoscopic.
3. CT
4. MRI
5. ERCP
6. Arteriography:
   a. Coeliac axis
   b. Superior mesenteric artery.

PLAIN FILMS

May be useful to demonstrate air within the biliary tree or portal venous system, opaque calculi or pancreatic calcification.

ULTRASOUND OF THE LIVER

Indications

1. Suspected focal or diffuse liver lesion
2. Jaundice
3. Abnormal liver function tests
4. Right upper-quadrant pain or mass
5. Hepatomegaly
6. Suspected portal hypertension
7. Staging known extrahepatic malignancy
8. Pyrexia of unknown origin
9. To facilitate the placement of needles for biopsy, etc.
10. Assessment of portal vein, hepatic artery or hepatic veins
11. Assessment of patients with surgical shunts or transjugular intrahepatic shunt (TIPS) procedures
12. Follow-up after surgical resection or liver transplant.

Contraindications

None.

Patient preparation

Not imperative, but fasting or restriction to clear fluids only required if the gallbladder is also to be studied.

Equipment

3–5-MHz transducer and contact gel. Selection of the appropriate pre-set protocol and positioning of focal zone will depend upon the type of machine, manufacturer and patient habitus.

Technique

1. Patient supine
2. Time-gain compensation set to give uniform reflectivity throughout the right lobe of the liver
3. Suspended inspiration
4. Longitudinal scans from epigastrium or left subcostal region across to right subcostal region. The transducer should be angled up to include the whole of the left and right lobes

5. Transverse scans, subcostally, to visualize the whole liver
6. If visualization is incomplete, due to a small or high liver, then right intercostal, longitudinal, transverse and oblique scans may be useful. Suspended respiration without deep inspiration may suffice for intercostal scanning. In patients who are unable to hold their breath, real-time scanning during quiet respiration is often adequate. Upright or left lateral decubitus positions are alternatives if visualization is still incomplete
7. Doppler studies:
   a. Pulsed Doppler
   b. Colour Doppler
   c. Power Doppler
   d. Doppler with US contrast media or 'US echo-enhancing agents'
   e. Second harmonic Doppler with contrast
   f. Pulse inversion Doppler with contrast.

Additional views

Hepatic veins

These are best seen using a transverse intercostal or epigastric approach. During inspiration, in real time, these can be seen traversing the liver to enter the inferior vena cava (IVC). Hepatic vein walls do not have increased reflectivity in comparison to normal liver parenchyma. The normal hepatic vein waveform on Doppler is triphasic reflecting right atrial pressures. Power Doppler may be useful to examine flow within the hepatic segment of the IVC since it is angle-independent.

Portal vein

The longitudinal view of the portal vein is shown by an oblique subcostal or intercostal approach. Portal vein walls are of increased reflectivity in comparison to parenchyma. The normal portal vein blood flow is towards the liver. There is usually continuous flow but the velocity may vary with respiration.

Hepatic artery

This may be traced from the coeliac axis, which is recognized by the 'seagull' appearance of the origins of the common hepatic artery and splenic artery. There is normally forward flow throughout systole and diastole with a sharp systolic peak.

Common bile duct

See below in 'Ultrasound of the gallbladder and biliary system'

Spleen

The spleen size should be measured in all cases of suspected liver disease or portal hypertension. 95% of normal adult spleens measure 12 cm or less in length, and less than 7×5 cm in thickness. The spleen size is commonly assessed by 'eyeballing' and measurement of the longest diameter.[1] In children, splenomegaly should be suspected if the spleen is more than 1.25 times the length of the adjacent kidney,[1] normal ranges have also been tabulated according to age and sex.[2]

References

1. Loftus, W.K. & Metreweli, C. (1998) Ultrasound assessment of mild splenomegaly: spleen/kidney ratio. *Pediatr. Radiol.* **28(2)**, 98–100.
2. Megremis, S.D., Vlachonikolis, I.G. & Tsilimigaki, A.M. (2004) Spleen length in childhood with US: normal values based on age, sex, and somatometric parameters. *Radiology* **231(1)**, 129–134.

Further reading

Albrecht, T., Hohmann, J., Oldenburg, A., et al. (2004) Detection and characterisation of liver metastases. *Eur. Radiol.* **14 Suppl 8**, 25–33.

Kim, T.K., Jang, H.J., Burns, P.N., et al. (2008) Focal nodular hyperplasia and hepatic adenoma: differentiation with low-mechanical-index contrast-enhanced sonography. *Am. J. Roentgenol.* **190(1)**, 58–66.

Kono, Y. & Mattrey, R.F. (2005) Ultrasound of the liver. *Radiol. Clin. North Am.* **43(5)**, 815–826.

Shapiro, R.S., Wagreich, J., Parsons, R.B., et al. (1998) Tissue harmonic imaging sonography: evaluation of image quality compared with conventional sonography. *Am. J. Roentgenol.* **171**, 1203–1206

Wilson, S.R. & Burns, P.N. (2006) An algorithm for the diagnosis of focal liver masses using microbubble contrast-enhanced pulse-inversion sonography. *Am. J. Roentgenol* **186(5)**, 1401–1412.

ULTRASOUND OF THE GALLBLADDER AND BILIARY SYSTEM

Indications

1. Suspected gallstones
2. Right upper quadrant pain
3. Jaundice
4. Fever of unknown origin
5. Acute pancreatitis
6. To assess gallbladder function
7. Guided percutaneous procedures.

Contraindications

None.

Patient preparation

Fasting for at least 6 h, preferably overnight. Water may be permitted.

Equipment

3–5-MHz transducer and contact gel. Selection of the appropriate pre-set protocol and positioning of focal zone will depend upon the type of machine, manufacturer and patient habitus. A stand-off may be used for a very anterior gallbladder.

Technique

1. The patient is supine.
2. The gallbladder can be located by following the reflective main lobar fissure from the right portal vein to the gallbladder fossa
3. Developmental anomalies are rare but the gallbladder may be intrahepatic or on a long mesentery
4. The gallbladder is scanned slowly along its long axis and transversely from the fundus to the neck leading to the cystic duct.
5. It must be re-scanned in the left lateral decubitus or erect positions because stones may be missed if only supine scans are used.
6. Visualization of the neck and cystic ducts may be improved by head down tilt.
   The normal gallbladder wall is never more than 3-mm thick.

Additional views

Assessment of gallbladder function

1. Fasting gallbladder volume may be assessed by measuring longitudinal, transverse and antero-posterior (AP) diameters.
2. Normal gallbladder contraction reduces the volume by more than 25%, 30 min after a standard fatty meal. Somatostatin, calcitonin, indometacin and nifedipine antagonize this contraction.

Intrahepatic bile ducts

1. Left lobe: transverse epigastric scan
2. Right lobe: subcostal or intercostal longitudinal oblique.

Normal intrahepatic ducts are visualized with modern scanners. Intrahepatic ducts are dilated if their diameter is more than 40% of the accompanying portal vein branch. There is normally acoustic enhancement posterior to dilated ducts but not portal veins. Dilated ducts have a beaded branching appearance.

Extrahepatic bile ducts

1. The patient is supine or in the right anterior oblique position.
2. The upper common duct is demonstrated on a longitudinal oblique, subcostal or intercostal scan running anterior to the portal vein. The right hepatic artery is often seen crossing transversely between the two.
3. The common duct may be followed downwards along its length through the head of the pancreas to the ampulla and, when visualized, transverse scans should also be performed to improve detection of intraduct stones.

The segment of bile duct proximal to the junction with the cystic duct (the common hepatic duct) is 4 mm or less in a normal adult; 5 mm is borderline and 6 mm is considered dilated. The lower bile duct (common bile duct) is normally 6 mm or less. Distinction of the common hepatic duct from the common bile duct depends on identification of the junction with the cystic duct. This is usually not possible with US. Colour-flow Doppler enables quick distinction of bile duct from ectatic hepatic artery. In less than one-fifth of patients the artery lies anterior to the bile duct.

Post-cholecystectomy

There is disagreement as to whether the normal common duct dilates after cholecystectomy. Symptomatic patients and those with abnormal liver function tests should have further investigations if the common duct measures more than 6 mm.

Further reading

Foley, W.D. & Quiroz, F.A. (2007) The role of sonography in imaging of the biliary tract. *Ultrasound Q.* **23(2)**, 123–135.

ULTRASOUND OF THE PANCREAS

Indications

1. Suspected pancreatic tumour
2. Pancreatitis or its complications
3. Epigastric mass
4. Epigastric pain
5. Jaundice
6. To facilitate guided biopsy and/or drainage.

Contraindications

None.

Patient preparation

Nil by mouth, preferably overnight.

Equipment

3–5-MHz transducer and contact gel. Selection of the appropriate pre-set protocol and positioning of focal zone will depend upon the type of machine, manufacturer and patient habitus. A stand-off may be required in thin patients.

Technique

1. The patient is supine.
2. The body of the pancreas is located anterior to the splenic vein in a transverse epigastric scan.
3. The transducer is angled transversely and obliquely to visualize the head and tail.
4. The tail may be demonstrated from a left intercostal view using the spleen as an acoustic window.
5. Longitudinal epigastric scans may be useful.
6. The pancreatic parenchyma increases in reflectivity with age, being equal to liver reflectivity in young adults.
7. Gastric or colonic gas may prevent complete visualization. This may be overcome by left and right oblique decubitus scans or by scanning with the patient erect. Water may be drunk to improve the window through the stomach and the scans repeated in all positions. One cup is usually sufficient. Degassed water is preferable.

The pancreatic duct should not measure more than 3 mm in the head or 2 mm in the body.

Endoscopic US (see p. 81) and intra-operative US are useful adjuncts to transabdominal US. EUS may be used to further characterize and biopsy pancreatic mass lesions. Intra-operative US is used to localize small lesions (e.g. islet cell tumours prior to resection).

Further reading

Eloubeidi, M.A., Jhala, D., Chhieng, D.C., et al. (2003) Yield of endoscopic ultrasound-guided fine-needle aspiration biopsy in patients with suspected pancreatic carcinoma. *Cancer* **99(5)**, 285–292.

Rizk, M.K. & Gerke, H. (2007) Utility of endoscopic ultrasound in pancreatitis: a review. *World J. Gastroenterol.* **13(47)**, 6321–6326.

COMPUTED TOMOGRAPHY OF THE LIVER AND BILIARY TREE

Indications

1. Suspected focal or diffuse liver lesion
2. Staging known primary or secondary malignancy
3. Abnormal liver-function tests
4. Right upper-quadrant pain or mass
5. Hepatomegaly
6. Suspected portal hypertension
7. Characterization of liver lesion
8. Pyrexia of unknown origin
9. To facilitate the placement of needles for biopsy, etc.
10. Assessment of portal vein, hepatic artery or hepatic veins
11. Assessment of patients with surgical shunts or transjugular intrahepatic portosystemic shunt (TIPS) procedures
12. Follow-up after surgical resection or liver transplant.

Contraindications

Pregnancy
Contraindication to iodinated intravenous (i.v.) contrast medium (contrast-enhanced computed tomography (CECT)) – see Chapter 2.

Technique
Single-phase (portal phase) contrast-enhanced CT

This is the technique for the majority of routine liver CT imaging. The liver is imaged during the peak of parenchymal enhancement, i.e. when contrast-medium-laden portal venous blood is perfusing the liver. This begins about 60–70 s after the start of a bolus injection. Oral contrast may be given but is not necessary if only the liver is being investigated. Slice thickness will depend upon the CT scanner specification but should be 5 mm or less.

Multi-phasic contrast-enhanced CT

The fast imaging times of helical/multi-slice CT enable the liver to be scanned multiple times after a single bolus injection of contrast medium. Most liver tumours receive their blood supply from the hepatic artery, unlike the hepatic parenchyma, which receives 80% of its blood supply from the portal vein. Thus liver tumours (particularly hypervascular tumours) will be strongly enhanced during the arterial phase (beginning 20–25 s after the start of a bolus injection) but of similar density to enhanced normal parenchyma during the portal venous phase. Some tumours are most conspicuous during early-phase arterial scanning (25 s after the start of a bolus injection), others later, during the late arterial phase 35 s after the start of a bolus injection. Thus a patient who is likely to have hypervascular primary or secondary liver tumours should have an arterial phase scan as well as a portal venous phase CT scan (see above). Early and late arterial phase with portal venous phase is appropriate for patients with suspected hepatocellular cancer (triple phase). In general, late arterial and portal venous scans are appropriate to investigate suspected hypervascular metastases, although an alternative strategy would be to perform an unenhanced scan followed by a portal venous phase scan.

Haemangiomas often show a characteristic peripheral nodular enhancement and progressive centripetal 'fill-in'. After the initial dual- or triple-phase protocol, delayed images at 5 and 10 min are obtained through the lesion.

COMPUTED TOMOGRAPHIC CHOLANGIOGRAPHY

Magnetic resonance (MR) cholangiography is non-invasive but sometimes fails to display the normal intra-hepatic ducts. Multidetector CT cholangiography can be useful in this instance. With this technique the biliary tree is opacified using an i.v. cholangiographic agent. Isotropic data from 0.625 mm section thickness can be reconstructed to provide high-resolution three-dimensional images.

Contraindications

Allergy to iodinated contrast agents.

Indications

1. Screening for cholelithiasis
2. Pre-operative screening of anatomy
3. Supected traumatic bile-duct injury
4. Other biliary abnormalities, e.g. cholesterol polyps, adenomyomatosis and congenital abnormalities.

Technique

1. Patient fasted for at least 6 h
2. 100 ml i.v. cholangiographic agent, e.g. meglumine iotroxate, infused for 50 min as a biliary contrast[1] or iodipamide meglumine 52%- 20 ml diluted with 80 ml of normal saline infused over 30 min.[2]
3. CT scans should be obtained at least 35 min after infusion of contrast agent.[2]

References
1. Hashimoto, M., Itoh, K., Takeda, K., et al. (2008) Evaluation of biliary abnormalities with 64-channel multidetector CT. *Radiographics* **28(1)**, 119–134.
2. Schindera, S.T., Nelson, R.C., Paulson, E.K., et al. (2007) Assessment of the optimal temporal window for intravenous CT cholangiography. *Eur. Radiol.* **17(10)**, 2531–2537.

Further reading
Francis, I.R., Cohan, R.H., McNulty, N.J., et al. (2003) Multidetector CT of the liver and hepatic neoplasms: effect of multiphasic imaging on tumor conspicuity and vascular enhancement. *Am. J. Roentgenol.* **180(5)**, 1217–1224. Erratum in: *Am. J. Roentgenol.* (2003) **181(1)**, 283.
Oto, A., Tamm, E.P. & Szklaruk, J. (2005) Multidetector row CT of the liver. *Radiol. Clin. North Am.* **43(5)**, 827–848.

COMPUTED TOMOGRAPHY OF THE PANCREAS

Indications

1. Epigastric pain
2. Obstructive jaundice
3. Suspected pancreatic malignancy
4. Acute pancreatitis and its complications
5. Chronic pancreatitis and its complications.

Contraindications

1. Pregnancy
2. Contraindication to iodinated intravenous contrast medium – see Chapter 2.

Technique

1. Negative (e.g. water) or positive (e.g. iodinated) oral contrast may be given. A positive oral contrast agent is contraindicated if CT angiography is to be performed. Volume and timing of oral contrast agent will depend upon whether it is necessary to opacify distal bowel loops.
2. Venous access is obtained.
3. The patient is supine on the CT scanner.
4. A scout view is obtained.
5. A non-contrast enhanced examination can be performed initially if detection of subtle calcification is required.

6. The volume of i.v. contrast used will depend upon the type of scanner. Faster acquisition will necessitate a smaller volume of contrast, generally 100 ml or less. The timing of the scan in relation to i.v. contrast will depend upon the clinical question. Pancreatic phase enhancement (40 s after commencement of bolus injection) is necessary for optimum contrast differences between pancreatic adenocarcinoma and normal pancreatic tissue, with portal venous phase scans included in the protocol to investigate hepatic metastatic disease. Islet cell tumours and their metastases may show avid enhancement on arterial phase scans and become isodense with normal pancreatic tissue on portal phase scans. A portal phase scan is generally necessary to investigate flow and the relationship of the tumour to the portal vein.
7. The volume and strength of the i.v. contrast will depend upon the speed of the scanner.
8. Slice thickness should be 3 mm or less.

Further reading

Fletcher, J.G., Wiersema, M.J., Farrell, M.A., et al. (2003) Pancreatic malignancy: value of arterial, pancreatic, and hepatic phase imaging with multi-detector row CT. *Radiology* **229(1)**, 81–90.

Goshima, S., Kanematsu, M., Kondo, H., et al. (2006) Pancreas: optimal scan delay for contrast-enhanced multi-detector row CT. *Radiology* **241(1)**, 167–174.

MAGNETIC RESONANCE IMAGING OF THE LIVER

Indications

1. Lesion detection particularly prior to hepatic resection for hepatic metastatic disease.
2. Lesion characterization following detection by CT or US.

Magnetic resonance (MRI) is rapidly emerging as the imaging modality of choice for detection and characterization of liver lesions. There is high specificity with optimal lesion-to-liver contrast and characteristic appearances on differing sequences and after contrast agents. Focal lesions may be identified on most pulse sequences. Most metastases are hypo- to isointense on T1 and iso- to hyperintense on T2-weighted images. However, multiple sequences are usually necessary for confident tissue characterization. The timing, degree and nature of tumour vascularity form the basis for liver lesion characterization based on enhancement properties. Liver metastases may be hypo or hyper-vascular.

Magnetic resonance imaging pulse sequences

Common pulse sequences are:

1. T1-weighted spoiled gradient echo (GRE)
   This has replaced the conventional spin-echo sequence. In and out of phase scans are used to investigate patients with suspected fatty liver.
2. Magnetization-prepared T1-weighted GRE
   A further breath-hold technique with very short sequential image acquisition.
3. T1-W GRE fat suppressed volume acquisition
   This sequence can be obtained rapidly following i.v. gadolinium.
4. T2-weighted spin echo (SE)

   T2-weighted fast spin-echo (FSE; General Electric) or turbo spin-echo (TSE; Siemens)

Compared with conventional T2-weighted SE images, FSE/TSE images show:

1. fat with higher signal intensity
2. reduced magnetic susceptibility effects which are of advantage in patients with embolization coils, IVC filters, etc., but disadvantageous after injection of superparamagnetic oxide contrast agent
3. increased magnetization transfer which may lower signal intensity for solid liver tumours. These sequences may be obtained with fat suppression.

Fat suppression:

1. decreases the motion artifact from subcutaneous and intra-abdominal fat
2. increases the dynamic range of the image
3. improves signal-to-noise and contrast-to-noise ratios of focal liver lesions.

Very heavily T2-weighted sequences can be used to show water content in bile ducts, cysts and some focal lesions. These may be obtained as:

1. gradient echo breath-hold sequences (e.g. fast imaging with steady state prescession (FISP), fast imaging employing steady state acquisition (FIESTA))
   or
2. as breath-hold very fast spin echo, e.g. half fourier acquisition single shot turbo spin echo (HASTE)
   or
3. as non-breath-hold respiratory gated sequences used for magnetic resonance cholangiopancreatographic (MRCP).

Fat suppression is also used to allow better delineation of fluid-containing structures.

Short tau inversion recovery (STIR) also suppresses fat, which has a short T1 relaxation time. Other tissues with short T1 relaxation (haemorrhage, metastases and melanoma) are also suppressed.

Contrast-enhanced magnetic resonance liver imaging

Gadolinium-enhanced T1-weighted MRI

These probably do not increase sensitivity for focal abnormalities but may help in tissue characterization. When used in conjunction with spoiled GRE sequences it is possible to obtain images during the arterial phase (ideal for metastatic disease and hepatocellular carcinoma), portal phase (hypovascular malignancies) and equilibrium phase (cholangiocarcinoma, slow-flow haemangiomas and fibrosis). Hepatic arterial phase and fast spin-echo T2-weighed sequences are the most sensitive sequences for the detection of hepatic metastases of neuroendocrine tumours.

Liver-specific contrast agents

Standard gadolinium extracellular agents are commonly used for liver MRI as described above, but other contrast agents have been developed to enhance the distinction between normal liver and lesions, especially malignant lesions. These are mostly used in patients who are potentially suitable for major liver surgery, e.g. resection or transplantation:

1. Reticuloendothelial (RE) cell agents, e.g. super paramagnetic iron oxides (SPIO), are taken up by the RE or Kuppfer cells in normal liver giving a decrease in signal on T2- and especially T2*-weighted sequences. They can also be used with T1-weighted sequences for characterization. On T2*-weighted images, malignant lesions without RE cells show as higher signal than the background normal liver.
   Examination with a SPIO agent may be combined with dynamic gadolinium enhancement in order to maximize the detection and characterization of metastases (and benign lesions) in a patient being considered for surgical resection of metastases. The same combination can be used in a patient with cirrhosis to maximize diagnosis and characterization of HCC v dysplastic or regenerative nodules.
2. Hepato-biliary agents are taken up by normal hepatocytes and excreted by normal liver into the bile. The normal liver shows increased signal on T1-weighted sequences for a prolonged period which varies according to the particular agent. Metastases, and other lesions not containing normal functioning hepatocytes, show as a lower signal than the background liver. Lesions containing hepatocytes will enhance to varying extents.

High signal contrast can be seen in the bile ducts. These agents are also excreted by the kidneys. Further details may be found in Chapter 2.

Magnetic resonance angiography

Contrast-enhanced spoiled GRE images may be obtained to give information with respect to the hepatic artery, portal vein and hepatic venous system.

Further reading

Catalano, O.A., Sahani, D.V., Kalva, S.P., et al. (2008) MR imaging of the gallbladder: a pictorial essay. *Radiographics* **28(1)**, 135–155.

Dromain, C., de Baere, T., Baudin, E., et al. (2003) MR imaging of hepatic metastases caused by neuroendocrine tumors: comparing four techniques. *Am. J. Roentgenol.* **180(1)**, 121–128.

Lutz, A.M., Willmann, J.K., Goepfert, K., et al. (2005) Hepatocellular carcinoma in cirrhosis: enhancement patterns at dynamic gadolinium – and superparamagnetic iron oxide-enhanced T1-weighted MR imaging. *Radiology* **237(2)**, 520–528. Epub 2005 Sep 28.

Onishi, H., Murakami, T., Kim, T., et al. (2006) Hepatic metastases: detection with multi-detector row CT, SPIO-enhanced MR imaging, and both techniques combined. *Radiology* **239(1)**, 131–138. Epub 2006 Feb 16.

Rappeport, E.D., Loft, A., Berthelsen, A.K., et al. (2007) Contrast-enhanced FDG-PET/CT vs. SPIO-enhanced MRI vs. FDG-PET vs. CT in patients with liver metastases from colorectal cancer: a prospective study with intraoperative confirmation. *Acta Radiol.* **48(4)**, 369–378.

Ward, J., Robinson, P.J., Guthrie, J.A., et al. (2005) Liver metastases in candidates for hepatic resection: comparison of helical CT and gadolinium – and SPIO-enhanced MR imaging. *Radiology* **237(1)**, 170–180. Epub 2005 Aug 26.

MAGNETIC RESONANCE CHOLANGIOPANCREATOGRAPHY (MRCP)

Indications

1. Investigation of obstructive jaundice
2. Suspected biliary colic/ bile duct stones
3. Suspected chronic pancreatitis
4. Suspected sclerosing cholangitis
5. Investigation of jaundice or cholangitis in patients who have undergone biliary enteric anastomosis
6. Prior to ERCP/PTC.

Contraindications

Those that apply to MRI – see Chapter 1.

Technique

MRCP is a non-invasive technique which uses heavily T2-weighted images to demonstrate the intra- and extra-hepatic biliary tree and pancreatic duct. Most commonly used to demonstrate the presence of stones and the level and cause of obstruction, especially combined with cross-sectional MRI, in cases of tumour or suspected tumour.

MAGNETIC RESONANCE IMAGING OF THE PANCREAS

Indications

1. Staging of pancreatic tumours
2. Suspected islet cell tumour
3. Other indications are similar to CT, although CT is generally preferred because of availability, cost and time implications.

Technique

Typical sequences in the axial plane include:

1. T1-weighted fat-suppressed gradient-echo. Normal pancreas hyperintense to normal liver.
2. T1-weighted spoiled gradient-echo (SPGR, GE Medical Systems; fast low-angle shot (FLASH), Siemens). Normal pancreas isointense to normal liver.
3. Gadolinium-enhanced T1-weighted fat suppressed spoiled gradient echo (GRE). Images are obtained immediately after the injection of contrast medium, after 45 s, after 90 s and after 10 min. Normal pancreas hyperintense to normal liver and adjacent fat on early images, fading on later images.

ENDOSCOPIC RETROGRADE CHOLANGIOPANCREATOGRAPHY

Diagnostic endoscopic retrograde cholangiopancreatography (ERCP) has almost been replaced by non-invasive investigations, e.g. CT and MRI. With the advances in non-invasive imaging of the biliary tree and pancreas, over 90% of ERCP procedures are performed with thera-peutic (interventional) intent. ERCP is performed by physicians most commonly, but surgeons and radiologists do perform this technique.

Indications

1. Diagnostic cholangography in patients unsuitable/intolerant of MRCP
2. Management of bile duct stones
3. Evaluation of ampullary lesions

4. Management of benign and malignant biliary strictures
5. Treatment and evaluation of chronic pancreatitis
6. Investigation of diffuse biliary disease, e.g. sclerosing cholangitis
7. Post-cholecystectomy syndrome.

Contraindications

1. Oesophageal obstruction; pyloric stenosis/gastric or duodenal obstruction
2. Previous gastric surgery that prevents access to the duodenum
3. Severe cardiac/respiratory disease.

Contrast medium

Pancreas
LOCM 240/300.

Bile ducts
LOCM 150; dilute contrast medium ensures that calculi will not be obscured.

Equipment

1. Side-viewing endoscope
2. Polythene catheters
3. Fluoroscopic unit with spot film facilities.

Patient preparation

1. Nil orally for 4–6 h prior to procedure
2. Premedication (see Chapter 18)
3. Antibiotic cover for patients with biliary obstruction, pseudocyst or high risk of endocarditis.

Preliminary film

Prone AP and left anterior oblique (LAO) of the upper abdomen, to check for opaque gallstones and pancreatic calcification/calculi.

Technique

The pharynx is anaesthetized with 50–100 mg Xylocaine spray and the patient is sedated until conscious sedation is achieved. The patient then lies on the left side and the endoscope is introduced. The ampulla of Vater is located and the patient is turned prone. A polythene catheter prefilled with contrast medium is inserted into the ampulla, having ensured that all air bubbles are excluded. A small test injection of contrast under fluoroscopic control is made to determine the position of the cannula. It is important to avoid over-filling of the pancreas. If it is desirable both to opacify the biliary tree and the pancreatic duct, the latter should be cannulated first. A sample of bile should be sent for culture and sensitivity if there is evidence of biliary obstruction.

Films

Pancreas (using fine focal spot)
Prone, both posterior obliques.

Bile ducts
1. Early filling films to show calculi:
   a. Prone – straight and posterior obliques
   b. Supine – straight, both obliques; Trendelenburg to fill intrahepatic ducts; semi-erect to fill lower end of common bile duct and gallbladder
2. Films following removal of the endoscope, which may obscure the duct
3. Delayed films to assess the gallbladder and emptying of the common bile duct.

Aftercare
1. Nil orally until sensation has returned to the pharynx (0.5–3 h)
2. Pulse, temperature and blood pressure half-hourly for 6 h
3. Maintain antibiotics if there is biliary or pancreatic obstruction
4. Serum/urinary amylase if pancreatitis is suspected.

Complications

Due to the contrast medium
1. Allergic reactions – rare
2. Acute pancreatitis – more likely with large volumes, high-pressure injections.

Due to the technique
Local
Damage by the endoscope, e.g. rupture of the oesophagus, damage to the ampulla, proximal pancreatic duct and distal common duct.

Distant
Bacteraemia, septicaemia, aspiration pneumonitis, hyperamylas-aemia (approx. 70%). Acute pancreatitis (0.7–7.4%).

Further reading
Canlas, K.R. & Branch, M.S. (2007) Role of endoscopic retrograde cholangiopancreatography in acute pancreatitis. *World J. Gastroenterol.* **13(47)**, 6314–6320.

INTRA-OPERATIVE CHOLANGIOGRAPHY

Indications

During cholecystectomy or bile duct surgery, to avoid surgical exploration of the common bile duct. This technique has been replaced in some centres by pre-operative MRCP.

Contraindications

None.

Contrast medium

High osmolar contrast material (HOCM) or low osmolar contrast material (LOCM) 150, i.e. low iodine content so as not to obscure any calculi; 20 ml.

Equipment

1. Operating table with CR/DR available or a film cassette tunnel
2. Mobile X-ray machine.

Patient preparation

As for surgery.

Technique

The surgeon cannulates the cystic duct with a fine catheter. This is prefilled with contrast medium to exclude air bubbles which might simulate calculi.

Films

1. After 5 ml have been injected
2. After 20 ml have been injected. Contrast medium should flow freely into the duodenum. Spasm of the sphincter of Oddi is a fairly frequent occurrence and may be due to anaesthetic agents or surgical manipulation. It can be relieved by glucagon, propantheline or amyl nitrite.

   The criteria for a normal operative choledochogram were given by Le Quesne[1] as:

1. common bile duct width not greater than 12 mm
2. free flow of contrast medium into the duodenum
3. the terminal narrow segment of the duct is clearly seen
4. there are no filling defects
5. there is no excess retrograde filling of the hepatic ducts.

Reference
1. Patey, D.H., Le Quesne, L.P., Whiteside, C.G., et al. (1960) Discussion on cholangiography. *Proc. R. Soc. Med.* **53**, 851–860.

POST-OPERATIVE (T-TUBE) CHOLANGIOGRAPHY

Indications

1. To exclude biliary tract calculi where (a) operative cholangiography was not performed, or (b) the results of operative cholangiography are not satisfactory or are suspect.
2. Assessment of biliary leaks following biliary surgery.

Contraindications
None.

Contrast medium
HOCM or LOCM 150; 20–30 ml.

Equipment
Fluoroscopy unit with spot film device.

Patient preparation
None.

Preliminary film
Coned supine PA of the right side of the abdomen.

Technique

1. The examination is performed on or about the 10th post-operative day, prior to removing the T-tube.
2. The patient lies supine on the X-ray table. The drainage tube is clamped off near to the patient and cleaned thoroughly with antiseptic.
3. A 23G needle, extension tubing and 20 ml syringe are assembled and filled with contrast medium. After all air bubbles have been expelled the needle is inserted into the tubing between the patient and the clamp. The injection is made under fluoroscopic control, the total volume depending on duct filling.

Films
PA and oblique views positioned under fluoroscopic control.

Aftercare
None.

Complications

Due to the contrast medium
The biliary ducts do absorb contrast medium and cholangiovenous reflux can occur with high injection pressures. Adverse reactions are, therefore, possible, but the incidence is small.

Due to the technique

Injection of contrast medium under high pressure into an obstructed biliary tract can produce septicaemia.

PERCUTANEOUS TRANSHEPATIC CHOLANGIOGRAPHY

Indications

1. Prior to therapeutic intervention, e.g. biliary drainage procedure to relieve obstructive jaundice, or to drain infected bile
2. Place a precutaneous biliary stent
3. Dilate a post-operative stricture
4. Stone removal (see below)
5. To facilitate ERCP by rendez-vous technique
6. Rarely for diagnostic purposes only.

Contraindications

1. Bleeding tendency:
   a. Platelets less than 100 000
   b. Prothrombin time >2s more than control.
      If patient requires urgent procedure then platelet transfusion and FFP can be used to correct. Vitamin K will correct abnormal prothrombin time due to biliary obstruction.
2. Biliary tract sepsis except to control the infection by drainage.

Contrast medium

LOCM 150; 20–60 ml.

Equipment

1. Fluoroscopy unit with digital spot film device (tilting table optional)
2. Chiba needle (a fine, flexible 22G needle, 15–20-cm long)
3. Appropriate catheters and wire for drainage or interventional procedure planned.

Patient preparation

1. Haemoglobin, prothrombin time and platelets are checked, and corrected if necessary
2. Prophylactic antibiotics, e.g. ciprofloxacin 500–750 mg oral before and after procedure
3. Nil by mouth or clear fluids only for 4 h prior to the procedure
4. Ensure patient well hydrated, by i.v. fluids if necessary
5. Sedation (i.v.) and analgesia with oxygen and monitoring.

Preliminary imaging

US to confirm position of liver and dilated ducts.

Technique

1. The patient lies supine. Using US a spot is marked over the right or left lobe of the liver as appropriate. On the right side this is usually intercostal between mid and anterior axillary lines. For the left lobe this is usually subcostal to the left side of the xiphisternum in the epigastrium.
2. Using aseptic technique the skin, deeper tissues and liver capsule are anaesthetized at the site of the mark.
3. During suspended respiration the Chiba needle is inserted into the liver, but once it is within the liver parenchyma the patient is allowed shallow respirations. It is advanced into the liver with real-time US or fluoroscopy control.
4. The stilette is withdrawn and the needle connected to a syringe and extension tubing prefilled with contrast medium. Contrast medium is injected under fluoroscopic control while the needle is slowly withdrawn. If a duct is not entered at the first attempt, the needle tip is withdrawn to approximately 2–3 cm from the liver capsule and further passes are made, directing the needle tip more cranially, caudally, anteriorly or posteriorly until a duct is entered. The incidence of complications is not related to the number of passes within the liver itself and the likelihood of success is directly related to the degree of duct dilatation and the number of passes made.
5. Excessive parenchymal injection should be avoided and when it does occur it results in opacification of intrahepatic lymphatics. Injection of contrast medium into a vein or artery is followed by rapid dispersion.
6. If the intrahepatic ducts are seen to be dilated, bile should be aspirated and sent for microbiological examination. (The incidence of infected bile is high in such cases.)
7. Contrast medium is injected to outline the duct system and allow access for a guidewire or selection of an appropriate duct for drainage.
8. Care should be taken not to overfill an obstructed duct system because septic shock may be precipitated.
9. For diagnostic PTC only the needle is removed after suitable images have been recorded.

Films

Contrast medium is heavier than bile and the sequence of duct opacification is, therefore, gravity-dependent and determined by the site of injection and the position of the patient.

Using the undercouch tube with the patient *horizontal*:

1. PA
2. LAO
3. RAO
4. If on a non-tilting table, rolling the patient onto the left side will fill the left ducts and common duct above an obstruction.

When the above films have shown an obstruction at the level of the porta hepatis, a further film after the patient has been tilted towards the erect position for 30 min may show the level of obstruction to be lower than originally thought.

Delayed films

Films taken after several hours, or the next day, may show contrast medium in the gallbladder if this was not achieved during the initial part of the investigation.

Aftercare

Bed rest, pulse and blood pressure half-hourly for 6 h.

Complications

Morbidity approximately 3%; mortality less than 0.1%.

Due to the contrast medium
Allergic/idiosyncratic reactions – very uncommon.

Due to the technique

Local

1. Puncture of extrahepatic structures – usually no serious sequelae
2. Intrathoracic injection
3. Cholangitis
4. Bile leakage – may lead to biliary peritonitis (incidence 0.5%). More likely if the ducts are under pressure and if there are multiple puncture attempts. Less likely if a drainage catheter is left in situ. (See 'Biliary drainage' below)
5. Subphrenic abscess
6. Haemorrhage
7. Shock – owing to injection into the region of the coeliac plexus.

Generalized

Bacteraemia, septicaemia and endotoxic shock. The likelihood of sepsis is greatest in the presence of choledocholithiasis because of the higher incidence of pre-existing infected bile.

BILIARY DRAINAGE

EXTERNAL DRAINAGE

This is achieved following transhepatic cannulation of the biliary tree as described above. The procedure may be performed to improve jaundice or sepsis prior to surgery or as a further percutaneous intervention.

INTERNAL DRAINAGE

This can be achieved following transhepatic (as above) or endoscopic cannulation of the biliary tree. A percutaneous drainage catheter may allow internal or external drainage with sideholes above and below the point of obstruction. At ERCP an endoprosthesis or stent is placed to drain bile from above a stricture or to prevent obstruction by a stone in the duct.

Indications

1. Malignant biliary stricture
2. Benign stricture following balloon dilatation.

Contraindications

As for percutaneous transhepatic cholangiography (PTC).

Contrast media

LOCM 200; 20–60 ml.

Equipment

1. Wide-channelled endoscope for introduction of endoprosthesis by ERCP
2. A biplane fluoroscope facility is useful but not essential for transhepatic puncture
3. Set including guidewires, dilators and endoprosthesis.

Patient preparation, see percutaneous transhepatic cholangiography above

Technique

Transhepatic

1. A percutaneous transhepatic cholangiogram is performed.
2. A duct in the right lobe of the liver is usually chosen that has a horizontal or caudal course to the porta hepatis. This duct is studied on US to judge its depth and then a 22G Chiba needle is inserted into the duct using US or fluoroscopic guidance. A coaxial introducer system is used over a 0.018 guidewire to allow 0.035 wire and catheter access into the bile ducts. If the

duct is not successfully punctured, the Chiba needle is withdrawn but remains within the liver capsule allowing a further puncture attempt. Once a 0.035 wire is established in the bile duct a sheath can be inserted, e.g. 7-F. Bile can be drained through the side arm of the sheath while a catheter is manipulated over the wire. For internal drainage or stent insertion the wire and catheter must be passed through the stricture into the duodenum or post-operative jejunal loop. For external drainage, a suitable catheter can be inserted over the wire after the sheath is withdrawn. A variety of wires and catheters may be needed to cross difficult strictures. Failing this, external drainage is instituted and a further attempt is made to pass the stricture a few days later.

3. An internal/external catheter may be placed across the stricture and secured to the skin with sutures.
4. A metal biliary stent may be positioned and deployed across a malignant stricture to facilitate internal drainage of bile. Balloon dilatation may be required before or after stent deployment in some cases. A temporary external drainage tube may be left in place for 24–48 h.

Endoscopic
1. Cholangiography following cannulation of the biliary tree
2. Endoscopic sphincterotomy
3. A guidewire is placed via the channel of the endoscope through the sphincter and pushed past the stricture using fluoroscopy to monitor progress
4. Following dilatation of the stricture the endoprosthesis (plastic stent) is pushed over the guidewire and sited with its side-holes above and below the stricture. Metal biliary stents can also be placed at ERCP when appropriate.

Aftercare
1. As for percutaneous transhepatic cholangiography
2. Antibiotics for at least 3 days
3. An externally draining catheter should be regularly flushed through with normal saline and exchanged at 3-monthly intervals. (It is rare to leave a drain in situ for such a long period.)

Complications
1. As for PTC, ERCP and sphincterotomy
2. Sepsis – particularly common with long-term, externally draining catheters
3. Dislodgement of catheters, endoprostheses
4. Blockage of catheters/endoprostheses
5. Perforation of bile duct above the stricture on passage of guidewires.

Further reading

Burke, D.R., Lewis, C.A., Cardella, J.F., et al. Society of Interventional Radiology Standards of Practice Committee (2003) Quality improvement guidelines for percutaneous transhepatic cholangiography and biliary drainage. *J. Vasc. Interv. Radiol.* **14 (9, part 2)**, S 234–236. Republished from (1997) *J. Vasc. Interv. Radiol.* **8,** 677–681.

PERCUTANEOUS EXTRACTION OF RETAINED BILIARY CALCULI (BURHENNE TECHNIQUE)

Indications

Retained biliary calculi seen on the T-tube cholangiogram (incidence 3%).

Contraindications

1. Small T-tube (<12-F)
2. Tortuous T-tube course in soft tissues
3. Acute pancreatitis
4. Drain in situ (cross connections exist between the drain tract and the T-tube tract).

Contrast medium

HOCM or LOCM 150. (Low-density contrast medium is used to avoid obscuring the calculus.)

Equipment

1. Fluoroscopy unit with spot film device
2. Steerable catheter system with wire baskets.

Patient preparation

1. Admission to hospital on the day prior to the procedure
2. Prophylactic antibiotics and pre-medication 1 h prior to the procedure
3. Analgesia during the procedure.

Technique

1. The patient lies supine on the X-ray table. A PTC is performed if a biliary drainage catheter is not already in situ.
2. The drainage catheter is removed over a guidewire and a sheath inserted in to the ducts (7 or 8-F).
3. Contrast is injected to identify stones and strictures.
4. If there is a stricture, advance a biliary manipulation catheter and guidewire (0.035) across it. Commence balloon dilatation over the guidewire (e.g. 8, 10 possibly 12 mm).

5. Attempt to dislodge stones with balloons into the Roux loop.
6. If this is unsuccessful pass Dormier basket through sheath and attempt to catch the stone in the basket.
7. Advance the basket into the Roux loop and release the stone into the loop.
8. Remove the basket.
9. Pass the guidewire, remove the sheath and place the biliary drainage catheter.
10. Intermittently inject the contrast media to clarify the position of the stones.

Aftercare
1. Pulse and blood pressure half-hourly for 6 h
2. Bed rest for 4–6 h.

Complications
Due to the contrast medium
1. Allergic reactions – rare
2. Pancreatitis.

Due to the technique
1. Fever
2. Perforation of the T-tube tract.

ANGIOGRAPHY

COELIAC AXIS AND SUPERIOR MESENTERIC
Indications
1. Suspected haemorrhage/haemobilia prior to intervention (embolization of bleeding point or aneurysm)
2. Prior to embolization and intervention, e.g. embolization, chemo-embolization, radio-embolization of tumours
3. Suspected polyarteritis nodosa
4. Demonstration of portal venous system (when cross sectional imaging is insufficient). This indication is rare with modern imaging.

Technique
See Chapter 3, page 80.

RADIONUCLIDE IMAGING OF LIVER AND SPLEEN

Indications

1. To assess liver for space-occupying lesions – essentially no longer performed because of greater utility of CT, MR and US
2. To characterize a focal liver lesion as possible focal nodular hyperplasia (these lesions contain Kupffer cells and hence take up colloid; other liver masses will be manifest as photopenic lesions)
3. To detect splenunculi (ectopic splenic tissue)
4. Assessment of liver function (displacement of activity of spleen and bone marrow).

Contraindications

None.

Radiopharmaceuticals

^{99m}Tc tin or sulphur colloid 80 MBq (ED 1 mSv), for SPECT 200 MBq (ED 2 mSv). Cleared by phagocytosis into the reticuloendothelial cells, where it is retained. Spleen is demonstrated as well as liver.

Equipment

1. Gamma-camera
2. Low-energy general purpose collimator.

Patient preparation

None.

Technique

1. Patient lies supine
2. Image at 20 min post injection
3. Films: anterior with costal margin markers, posterior, left and right laterals.

500 kilocounts are used for each view. SPECT can be used when necessary.

An additional technique is first-pass dynamic flow study, which may occasionally be performed to improve differential diagnosis of liver masses.

Aftercare

None.

Complications

None.

Alternative investigative imaging modalities

1. Multidetector CT
2. MRI with reticuloendothelial contrast agent
3. [18]FDG-PET for investigation of primary or secondary malignancy (see Chapter 11)
4. Platelet or denatured red-cell scan for splenunculi.

Further reading

Harding, L.K. & Notghi, A. (2005) Gastrointestinal tract and liver. In: Sharp, P.F., Gemmell, H.G. & Murray, A.D. (eds) *Practical Nuclear Medicine.* 3rd edn. London: Springer-Verlag; 273–304.

RADIONUCLIDE HEPATOBILIARY AND GALLBLADDER RADIONUCLIDE IMAGING

Indications

1. Suspected acute cholecystitis
2. Assessment of gallbladder, common bile duct and sphincter of Oddi function[1,2]
3. Assessment of neonatal jaundice where biliary atresia is considered
4. Suspected bile leaks after trauma or surgery[3]
5. Investigation of biliary drainage.

Contraindications

None.

Radiopharmaceuticals

[99m]Tc-trimethylbromo-iminodiacetic acid (TBIDA) or other imino-diacetic acid (IDA) derivative; 80 MBq typical (1 mSv ED), 150 MBq max (2 mSv ED). ^{99m}Tc-pertechnetate 10 MBq (0.13 mSv ED) to demonstrate stomach outline.

These ^{99m}Tc-labelled IDA derivatives are rapidly cleared from the circulation by hepatocytes and secreted into bile in a similar way to bilirubin;[4] this allows the assessment of biliary drainage and gallbladder function. A number have been developed with similar kinetics, but the later ones, such as TBIDA, have high hepatic uptake and low urinary excretion, giving better visualization of the biliary tract at high bilirubin levels than the early agents.

Equipment

1. Gamma-camera
2. Low-energy general purpose collimator.

Patient preparation

1. Nil by mouth for 4–6 h
2. For the investigation of biliary atresia, infants are given Phenobarbital orally $5\,\text{mg}\,\text{kg}^{-1}\,\text{day}^{-1}$ in two divided doses for 3–5 days prior to the study to enhance hepatic excretion of radiopharmaceutical.

Technique

The imaging protocol depends upon the clinical question being asked. A dynamic study should be performed where it is important to visualize the progress of the bile in detail, e.g. post-surgery:

1. The patient lies supine with the camera anterior and liver at the top of the field of view
2. The radiopharmaceutical is injected i.v.

Films

1. 1-min 128×128 dynamic images are acquired for 45 min after injection.
2. 30–45 min post-injection when the gallbladder is well visualized, a liquid fatty meal (e.g. 300 ml full cream milk) is given through a straw to stimulate gallbladder contraction and imaging continued for a further 45 min. A gallbladder ejection fraction can be calculated.
3. If the gallbladder and duodenum are not seen, static images are obtained at intervals up to 4–6 h.
4. If images are suggestive of reflux, 100–200 ml of water is given through a straw to diffuse any activity in the stomach and thereby differentiate it from nearby bowel activity. 4 min before the end of imaging, 100 ml of water containing 10 MBq ^{99m}Tc-pertechnetate may be given to delineate the stomach.
5. If no bowel activity is seen by 4–6 h and it is important to detect any flow of bile at all, e.g. in suspected biliary atresia, a 24-h image should be taken.

Additional techniques

Cholecystokinin (CCK) and morphine provocation[1]

Pharmacological intervention can be used in combination with TBIDA scanning to improve diagnosis of diseases affecting the gallbladder, common bile duct or sphincter of Oddi. CCK causes gallbladder contraction and sphincter of Oddi relaxation. An i.v. infusion of CCK is given over 2–3 min when the gallbladder is visualized 30–45 min after TBIDA administration. Dynamic imaging is continued for a further 30–40 min.

Quantitative measures of gallbladder ejection fraction and emptying rate can be calculated. It has been suggested that a slow CCK infusion over 30–60 min may improve specificity.[5]

Morphine causes sphincter of Oddi contraction. In a clinical setting of suspected acute cholecystitis, if the gallbladder is not observed by 60 min, an infusion of $0.04\,mg\,kg^{-1}$ over 1 min can be given and imaging continued for a further 30 min. Continued non-visualization of the gallbladder up to 90 min is considered to confirm the diagnosis. Morphine provocation has also found success in diagnosis of elevated sphincter of Oddi basal pressure.[2]

Quantitative analysis
Some investigators have calculated liver function parameters from dynamic studies, e.g. in order to attempt to differentiate between transplant rejection and hepatocyte dysfunction.

Aftercare
None.

Complications
Monitor for adverse reactions to CCK and morphine.

References
1. Krishnamurthy, S. & Krishnamurthy, G.T. (1996) Cholecystokinin and morphine pharmacological intervention during ^{99m}Tc-HIDA cholescintigraphy: a rational approach. *Semin. Nucl. Med.* **26**, 16–24.
2. Thomas, P.D., Turner, J.G., Dobbs, B.R., et al. (2000) Use of ^{99m}Tc-DISIDA biliary scanning with morphine provocation for the detection of elevated sphincter of Oddi basal pressure. *Gut* **46(6)**, 838–841.
3. Rayter, Z., Tonge, C., Bennett, C., et al. (1991) Ultrasound and HIDA: scanning in evaluating bile leaks after cholecystectomy. *Nucl. Med. Commun.* **12**, 197–202.
4. Krishnamurthy, G.T. & Turner, F.E. (1990) Pharmacokinetics and clinical application of technetium 99m-labeled hepatobiliary agents. *Semin. Nucl. Med.* **20**, 130–149.
5. Ziessman, H.A. (1999) Cholecystokinin cholescintigraphy: victim of its own success? *J. Nucl. Med.* **40**, 2038–2042.

Further reading
Harding, L.K. & Notghi, A. (2005) Gastrointestinal tract and liver. In: Sharp, P.F., Gemmell, H.G. & Murray, A.D. (eds) *Practical Nuclear Medicine*. 3rd edn. London: Springer-Verlag; 273–304.

INVESTIGATION OF SPECIFIC CLINICAL PROBLEMS

THE INVESTIGATION OF LIVER TUMOURS

Investigation

This falls into three stages:

1. Detection
2. Characterization of the tumour
3. Assessment for surgical resection or staging for chemotherapy.

The clinical context and proposed management course usually determine the extent of investigation. Liver metastases are much commoner than primary liver cancers. Benign haemangiomas are also common, being present in 5–10% of the population. Other benign liver lesions, except cysts, are less common.

The clinical data correlated with the radiological investigations usually enable the character of a liver tumour to be determined with a high degree of probability. This can be confirmed with image-guided or surgical biopsy when appropriate. Many surgeons are averse to pre-operative biopsy in a patient with a potentially resectable/cureable lesion because of the small risk of disseminating malignant cells and the possibility of misleading sampling error. If biopsy is performed, it is sometimes important to sample the 'normal' liver as well as the lesion. The presence of cirrhosis may have a major impact on management. Hepatic resection is an established procedure for the management of selected hepatic metastases and primary liver tumours. Imaging is used to assess the number and location of tumours.

Ultrasound

Often the first modality to detect an unsuspected focal liver lesion or lesions, but no longer appropriate for screening all patients for liver metastases.

Computed tomography

Widely used for general screening and staging. The remainder of the abdomen and chest may also be imaged for full staging.

Magnetic resonance imaging

Very useful for determining the nature of an unknown liver lesion and for characterizing and staging patients who are considered to be suitable for surgical resection based on CT findings.

THE INVESTIGATION OF JAUNDICE

The aim is to separate haemolytic causes of jaundice from obstructive jaundice or hepatocellular jaundice. Clinical history and examination are followed by biochemical tests of blood and urine, and haematological tests.

Investigations

Obstructive jaundice

US is the primary imaging investigation. The presence of dilated ducts suggests obstructive jaundice. The bile ducts, gallbladder and pancreas should be examined to determine the level and cause of obstruction. MRCP or CT is often required to confirm the cause of the obstruction. If the suspected cause is tumour, a CT or MRI scan is performed to stage the tumour. MRCP is a non-invasive method of imaging the ducts to demonstrate the presence of stones and the level and cause of obstruction, especially combined with cross-sectional MRI in cases of tumour or suspected tumour. Endoscopic ultrasound also can be very helpful in cases where the diagnosis is in doubt after cross-sectional imaging and to confirm or exclude small tumours or very small stones.

ERCP and/or PTC for higher level obstruction should be reserved for those cases where a non-operative management strategy has been determined or in cases with severe jaundice requiring drainage before definitive treatment.

Non-obstructive jaundice

When US shows no dilated ducts and hepatocellular jaundice is suspected, liver biopsy is considered. There may be other US evidence of parenchymal liver disease or signs of portal hypertension.

If obstructive jaundice is still suspected despite the US result, then MRCP is required. Extrahepatic obstruction may be present in the absence of duct dilatation, and patients with primary sclerosing cholangitis or widespread intrahepatic metastases may have obstruction without duct dilatation.

THE INVESTIGATION OF PANCREATITIS

US can be the first investigation, but in acute pancreatitis the presence of a sentinel loop of bowel will often obscure the pancreas and prevent good visualization. Even if the pancreas is seen, it can appear normal in acute pancreatitis. The gallbladder and biliary tree should always be examined in the fasted patient to exclude the presence of gallstones which may be causing the pancreatitis.

CT is the next investigation. It should be performed initially without oral or i.v. contrast enhancement to look for the presence of calcification within the pancreas itself and to look for small gallstones, which can be obscured by the presence of oral contrast medium. Scans of the pancreas should then be obtained during portal venous phase enhancement. This will enable identification of non-perfused areas of pancreas, and the presence of pseudocysts, abscesses and phlegmons should be sought.

PANCREATIC PSEUDOCYSTS

Initial investigation can be with US. It should be remembered that pseudocysts can occur anywhere in the abdomen or pelvis and can even be found in the thorax. The spleen and left kidney provide acoustic windows to visualize the region of the tail of the pancreas.

CT scanning may also be performed if bowel loops prevent adequate visualization and should always be performed prior to radiologically guided intervention to prevent drainage of a pseudoaneurysm. (During ultrasonography supposed fluid collections can be interrogated with colour or duplex Doppler.)

Further reading

Burns, P.N. & Wilson, S.R. (2007) Focal liver masses: enhancement patterns on contrast-enhanced images - concordance of US scans with CT scans and MR images. *Radiology* **242(1)**, 162–174. Epub 2006 Nov 7.

Hussain, S.M. & Semelka, R.C. (2005) Hepatic imaging: comparison of modalities. *Radiol. Clin. North Am.* **43(5)**, 929–947.

Rubens, D.J. (2004) Hepatobiliary imaging and its pitfalls. *Radiol. Clin. North. Am.* **42(2)**, 257–278.

Siddiqi, A.J. & Miller, F. (2007) Chronic pancreatitis: ultrasound, computed tomography, and magnetic resonance imaging features. *Semin. Ultrasound CT MR* **28(5)**, 384–394. Review.

Wilson, S.R., Kim, T.K., Jang, H.J., et al. (2007) Enhancement patterns of focal liver masses: discordance between contrast-enhanced sonography and contrast-enhanced CT and MRI. *Am. J. Roentgenol.* **189(1)**, W7–W12.

Urinary tract

Methods of imaging the urinary tract

1. Plain films
2. Excretion urography
3. Ultrasound (US)
4. Computed tomography (CT) – CT KUB, CT urography, 'staging CT', CT angiography
5. Magnetic resonance imaging (MRI) – MR urography, MR prostate, MR bladder, MR angiography
6. Micturating cystourethrography
7. Ascending urethrography
8. Retrograde pyeloureterography
9. Percutaneous renal puncture – nephrostomy, biopsy, antegrade pyelography, cyst puncture
10. Arteriography
11. Venography – including renal vein sampling
12. Conduitogram
13. Radionuclide imaging:
    a. Static
    b. Dynamic
    c. Radionuclide cystography – direct and indirect.

Further reading

Akin, O. & Hricak, H. (2007) Imaging of prostate cancer. *Radiol. Clin. North Am.* **45(1)**, 207–222.

Zhang, J., Gerst, S., Lefkowitz, R.A., et al. (2007) Imaging of bladder cancer. *Radiol. Clin. North Am.* **45(1)**, 183–205.

Zhang, J., Lefkowitz, R.A. & Bach, A. (2007) Imaging of kidney cancer. *Radiol. Clin. North Am.* **45(1)**, 119–147.

EXCRETION UROGRAPHY

Also known as intravenous urography (IVU). The technique is much less frequently used than in the past, being largely replaced by CT, MRI or US.

Indications

1. Haematuria
2. Renal colic
3. Recurrent urinary tract infection
4. Suspected urinary tract pathology.

Contraindications

See Chapter 2 – general contraindications to intravenous (i.v.) water-soluble contrast media and ionizing radiation. Pre-medication with steroids (see Chapter 2) may be considered but information regarding the renal size, presence of calcification and pelvicalyceal systems may be gained by using a combination of plain film, US, unenhanced CT and MRI.

Contrast medium

Low osmolar contrast material (LOCM) 370

Adult dose
50–100 ml

Paediatric dose
1 ml kg^{-1}

Patient preparation

1. No food for 5 h prior to the examination. Dehydration is not necessary and does not improve image quality.
2. Patients should, preferably, be ambulant for 2 h prior to the examination to reduce bowel gas.
3. The routine administration of bowel preparation fails to improve the diagnostic quality of the examination and its use makes the examination more unpleasant for the patient.

Preliminary film

1. Supine, full-length anterior posterior (AP) of the abdomen, in inspiration. The lower border of the cassette is at the level of the symphysis pubis and the X-ray beam is centred in the mid-line at the level of the iliac crests.

If necessary, the position of overlying opacities may be further determined by:

a. supine AP of the renal areas, in expiration. The X-ray beam is centred in the mid-line at the level of the lower costal margin

or

b. 35° posterior oblique views

or

c. tomography of the kidneys at the level of a third of the AP diameter of the patient (approx. 8–11 cm). The optimal angle of swing is 25–40°.

The examination should not proceed further until these films have been reviewed by the radiologist and deemed satisfactory.

Technique

Venous access via the median antecubital vein is the preferred injection site because flow is retarded in the cephalic vein as it pierces the clavipectoral fascia. The gauge of the cannula/needle should allow the injection to be given rapidly as a bolus to maximize the density of the nephrogram.

Upper arm or shoulder pain may be due to stasis of contrast medium in the vein. This is relieved by abduction of the arm.

Films

1. *Immediate film.* AP of the renal areas. This film is exposed 10–14 s after the injection (approximate arm-to-kidney time). It aims to show the nephrogram, i.e. the renal parenchyma opacified by contrast medium in the renal tubules.

2. *5-min film.* AP of the renal areas. This film is taken to determine if excretion is symmetrical and is invaluable for assessing the need to modify technique, e.g. a further injection of contrast medium if there has been poor initial opacification.
   A compression band is now applied around the patient's abdomen and the balloon positioned midway between the anterior superior iliac spines, i.e. precisely over the ureters as they cross the pelvic brim. The aim is to produce better pelvicalyceal distension. Compression is contraindicated:
   a. after recent abdominal surgery
   b. after renal trauma
   c. if there is a large abdominal mass or aortic aneurysm
   d. when the 5-min film shows already distended calyces.

3. *10-min film.* AP of the renal areas. There is usually adequate distension of the pelvicalyceal systems with opaque urine by this time. Tomography may be useful to improve visualization of the pelvicalyceal systems if these are obscured by bowel. Compression is released when satisfactory demonstration of the pelvicalyceal system has been achieved.

4. *Release film*. Supine AP abdomen. This film is taken to show the whole urinary tract. If this film is satisfactory, the patient is asked to empty their bladder.
5. *After micturition film*. Based on the clinical findings and the radiological findings on the earlier films, this will be either a full-length abdominal film or a coned view of the bladder with the tube angled 15° caudad and centred 5 cm above the symphysis pubis. The aims of this film are to assess bladder emptying, to demonstrate a return to normal of dilated upper tracts with relief of bladder pressure, to aid the diagnosis of bladder tumours, to confirm ureterovesical junction calculi and, uncommonly, to demonstrate a urethral diverticulum in females.

Additional films

1. 35° posterior obliques of the kidneys, ureters or bladder
2. Tomography – when there are confusing overlying shadows
3. 30° caudad angulation of the tube for the renal area. This may throw a faecal laden transverse colon clear of the kidneys
4. Prone abdomen – may improve visualization of ureters by making them more dependent
5. Delayed films – may be necessary for up to 24 h after injection in obstructive uropathy.

ULTRASOUND OF THE URINARY TRACT IN ADULTS

Indications

1. Suspected renal mass lesion
2. Suspected renal parenchymal disease
3. Possible renal obstruction
4. Haematuria
5. Hypertension resistant to conventional medical treatment
6. Renal cystic disease
7. Renal size measurement
8. To facilitate accurate needle placement in interventional procedures
9. Prostatism
10. Bladder volume before and after micturition
11. Bladder tumour
12. Following renal transplant to assess the pelvicalyceal system and patency of vessels, and to investigate perirenal collections.

Contraindications

None.

Patient preparation

None – unless full bladder is required.

Equipment

3.5–5 MHz transducer. Contact gel. The choice of pre-set protocol and positioning of focal zones will depend upon the type of US machine.

Technique

1. Patient supine, right (RAO) and left anterior oblique (LAO) positions or prone for kidneys. The kidneys are scanned longitudinally and transversely. The right kidney may be scanned through the liver and posteriorly in the right loin. The left kidney is harder to visualize anteriorly unless the spleen is large, but can be visualized from the left loin.
2. The length of the kidney measured by US is smaller than that measured at excretion urography because there is no geometric magnification and no change in size related to contrast-induced osmotic diuresis. With US measurement, care must be taken to ensure that the true longitudinal diameter is scanned. The mean length of the normal adult right kidney is 10.7 cm and the left 11.1 cm (range 9–12 cm).
3. The bladder is scanned suprapubically in transverse and longitudinal planes. Measurements taken of three diameters before and after micturition enable an approximate volume to be calculated.
4. Colour flow and duplex Doppler may be used to examine the renal arteries and veins.
5. Renal transplants are usually located in the right or left iliac fossa. These usually lie fairly superficially. Attention should be paid to the pelvicalyceal system and renal vessels.

ULTRASOUND OF THE URINARY TRACT IN CHILDREN

The availability of high-resolution real-time US has revolutionized the investigation of paediatric renal disease. It demonstrates anatomy without the necessity for adequate renal function but, because it gives no functional information, it is the ideal complement to nuclear medicine imaging. It should be stressed that the technique is only as good as the effort put in to obtain the images.

Indications (after Lebowitz, 1985)[1]

1. Urinary tract infection – to document scarring, elicit signs of acute upper tract infection and to exclude an underlying structural abnormality.
2. An abdominal or pelvic mass. Ultrasonography will demonstrate the relationship of the mass to other organs, its possible site of origin and its characteristics, i.e. solid or cystic and the presence of calcification.
3. Renal failure – to differentiate medical from surgical causes.
4. Abnormal antenatal US – to confirm or refute an antenatal diagnosis of hydronephrosis or multicystic dysplasia. The role of US should be to help in the efficient planning of the postnatal management before infection occurs and plasma creatinine rises, rather than to provoke antenatal intervention. It must be remembered that, because urine output falls rapidly after birth when compared with in utero, US on day 1 may show considerably less pelvicalyceal dilatation than was observed on the antenatal scans. Further follow-up scans are mandatory.
5. Conditions associated with a high likelihood of renal abnormalities, e.g. imperforate anus and genital anomalies. The most frequently found abnormalities are a single or ectopic kidney.
6. Genetic conditions, such as Beckwith–Wiedemann, which predispose to >5% risk of developing Wilms' tumour.[2] US surveillance should be performed every 3–4 months.
7. Screening of family members for genetically linked renal diseases, e.g. dominant polycystic renal disease.
8. Periodic follow-up of kidneys which are at risk of deterioration, e.g. children with myelomeningocele or urinary diversion. Patients on chronic dialysis have a high incidence of acquired cystic disease and may develop adenomas or adenocarcinomas.
9. To assess the patency of the IVC and renal vein in patients with Wilms' tumour.
10. To assess residual bladder volume.
11. To facilitate the accurate placement of needles for renal biopsy, antegrade pyelography, percutaneous nephrostomy, cyst aspiration and drainage of perinephric collections.

When assessing possible renal disease by ultrasonography, a number of normal 'variants' may be confused with disease. These include increased parenchymal echogenicity in the neonatal period, echo-poor papillae which may mimic dilated calyces and persistent fetal lobulation, hepatic and splenic impressions, and parenchymal junctional lines, which may mimic scarring.

Equipment

3.5–7.5 MHz transducer – dependent on age.

Patient preparation

Full bladder. Patients with an indwelling catheter should have this clamped 1 h before the examination is scheduled.

Technique

1. Begin by examining the bladder, because contact of the transducer and jelly against the skin may promote bladder emptying. You may have only one chance to image the bladder.
2. It may be necessary to examine uncooperative children while they sit on a carer's lap. Otherwise the technique is as for adults.
3. If possible the kidneys are examined in full inspiration or with the child being asked to 'push the tummy out'.

References
1. Lebowitz, R.L. (1985) Pediatric uroradiology. *Pediatr. Clin. North Am.* **32**, 1353–1362.
2. Scott, R.H., Walker, L., Olsen, Ø.E., et al. (2006) Surveillance for Wilms tumour in at-risk children: pragmatic recommendations for best practice. *Arch. Dis. Child.* **91**, 995–999.

COMPUTED TOMOGRAPHY OF THE URINARY TRACT

Indications

1. Renal colic/suspected renal stone disease
2. Suspected renal tumour
3. Suspected renal/perirenal collection
4. Loin mass
5. Staging and follow-up of renal, transitional cell or prostatic cancer. Local staging of prostatic cancer is performed using high-resolution MRI or endorectal US. Local staging of bladder cancer may be performed using MRI or CT
6. Investigation of obstructive uropathy
7. CT angiography may be used to assess renal vessels for suspected renal artery stenosis or arterio-venous fistula or malformation.

Technique
Computed tomography of kidneys, ureters and bladder

CT KUB (non-contrast enhanced CT of kidneys, ureters and bladder) is useful to determine the number and location of urinary tract calculi. It is used in some centres as the primary investigation of renal colic:

1. The patient lies in prone position on CT scanner table.
2. A scout view is obtained.
3. A low-radiation-dose technique is used to scan from the top of the kidneys to include the bladder base with a slice thickness of 5 mm or less, as determined by CT scanner. An i.v. contrast is not given.

CT urogram

This technique uses a combination of unenhanced, nephrographic and delayed scans following i.v. contrast to allow examination of renal parenchyma and collecting systems. This is one suggested method:

1. Venous access is obtained
2. Patient lies in supine position
3. Scanogram is obtained
4. Initial low-dose unenhanced scans of urinary tract if renal stone disease is suspected
5. Low osmolar contrast material (LOCM) 300 (100–150 ml) is given as bolus intravenously
6. 3 mm or less thickness scans are obtained from diaphragm to lower poles of kidneys during nephrographic/parenchymal enhancement phase (100–120 s following start of bolus injection)
7. If possible, the patient is then encouraged to walk freely within the scan room or department for a few minutes
8. 3 mm or less thickness scans are obtained from upper pole of kidneys to bladder base 10 min after contrast injection, to examine collecting systems and ureters
9. Reconstructions can then be made of the pelvi-calyceal systems and ureters in appropriate planes.

'Staging CT'

This technique is used to stage and follow-up known renal-tract malignancy or to investigate more non-specific signs attributed to the renal tract. Examination of the thorax in addition to the abdomen and pelvis is often appropriate in conditions where pulmonary metastatic disease or mediastinal nodal spread is a possibility:

1. Venous access is obtained
2. Patient lies supine on the scanner
3. Scanogram of chest, abdomen and pelvis as appropriate
4. 100 ml i.v. LOCM given
5. Scans obtained approximately 70 s after i.v. contrast at 5 mm slice thickness or less, depending upon scanner. Arterial phase scans of the liver (20–25 s after i.v. contrast) may be appropriate in those patients with suspected metastatic renal cancer who may have hypervascular liver metastases.

CT angiography

Indications
1. Renal artery stenosis
2. Renal artery aneurysm, arteriovenous malformation, dissection or thrombosis
3. Delineation of vascular anatomy prior to laparoscopic surgery, e.g. nephrectomy
4. Renal vein thrombosis or renal vein/IVC tumour.

Technique
1. No oral iodinated contrast used.
2. Localize the renal hilum accurately using non-enhanced images.
3. Use narrow collimation (1–3 mm).
4. 100–150 ml i.v. contrast medium (LOCM 300) injected at 3–4 ml s^{-1}.
5. Use of bolus triggering devices is recommended to ensure appropriate timing. Otherwise scans are initiated after a preset empiric delay of 20–25 s from start of contrast material injection.
6. Examination of the inferior vena cava requires scanning at a later time (90–120 s delay).

Further reading
Kluner, C., Hein, P.A., Gralla, O., et al. (2006) Does ultra-low-dose CT with a radiation dose equivalent to that of KUB suffice to detect renal and ureteral calculi? *J. Comput. Assist. Tomogr.* **30(1)**, 44–50.

Van Der Molen, A.J., Cowan, N.C., Mueller-Lisse, U.G., et al. CT Urography Working Group of the European Society of Urogenital Radiology (ESUR). (2008) CT urography: definition, indications and techniques. A guideline for clinical practice. *Eur. Radiol.* **18(1)**, 4–17.

MAGNETIC RESONANCE IMAGING OF THE URINARY TRACT

Indications
1. Local staging of prostatic cancer
2. Local staging of bladder cancer
3. Staging of pelvic lymph nodes
4. Suspected renal mass
5. Screening of patients with von Hippel–Lindau disease or their relatives
6. Suspected renal obstruction in patients with poor renal function
7. MR angiography: of potential living related donors, suspected renal artery stenosis.

Technique

Technique will be tailored to the clinical question with MR urography used to investigate the renal tract as a whole. MRI of the abdomen and pelvis can be obtained to assess retroperitoneal adenopathy as part of the staging investigations for patients with bladder and prostate cancer, but CT is often used for this purpose with MRI used for local staging.

MAGNETIC RESONANCE UROGRAPHY

The two most common MR urographic techniques are:

1. static (fluid-filled) urography using heavily T2-weighted MRI techniques to display fluid-filled structures in a similar fashion to magnetic resonance cholangiopancreatography (MRCP) (see Chapter 4)
2. excretory MR urography using T1-weighted gadolinium enhanced scans.

In and out of phase T1-weighted gradient echo scans can be performed to characterize adrenal mass lesions or identify lipid within angiomyolipomas and clear cell carcinoma of the kidney.

Indications

1. To demonstrate the collecting system/determine level of obstruction in a poorly functioning/obstructed kidney
2. Urinary tract obstruction unrelated to urolithiasis. Suspected renal colic from calculus is probably better imaged with CT KUB/ IVU
3. Congenital anomalies
4. Potential renal transplant donors (combined with MR angiography and standard MR imaging of renal parenchyma).

Technique

1. The patient is supine with an empty bladder.
2. Scout views are obtained.
3. Static MR urography may be performed prior to excretory urography. Thick-slab, single-shot, fast-spin echo or a similar thin-section technique, e.g. half-Fourier rapid acquisition with relaxation enhancement; single-shot, fast-spin echo; single-shot, turbo-spin echo. Three-dimensional respiratory triggered sequences may be used to obtain thin-section data sets that may be further manipulated.

   The use of hydration, compression or diuretics may be used to improve visualization of non-dilated collecting systems.
4. Diuretic administration (e.g. 5–10 mg furosemide for adults) given prior to i.v. contrast, can improve the distension of the collecting system and dilute the contrast within the collecting system improving the quality. This may be omitted in patients shown to have obstruction on static MR urography.

5. Excretory MR urography uses pre- and post-contrast scans in the same position. A gadolinium-based contrast agent is administered i.v. using a dose of 0.1 mmol gadolinium/kg body weight. The collecting systems are imaged during the excretory phase using a breath-hold, three-dimensional gradient echo, T1-weighted sequence. Nephrographic phase images may be obtained to image renal parenchyma. Fat suppression will improve the conspicuity of the ureters. Sequences, such as VIBE (volumetric interpolated breath-hold examination) or LAVA (liver acquisition with volume acceleration) can be used. T2* effects from a sufficient concentration of contrast agent may reduce the signal intensity of urine and potentially obscure small masses within the collecting system. This can be overcome, to a certain extent, by using lower concentration of i. v. contrast (e.g. 0.01 mmol kg) but this technique will not distend the collecting system and may compromise soft-tissue imaging. The optimum concentration of contrast has not been established as yet.

5

Further reading

Leyendecker, J.R., Barnes, C.E. & Zagoria, R.J. (2008) MR urography: techniques and clinical applications. *Radiographics* **28(1)**, 23–46; discussion 46–47.

Nikken, J.J. & Krestin, G.P. (2007) MRI of the kidney - state of the art. *Eur. Radiol.* **17(11)**, 2780–2793.

Takahashi, N., Kawashima, A., Glockner, J.F., et al. (2008) Small (<2-cm) upper-tract urothelial carcinoma: evaluation with gadolinium-enhanced three-dimensional spoiled gradient-recalled echo MR urography *Radiology* **247(2)**, 451–457.

MAGNETIC RESONANCE IMAGING OF THE PROSTATE

Technique

1. Patient supine
2. Scout views
3. High-resolution T2-weighted spin echo (SE) scans in axial sagittal and coronal plane orthogonal to the prostate
4. T2 and /or T1-weighted scans are performed to evaluate pelvic nodes if these have not been staged with CT.

Further reading

Ramchandai, P. (ed.) (2006) Prostate imaging. *Radiol. Clin. North Am.* **44(5)** (The entire issue is dedicated to prostate imaging.)

MAGNETIC RESONANCE IMAGING OF THE BLADDER

Technique

1. Patient supine with bladder not emptied before scan and any urinary catheter clamped
2. Scout views
3. High-resolution T2-weighted SE scans in axial sagittal and coronal plane orthogonal to the bladder
4. T2 and /or T1-weighted scans are performed to evaluate pelvic/abdominal nodes if these have not been staged with CT.

MAGNETIC RESONANCE RENAL ANGIOGRAPHY

TECHNIQUE

Three-dimensional spoiled gradient echo sequences are performed before and following i.v. injection (2 ml/s) of 0.1 mmol/kg gadolinium. A saline flush (20 ml) at the same rate is given. Accurate timing of injection is determined by bolus tracking with ROI (region of interest) positioned over abdominal aorta. The scan is triggered when signal intensity at the ROI reaches a preset value.

Further reading

Soulez, G., Pasowicz, M., Benea, G., et al. (2008) Renal artery stenosis evaluation: diagnostic performance of gadobenate dimeglumine-enhanced MR angiography - comparison with DSA. *Radiology* **247(1)**, 273–285.

Willmann, J.K., Wildermuth, S., Pfammatter, T., et al. (2003) Aortoiliac and renal arteries: prospective intraindividual comparison of contrast-enhanced three-dimensional MR angiography and multi-detector row CT angiography. *Radiology* **226(3)**, 798–811.

MICTURATING CYSTOURETHROGRAPHY

Indications

1. Vesicoureteric reflux
2. Study of the urethra during micturition
3. Abnormalities of the bladder
4. Stress incontinence.

Contraindications

Acute urinary tract infection.

Contrast medium

High osmolar contrast material (HOCM) or LOCM 150.

Equipment

1. Fluoroscopy unit with spot film device and tilting table
2. Video recorder
3. Jaques or Foley catheter. In small infants a fine (5–7-F) feeding tube is adequate.

Patient preparation

The patient micturates prior to the examination.

Preliminary film

Coned view of the bladder, using the undercouch tube.

Technique

To demonstrate vesico-ureteric reflux

1. This indication is almost exclusively confined to children.
2. The patient lies supine on the X-ray table. Using aseptic technique a catheter, lubricated with a sterile gel containing a local anaesthetic and antiseptic, is introduced into the bladder. Residual urine is drained. Contrast medium is slowly dripped in and bladder filling is observed by intermittent fluoroscopy. It is important that initial filling is monitored by fluoroscopy in case the catheter is in the distal ureter (thereby mimicking vesico-ureteric reflux) or vagina. It is also important to look for a ureterocele at this stage, as it may be masked by contrast media when the bladder is full.
3. Any reflux is recorded on spot films.
4. The catheter should not be removed until the radiologist is convinced that the patient will micturate or until no more contrast medium will drip into the bladder. The examination is expedited if the catheter remains in situ until micturition commences and then is quickly withdrawn. Small feeding tubes do not obstruct micturition.
5. Older children and adults are given a urine receiver but smaller children should be allowed to micturate onto absorbent pads on which they can lie. Children can lie on the table but adults will probably find it easier to micturate while standing erect.
6. In infants and children with a neuropathic bladder, micturition may be accomplished by suprapubic pressure.
7. Spot films are taken during micturition and any reflux recorded. A video recording may be useful. The lower ureter is best seen in the anterior oblique position of that side. Boys

should micturate in an oblique or lateral projection, so that spot films can be taken of the *entire* urethra.

8. Finally, a full-length view of the abdomen is taken to demonstrate any reflux of contrast medium that might have occurred unnoticed into the kidneys and to record the post-micturition residue.

To demonstrate a vesico-vaginal or recto-vesical fistula
As above, but films are taken in the lateral position.

To demonstrate stress incontinence
Initially the technique is as for demonstrating vesico-ureteric reflux. However, the catheter is left in situ until the patient is in the erect position.

Films
These should include sacrum and symphysis pubis because bony landmarks are used to assess bladder neck descent:

1. Lateral bladder
2. Lateral bladder, straining – the catheter is then removed
3. Lateral bladder during micturition.

Aftercare
1. No special aftercare is necessary, but patients and parents of children should be warned that dysuria, possibly leading to retention of urine, may rarely be experienced. In such cases a simple analgesic is helpful and children may be helped by allowing them to micturate in a warm bath.
2. Most children will already be receiving antibiotics for their recent urinary tract infection. However, if reflux is demonstrated in a child who is not receiving antibiotics, they should be prescribed.

Complications
Due to the contrast medium
1. Adverse reactions may result from absorption of contrast medium by the bladder mucosa. The risk is small when compared with excretion urography.
2. Contrast medium-induced cystitis.

Due to the technique
1. Acute urinary tract infection
2. Catheter trauma – may produce dysuria, frequency, haematuria and urinary retention
3. Complications of bladder filling, e.g. perforation from overdistension – prevented by using a non-retaining catheter, e.g. Jaques
4. Catheterization of vagina or an ectopic ureteral orifice
5. Retention of a Foley catheter.

ASCENDING URETHROGRAPHY IN THE MALE

Indications

1. Strictures
2. Urethral tears
3. Congenital abnormalities
4. Periurethral or prostatic abscess
5. Fistulae or false passages.

Contraindications

1. Acute urinary tract infection
2. Recent instrumentation.

Contrast medium

HOCM or LOCM 200–300, 20 ml. Pre-warming the contrast medium will help reduce the incidence of spasm of the external sphincter.

Equipment

1. Tilting radiography table with fluoroscopy unit and spot film device
2. Foley catheter 8-F.

Patient preparation

Consent.

Preliminary film

Coned supine postero-anterior (PA) of bladder base and urethra.

Technique

1. The patient lies supine on the X-ray table.
2. Using aseptic technique the tip of the catheter is inserted so that the balloon lies in the fossa navicularis and its balloon is inflated with 1–2 ml of water. Contrast medium is injected under fluoroscopic control and films are taken in the following positions:
   a. 30° LAO, with right leg abducted and knee flexed
   b. supine PA
   c. 30° RAO, with left leg abducted and knee flexed.
3. Ascending urethrography should be followed by micturating cystourethrography or excretory micturating cystourethrography to demonstrate the proximal urethra. Occasionally, a urethral fistula or periurethral abscess is seen only on the voiding examination; reflux of contrast medium into dilated prostatic ducts is also better seen during micturition.

Aftercare

None.

Complications

Due to the contrast medium

Adverse reactions are rare.

Due to the technique

1. Acute urinary tract infection
2. Urethral trauma
3. Intravasation of contrast medium, especially if excessive pressure is used to overcome a stricture.

Further reading

McCallum, R.W. (1979) The adult male urethra: normal anatomy, pathology and method of urethrography. *Radiol. Clin. North Am.* **17 (2)**, 227–244.

RETROGRADE PYELOURETEROGRAPHY

Indications

1. Demonstration of the site, length, lower limit and, if possible, the nature of an obstructive lesion.
2. Demonstration of the pelvicalyceal system after an unsatisfactory excretion urogram. Seldom necessary with modern imaging methods.

Contraindications

Acute urinary tract infection.

Contrast medium

HOCM or LOCM 150–200, i.e. not too dense to obscure small lesions, 10 ml.

Equipment

Fluoroscopy unit.

Patient preparation

As for surgery.

Preliminary film

Full-length supine anterior posterior (AP) abdomen when the examination is performed in the X-ray department.

Technique

In the operating theatre

The surgeon catheterizes the ureter via a cystoscope and advances the ureteric catheter to the desired level. Contrast medium is injected under fluoroscopic control and spot films are exposed.

In the X-ray department

1. With ureteric catheter(s) in situ, the patient is transferred from the operating theatre to the X-ray department.
2. Urine is aspirated and, under fluoroscopic control, contrast medium is slowly injected. About 3–5 ml are usually enough to fill the pelvis but the injection should be terminated before this if the patient complains of pain or fullness in the loin.
3. If there is pelviureteric junction obstruction, the contrast medium in the pelvis is aspirated. The films are examined and, if satisfactory, the catheter is withdrawn, first to 10 cm below the renal pelvis, and then to lie just above the ureteric orifice.

About 2 ml of contrast medium are injected at each of these levels and films taken.

Films

Using the undercouch tube:

1. supine PA of the ureter
2. both 35° anterior obliques of the ureter.

N.B. The catheter may be left in the renal pelvis to drain a pelviureteric obstruction. In this case withdrawal ureterograms are not possible.

Aftercare

1. Post-anaesthetic observations
2. Prophylactic antibiotics may be used.

Complications

Due to the anaesthetic

Complications of general anaesthesia.

Due to the contrast medium

1. Contrast medium can be absorbed from the intact renal pelvis, giving rise to adverse reactions. However, the risks are much less than with excretion urography.
2. Chemical pyelitis – if there is stasis of contrast medium.
3. Extravasation due to overdistension of the pelvis. This is usually asymptomatic, but may result in pain, fever and rigors.

Due to the technique

1. Introduction of infection.
2. Mucosal damage to the ureter.
3. Perforation of the ureter or pelvis by the catheter.

PERCUTANEOUS NEPHROSTOMY

The introduction of a drainage catheter into the collecting system of the kidney.

Indications

1. Obstructive uropathy
2. Pyonephrosis
3. Prior to percutaneous nephrolithotomy
4. Ureteric fistulae; external drainage may allow closure.

Contraindications

Uncontrolled bleeding diathesis.

Contrast medium

As for percutaneous renal puncture.

Equipment

1. Puncturing needle: coaxial needle/catheter set or sheathed 18G needle.
2. Drainage catheter: at least 7-F pigtail with multiple side holes.
3. Guidewires: conventional angiographic ± stiff wire.
4. US and/or fluoroscopy.

Patient preparation

1. Fasting for 4 h
2. Premedication
3. Prophylactic antibiotic
4. Surgical backup in view of clinical workup, possible complications and further management.

Technique

Patient position

With the patient lying in the prone position on the fluoroscopic table, a foam pad or non-opaque pillow is placed under the abdomen so that the kidney lies in a fixed posterior position. An oblique position with the side to be punctured raised is often used.

Identifying the collecting system

1. US may be used to identify the renal collecting system for antegrade pyelography and to determine the plane of definitive puncture of the collecting system. Freehand or with a biopsy needle attachment, US may be used to guide the puncturing needle into the collecting system. US guidance is the most common method for localizing the kidney and guiding the initial needle puncture.

2. Excretion urography, if adequate residual function.
3. Antegrade pyelography.

Site/plane of puncture

A point on the posterior axillary line is chosen below the twelfth rib. Having identified the mid/lower pole calyces with US or contrast, the plane of puncture is determined. This will be via the soft tissues and renal parenchyma, so that vessels around the renal pelvis will be avoided and the drainage catheter will gain some purchase on the renal parenchyma. The drainage catheter is also more comfortable for the patient in this position, and is less likely to be kinked when he/she lies supine.

Techniques of puncture, catheterization

The skin and soft tissues are infiltrated with local anaesthetic using a spinal needle. Puncture may then be made using one of the following systems (depending on preference):

1. *An 18G sheathed needle, a cyst puncture or a Longdwell needle or Kellett needle*, in conjunction with the Seldinger technique for catheterization. Upon successful puncture a J guidewire is inserted and coiled within the collecting system; the sheath is then pushed over the wire, which may be exchanged for a stiffer wire. If possible the guidewire is manipulated into the ureter. Dilatation is then performed to 1-F greater than the size of the drainage catheter, which is then inserted. During all manipulation, care must be taken not to kink the guidewire within the soft tissues. A substantial amount of guidewire should be maintained within the collecting system so that position is not lost and if kinking does occur, then the kinked portion of the wire can be withdrawn outside the skin.
2. *Coaxial needle puncture systems, e.g. Neff or Accustik*, using a 22/21G puncturing needle that takes a special 0.018 guidewire. This affords a single puncture with a fine needle, with insertion of a 3-part coaxial system to allow insertion of 0.035 guidewire and then proceed as in 1 above.
3. *The trocar-cannula system*, in which direct puncture of the collecting system is made with the drainage catheter already assembled over a trocar. On removal of the trocar the drainage catheter is pushed further into the collecting system.

Having successfully introduced a catheter, the latter is securely fixed to the skin and drainage commenced.

Aftercare

1. Bed rest for 6 h
2. Pulse, blood pressure and temperature half-hourly for 6 h
3. Urine cultures and sensitivity.

Complications

1. Septicaemia
2. Haemorrhage
3. Perforation of the collecting system with urine leak
4. Unsuccessful drainage
5. Later catheter dislodgement.

PERCUTANEOUS RENAL PUNCTURE AND BIOPSY

Indications

1. Diagnostic biopsy: unexplained renal failure, mass, etc.
2. Renal cyst puncture to relieve local symptoms attributable to a cyst
3. Antegrade pyelography:
   a. When other less invasive imaging modalities fail to delineate the cause and/or level of an obstruction
   b. When retrograde pyelography is unsuccessful or not possible, e.g. internal ureteral diversion
   c. Prior to, or as part of *percutaneous nephrostomy* (see p. 150).

Contraindications

1. As for water-soluble contrast medium in the radiographic method (see tables 2.3 and 2.4)
2. Bleeding diathesis
3. The possibility of renal hydatid disease.

Contrast medium

US guidance is generally used for preliminary visualization of the kidneys:

1. To outline the pelvicalyceal system or renal cyst by direct injection into the collecting system – any HOCM or LOCM 200. Volume is dependent on the size of the cyst or collecting system.
2. Indirect opacification of pelvicalyceal system by intravenous injection – LOCM 370 50 ml.

Equipment

1. Fluoroscopy unit, US machine or CT scanner
2. Overcouch tube
3. 22G needle, e.g. Chiba or Greenburg or core biopsy needle.

Patient preparation

1. Confirm normal blood coagulation
2. Nervous patients may need sedation; children will need general anaesthesia.

Preliminary film

Supine AP of the renal area for the radiographic method.

Technique

RENAL CYST PUNCTURE OR BIOPSY

Insertion of the needle can be controlled by either fluoroscopy after i.v. contrast, ultrasonography or CT:

1. The patient is placed in the prone position. A radiolucent pad is placed under the abdomen to limit anterior movement of the kidney.
2. The mass or cyst is located directly with US or CT or indirectly after opacification of the kidneys with i.v. contrast medium. The optimum site for puncture is marked on the skin.
3. The skin and subcutaneous tissues are infiltrated with 1% lidocaine.
4. The needle is passed directly into the lesion during suspended respiration. US or CT, or intermittent fluoroscopy, is used to monitor the path of the needle. The needle may be deflected around the cyst or mass and, if this happens, it will be necessary to advance it into the cyst or mass with a quick thrust.
5. For cyst puncture the stilette is removed. The cyst contents are aspirated and examined. For biopsy the biopsy needle is 'fired' with due consideration given to the length of throw of the needle biopsy system and adjacent structures.

If no fluid can be aspirated, the position of the needle can be confirmed with US or CT, and adjustment of position made. If the procedure is performed with fluoroscopy only, the needle is withdrawn until fluid is obtained. If that is unsuccessful, a further attempt at puncture is made.

ANTEGRADE PYELOGRAPHY

1. The needle is introduced as for cyst puncture but directed through the renal parenchyma into a minor calyx, posterior lower pole preferred. This reduces the risk of laceration of the pelvis and extravasation of urine.
2. Contrast medium is introduced until the level of obstruction is outlined.

Films

1. AP
2. both 35° posterior obliques.

This is generally followed by drainage with nephrostomy tube insertion if the system is found to be obstructed. This allows contrast medium to be removed from an obstructed pelvis to prevent the development of chemical pyelitis.

PERCUTANEOUS NEPHROLITHOTOMY

This is the removal of renal calculi through a nephrostomy tract. It is often reserved for large complicated calculi which are unsuitable for extracorporeal shock-wave lithotripsy.

Indications

1. Removal of renal calculi
2. Disintegration of large renal calculi.

Contraindications

Uncontrolled bleeding diathesis.

Contrast medium

As for percutaneous renal puncture.

Equipment

1. Puncturing needle (18G): Kellett (15–20 cm length) or equivalent
2. Guidewires, including hydrophilic (Terumo) and superstiff Amplatz
3. Tract dilating equipment; Teflon dilators (from 7–30-F), metal coaxial dilators or a special angioplasty type balloon catheter
4. US machine
5. Fluoroscopy facilities with rotating C arm if possible.

Patient preparation

1. Full discussion between radiologist/urologist concerning indications, etc.
2. Imaging (IVU, CT KUB, CTU) to demonstrate position of calculus and relationship to calyces
3. Admission on the day prior to the procedure – general anaesthetic is usually required
4. Coagulation screen
5. Two units of blood cross matched
6. Antibiotic cover
7. Premedication
8. Bladder catheterization, as large volumes of irrigation fluid will pass down the ureter during a prolonged procedure.

Technique

Patient position

As for a percutaneous nephrostomy, usually prone (see p. 150).

Methods of opacification of the collecting system

1. Retrograde ureteric catheterization; distension of the collecting system may be achieved. In addition, a retrograde occlusion balloon catheter in the ureter will prevent large fragments of stone passing down the ureter
2. Excretion urography
3. Antegrade pyelography; this also enables distension of the collecting system.

Puncture of the collecting system

A lower pole posterior calyx is ideally chosen if the calculus is situated in the renal pelvis. Otherwise the calyx in which the calculus is situated must be punctured. Special care must be taken if puncturing above the twelfth rib because of the risk of perforating the diaphragm and pleura. Puncture is in an oblique plane from the posterior axillary line through the renal parenchyma. Puncture of the selected calyx is made using a combination of US and a rotating C-arm fluoroscopic facility. On successful puncture a guidewire is inserted through the cannula and as much wire as possible is guided into the collecting system. The cannula is then exchanged for an angled catheter and the wire and catheter are manipulated into the distal ureter. At this stage full dilatation may be performed (single stage) or a nephrostomy tube left in situ with dilatation later (two-stage procedure).

Dilatation

This is carried out under general anaesthesia. It is performed using Teflon dilators from 7-F to 30-F, which are introduced over the guidewire. Alternatively, metal coaxial dilators or a special angioplasty balloon (10 cm long) are used. A sheath is inserted over the largest dilator or balloon through which the nephroscope is passed followed by removal of the calculus or disintegration.

Removal/disintegration

Removal of calculi of less than 1 cm is possible using a nephroscope and forceps. Larger calculi must be disintegrated using an ultrasonic or electrohydraulic disintegrator.

Aftercare

1. Usually determined by the anaesthetist/urologist
2. Plain radiograph of renal area to ensure that all calculi/fragments have been removed.

Complications

Immediate

1. Failure of access, dilatation or removal
2. Perforation of the renal pelvis on dilatation
3. Inadvertent access to renal vein and IVC
4. Haemorrhage. Less than 3% of procedures should require transfusion. Rarely, balloon tamponade of the tract or embolization may be required
5. Damage to surrounding structures, i.e. diaphragm, colon, spleen and liver
6. Problems related to the irrigating fluid, i.e. haemolysis.

Delayed

1. Pseudo-aneurysm of an intrarenal artery
2. Arterio-venous fistula.

RENAL ARTERIOGRAPHY

INDICATIONS

1. Renal artery stenosis prior to angioplasty or stent placement. Diagnostic arteriography has been replaced generally by MR or CT angiography (MRA or CTA (see p 140))
2. Renal tumour prior to embolization
3. Assessment of living related renal transplant donors – replaced generally by MRA
4. Haematuria particularly following trauma, including biopsy or other intervention when vascular trauma is possible. This may precede embolization.

Contrast medium

Selective renal artery injection
LOCM 300, 10 ml at 5 ml s^{-1}, or by hand injection – consider use of Visipaque.

Flush aortic
LOCM 300/320, 45 ml at 15 ml s^{-1}.

Equipment

1. Digital fluoroscopy unit
2. Pump injector
3. Catheters:
   a. Selective injection – Sidewinder or Cobra
   b. Flush aortic injection – pigtail 4-F.

5

Technique

Flush aortography
Femoral artery puncture. The catheter is placed proximal to the renal vessels (i.e. approx. T12) and AP and oblique runs are performed (the oblique run demonstrating the renal origins). Selective catheterization may overlook a stenosis at the origin of the renal artery or convert a stenosis into an occlusion, but is occasionally required to define the renal vasculature better.

CONDUITOGRAM

Indications

1. Suspected stricture at anastomosis of ureter and urinary conduit
2. Suspected narrowing of conduit.

Contrast

LOCM or HOCM 150

Technique

The conduit is catheterized using a sterile technique with a 18–20-F Foley catheter. The catheter balloon is inflated and minimal traction applied to the catheter to occlude the stoma. Contrast is gently hand injected under fluoroscopic control into the lumen of the conduit. The aim is to visualize the conduit and ureters.

STATIC RENAL SCINTIGRAPHY

Indications

1. Assessment of individual renal function
2. Investigation of urinary tract infections, particularly in children
3. Assessment of reflux nephropathy
4. Investigation of horseshoe, solitary or ectopic kidney
5. Space-occupying lesions.

^{99m}Tc-dimercaptosuccinic acid (DMSA) gives the best morphological images of any renal radiopharmaceutical and is used for assessment of scarring, and the most accurate assessment of differential renal function.

Contraindications

None.

Radiopharmaceuticals

^{99m}Tc-dimercaptosuccinic acid (DMSA), 80 MBq max (0.7 mSv ED), which is bound to plasma proteins and cleared by tubular absorption. DMSA is retained in the renal cortex, with an uptake of 40–65% of the injected dose within 2 h, and no significant excretion during the imaging period.

Equipment

1. Gamma-camera
2. Low-energy high-resolution collimator.

Patient preparation

None.

Technique

1. The radiopharmaceutical is administered i.v.
2. Images are acquired at any time 1–6 h later. Imaging in the first hour is to be avoided because of free ^{99m}Tc in the urine.

Images

1. Posterior, right (RPO) and left posterior oblique (LPO) views, 256×256 resolution, 300–500000 counts
2. Zoomed or pinhole views may be useful in children.

Additional images

Anterior images may be taken in cases of suspected pelvic or horse-shoe kidney and severe scoliosis, or if relative function is to be calculated by geometric mean method.

Analysis

1. Relative function is best calculated from the geometric mean of posterior and anterior computer images. A single posterior view is often used, but this requires assumptions about kidney depth, unless depth information is available to enable attenuation correction.
2. Absolute uptake can be estimated if required with additional information on patient and kidney size from lateral images.

Additional techniques

1. Single photon emission computed tomography (SPECT) – in the assessment of scarring and renal masses/ 'pseudotumours'.
2. ^{99m}Tc-mercaptoacetyltriglycine (MAG-3) (max. 100 MBq, 0.7 mSv ED) may be considered as a possible alternative to DMSA; it gives inferior kidney visualization, but has the advantage of additional dynamic assessment of excretion in the same study and a lower radiation dose.
3. Fast dynamic frames with motion correction may be useful to reduce movement artefact, particularly in young children.

Aftercare

None.

Complications

None.

Further reading

Blaufox, M.D. (1991) Procedures of choice in renal nuclear medicine. *J. Nucl. Med.* **32**, 1301–1309.

Cosgriff, P.S. (2005) The urinary tract. In: Sharp, P.F., Gemmell, H.G. & Murray, A.D. (eds) *Practical Nuclear Medicine*. 3rd edn. London: Springer-Verlag; 205–229.

Hilson, A.J. (2003) Functional renal imaging with nuclear medicine *Abdom. Imaging* **28**, 176–179.

DYNAMIC RENAL SCINTIGRAPHY

Indications[1]

1. Diagnosis of obstructed v non-obstructed dilatation
2. Diagnosis of renal artery stenosis[2]
3. Assessment of perfusion in acute native or transplant renal failure
4. Assessment of renal function following drainage procedures to the urinary tract
5. Demonstration of vesicoureteric reflux
6. Assessment of renal transplantation
7. Renal trauma.

Contraindications

None.

Radiopharmaceuticals

1. *99mTc-MAG-3 (mercaptoacetyltriglycine)*, 100 MBq max (0.7 mSv ED); (200 MBq max (1 mSv ED) for first-pass blood flow imaging). Highly protein-bound, so mainly cleared by tubular secretion (80%), but with around 20% glomerular filtration (mean normal clearance is approx. 370 ml min^{-1}). Good-quality images due to fast clearance and greater kidney/background ratio than ^{99m}Tc-diethylene triamine pentacetic acid (DTPA), therefore better for poor renal function although more expensive. It is now the radiopharmaceutical of choice owing to its providing the best image quality.
2. *99mTc-DTPA*, 150 MBq typical (1 mSv ED), 300 MBq max (2 mSv ED); (800 MBq max (5 mSv ED) for first-pass blood flow imaging). Cleared by glomerular filtration (mean normal clearance is approx. 120 ml min^{-1}). There is a lower kidney/background ratio than MAG-3 or hippuran, and so a poorer image quality and noisier clearance curves. However, it is cheap and widely available.
3. *123I-orthoiodohippurate (hippuran)*, 20 MBq max (0.2 mSv ED). Almost entirely cleared by tubular secretion (mean normal clearance is approx. 500 ml min^{-1}). High kidney/background ratio, but image quality is limited by the recommended maximum activity. For many years it has been the gold standard, but there is a high cost and limited availability due to ^{123}I being a cyclotron product.

Equipment

1. Gamma-camera
2. Low-energy general purpose collimator.

Patient preparation

1. The patient should be well hydrated with around 500 ml of fluid immediately before administration of tracer
2. The bladder should be voided before injection.

Technique

1. The patient lies supine or sits reclining with their back against the camera.
2. The radiopharmaceutical is injected i.v. and image acquisition is started simultaneously.
3. Perform dynamic 128×128 acquisition with 10–15 s frames for 30–40 min. (For quantitative perfusion studies, e.g. in the transplanted kidney, 1–2-s frames over the 1st minute are acquired.)
4. If poor excretion is seen from one or both kidneys after 10–20 min, a diuretic (furosemide 40 mg) is administered slowly during imaging. Imaging should be continued for at least a further 15 min. Since maximum diuresis does not occur until 15 min after administration of furosemide, as an alternative it may be given 15 min before the radiopharmaceutical (the so-called 'F − 15' renogram), which can be useful after equivocal standard 'F + 20' studies.
5. If significant retention in the kidneys is apparent at the end of the imaging period, ask the patient to void and walk around for a minute, then take a further short image.

Films

1. All posterior
2. *Hard copy*: 2–5-min images for duration of study.

Analysis

The following information is produced using standard computer analysis:

1. Kidney time-activity ('renogram') curves, background-subtracted
2. Relative function figures.
   Additional figures are sometimes calculated:
3. Perfusion index, especially in renal transplant assessment
4. Parenchymal and whole kidney transit times.

Additional techniques

1. Pre- and 1 h post-captopril (25–50 mg) study for diagnosis of renal artery stenosis (RAS). Radionuclide techniques have the advantage of showing the functional effect of a stenotic renal artery, as opposed to the anatomical demonstration as provided by angiographic techniques. This, therefore, helps identify

patients in whom RAS is the cause of hypertension (renovascular). The patient should, ideally, stop diuretic and ACE inhibitor medication 3–5 days prior to the test.[2]

2. Indirect micturating cystography following renography to demonstrate vesicoureteric reflux. The bladder must not have been emptied and the kidneys should be reasonably clear of activity. Continuous dynamic 5-s images are acquired for 2 min before and up to 3 min after micturition, with generation of bladder and kidney time–activity curves.

3. Glomerular filtration rate (GFR) measurement and individual kidney GFR with DTPA studies by taking blood samples for counting. Similarly, effective renal plasma flow (ERPF) measurement with hippuran and a MAG-3 clearance index may be obtained.[3]

4. The images obtained with MAG-3 can be analysed for the presence of renal scarring and there is good correlation with the results obtained with DMSA (MAG-3 is 80% tubular secreted). DMSA remains the gold standard for cortical scarring because of the higher information density and ability to obtain multiple projections, but simultaneous renal clearance information can be gained with MAG-3.[4]

5. With the appropriate computer software and fast-frame acquisition, compressed images may be generated to demonstrate and quantify ureteric peristalsis and show reflux (best with MAG-3 or hippuran), although the technique has not yet found a widely accepted clinical role.

Aftercare

1. The patient is warned that the effects of diuresis may last a couple of hours. The patient may feel faint because of hypotension when standing erect at the end of the procedure.

2. After captopril administration, blood pressure monitoring should be carried out until back to normal.

3. Normal radiation safety precautions (see Chapter 1).

Complications

None, except after captopril, when care must be taken in patients with severe vascular disease to avoid hypotension and renal failure.

References

1. Woolfson, R.G. & Neild, G.H. (1997) The true clinical significance of renography in nephro-urology. *Eur. J. Nucl. Med.* **24**, 557–570.
2. Taylor, A., Nally, J., Aurell, M., et al. (1996) Consensus report on ACE inhibitor renography for detecting renovascular hypertension. *J. Nucl. Med.* **37**, 1876–1882.

3. Blaufox, M.D., Aurell, M., Bubeck, B., et al. (1996) Report of the Radionuclides in Nephrourology Committee on renal clearance. *J. Nucl. Med.* **37**, 1883–1890.
4. Pickworth, F.E., Vivian, G.C., Franklin, K., et al. (1992) ^{99}Tc^m-mercapto acetyl triglycine in paediatric renal tract disease. *Br. J. Radiol.* **65**, 21–29.

Further reading

Blaufox, M.D. (1991) Procedures of choice in renal nuclear medicine. *J. Nucl. Med.* **32**, 1301–1309.
Cosgriff, P.S. (2005) The urinary tract. In: Sharp, P.F., Gemmell, H.G. & Murray, A.D. (eds) *Practical Nuclear Medicine*. 3rd edn. London: Springer-Verlag; 205–229.
Hilson, A.J. (2003) Functional renal imaging with nuclear medicine *Abdom. Imaging* **28**, 176–179.

DIRECT RADIONUCLIDE MICTURATING CYSTOGRAPHY

Indications

Vesicoureteric reflux.

Contraindications

Acute urinary tract infection.

Radiopharmaceuticals

^{99m}Tc-pertechnetate, 25 MBq max (0.3 mSv ED), administered into the bladder. Some pertechnetate is absorbed in the urinary tract and gastric activity may be seen.

Equipment

1. Gamma-camera
2. Low-energy general purpose collimator
3. Sterile saline infusion
4. Commode or plastic urinal
5. Screens for patient privacy.

Patient preparation

The patient micturates prior to the investigation.

Technique[1]

This examination is most frequently performed on children. Direct radionuclide cystography is considered to be at least as sensitive as conventional X-ray micturating cystourethrography (MCU) for the detection of vesicoureteric reflux.[1] The examination enables continuous imaging and quantification of bladder, ureter and kidney activity to be performed and delivers a much smaller radiation dose than conventional cystography.

The technique requires catheterization and is similar to that for MCU except that:

1. ^{99m}Tc-pertechnetate is administered using one of two methods:
   a. Diluted in 500 ml sterile saline solution at body temperature and then infused into the bladder via the catheter
   b. Injected directly into the bladder via the catheter and continuously diluted with sterile saline solution infusion at body temperature.
2. During infusion, the patient lies supine with the gamma-camera posterior. Ensure that both of the kidneys and the ureters and bladder are in the field of view for all imaging. Dynamic image acquisition is performed for the duration of bladder filling at 5–10 s per frame with a 128×128 matrix size to demonstrate any reflux during this phase.
3. When the bladder is as full as tolerable, the infusion is stopped, but imaging is continued for a further 30 s. The patient then sits in front of the gamma-camera on a commode or child's plastic urinal.
4. Dynamic imaging with 5–10-s frames is performed during micturition, continuing for 2–5 min after to evaluate bladder re-filling. If the patient is capable, the embarrassment of the procedure may be reduced by giving them a remote control to start computer acquisition just before they micturate, and leaving them in private.

Analysis

1. Time–activity curves are produced from regions over the bladder, kidneys and ureters.
2. If the voided volume is measured, residual and reflux volumes can be calculated.
3. Viewing the image set cinematically may aid identification of reflux.
4. Images may be summed to highlight any reflux episodes.

Additional techniques

1. If vesico-ureteric reflux is not seen during a single filling and voiding cycle, the sensitivity of the test may be improved by immediately repeating the procedure.[2] The first voiding is performed, if possible, without removing the catheter, and re-filling is commenced shortly after.

2. Indirect radionuclide cystography may be performed after conventional radionuclide renography (see Dynamic renal scintigraphy, p. 160).

3. Intrarenal reflux has been investigated with delayed imaging of radiocolloid reflux at 5 and 20 h.

Aftercare

As for conventional cystography.

Complications

As for conventional cystography.

References

1. Mandell, G.A., Eggli, D.F., Gilday, D.L., et al. (1997) Procedure guideline for radionuclide cystography in children. *J. Nucl. Med.* **38**, 1650–1654.
2. Fettich, J.J. & Kenda, R.B. (1992) Cyclic direct radionuclide voiding cystography: increasing reliability in detecting vesicoureteral reflux in children. *Pediatr. Radiol.* **22**, 337–338.

Further reading

Treves, S.T., Gelfand, M., Willi, U.V., et al. (1995) Vesicoureteric reflux and radionuclide cystography. In: Treves, S.T. (ed) *Pediatric Nuclear Medicine*. 2nd edn. New York: Springer-Verlag; 411–429.

Reproductive system

Methods of imaging the female reproductive system

1. Plain abdominal film
2. Hysterosalpingography
3. Ultrasound (US) – transabdominal/transvaginal
4. Computerized tomography (CT)
5. Magnetic resonance imaging (MRI)
6. Arteriography (including embolization of fibroids).

Methods of imaging the scrotum and testes

1. US
2. MRI
3. Radionuclide imaging
4. Arteriography
5. Venography (including embolization of varices).

Further reading

Akin, O., Mironov, S., Pandit-Taskar, N., et al. (2007) Imaging of uterine cancer. *Radiol. Clin. North Am.* **45(1)**, 167–182.

Barakat, R.R. & Hricak, H. (2002) What do we expect from imaging? *Radiol. Clin. North Am.* **40(3)**, 521–526, vii.

Fütterer, J.J, Heijmink, S.W. & Spermon, J.R. (2008) Imaging the male reproductive tract: current trends and future directions. *Radiol. Clin. North Am.* **46(1)**, 133–147, vii.

HYSTEROSALPINGOGRAPHY

Indications

1. Infertility
2. Recurrent miscarriages: investigation of suspected incompetent cervix, suspected congenital anomaly
3. Following tubal surgery, post sterilization to confirm obstruction and prior to reversal of sterilization
4. Assessment of the integrity of a caesarean uterine scar (rare).

Contraindications

1. During menses
2. Pregnancy
3. A purulent discharge on inspection of the vulva or cervix, or diagnosed pelvic inflammatory disease (PID) in the preceding 6 months
4. Contrast sensitivity (relative).

Contrast medium

High osmolar contrast material (HOCM) or low osmolar contrast material (LOCM) 300/320. Volume 10–20 ml.

Equipment

1. Fluoroscopy unit with spot film device
2. Vaginal speculum
3. Vulsellum forceps
4. Uterine cannula, Leech-Wilkinson cannula, olive or 8-F paediatric Foley catheter or hysterosalpingography balloon catheter 5-F or 7-F.

Patient preparation

1. The patient should abstain from intercourse between booking the appointment and the time of the examination, unless she uses a reliable method of contraception and the appointment is made before day 21, *or* the examination can be booked between the 4th and 10th days in a patient with a regular 28-day cycle.
2. Apprehensive patients may need premedication.
3. Consent should be obtained.[1]

Preliminary film

Coned postero-anterior (PA) view of the pelvic cavity.

Technique

1. The patient lies supine on the table with knees flexed, legs abducted.
2. Using aseptic technique the operator inserts a speculum and cleans the vagina and cervix with chlorhexidine.
3. The anterior lip of the cervix is steadied (vulsellum forceps may be used but positioning the speculum can often achieve this) and the cannula is inserted into the cervical canal. If a Foley catheter is used, there is usually no need to grasp the cervix with the vulsellum forceps. The catheter should be left within the lower cervical canal if cervical incompetence is suspected.
4. Care must be taken to expel all air bubbles from the syringe and cannula, as these would otherwise cause confusion in interpretation. Contrast medium is injected slowly into the uterine cavity under intermittent fluoroscopic control.
5. Spasm of the uterine cornu may be relieved by intravenous (i.v.) glucagon.

N.B. Opiates increase pain by stimulating smooth muscle contraction.

Films

Using the undercouch tube:

1. Early, mid and full uterine filling
2. As the tubes begin to fill: isthmic and ampullary phases
3. When peritoneal spill has occurred and with all the instruments removed
4. If a balloon has been inflated in the cavity then this should be deflated or withdrawn and a further film taken to show the lower uterine cavity.

Aftercare

1. It must be ensured that the patient is in no serious discomfort nor has significant bleeding before she leaves.
2. The patient must be advised that she may have bleeding per vaginam for 1–2 days and pain may persist for up to 2 weeks.
3. Prophylactic antibiotics should be given for at-risk groups, e.g. hydrosalpinx or tubal adhesions.

Complications

Due to the contrast medium
Allergic phenomena – especially if contrast medium is forced into the circulation.

Due to the technique
1. Pain may occur at the following times:
   a. Using the vulsellum forceps
   b. During insertion of the cannula
   c. With tubal distension proximal to a block

    d. With distension of the uterus if there is tubal spasm

    e. With peritoneal irritation during the following day, and up to 2 weeks.

2. Bleeding from trauma to the uterus or cervix.

3. Transient nausea, vomiting and headache.

4. Intravasation of contrast medium into the venous system of the uterus results in a fine lace-like pattern within the uterine wall. When more extensive, intravasation outlines larger veins. It is of little significance when water-soluble contrast media are used. The following factors predispose to intravasation:

    a. Direct trauma to the endometrium

    b. Timing of the procedure near to menstruation

    c. Timing of the procedure within a few days after curettage

    d. Tubal occlusion because of the high pressures generated within the uterine cavity

    e. Uterine abnormalities, e.g. uterine tuberculosis, carcinoma and fibroids.

5. Infection – which may be delayed. Occurs in up to 2% of patients and more likely when there is a previous history of pelvic infection.

6. Abortion. The operator must ensure that the patient is not pregnant.

ULTRASOUND OF THE FEMALE REPRODUCTIVE SYSTEM

Indications

1. Pelvic mass

2. Pregnancy – normal and suspected ectopic

3. Precocious puberty or delayed puberty

4. Pelvic pain

5. Assessment of tubal patency

6. In assisted fertilization techniques

7. Postmenopausal bleeding

8. Menstrual problems.

Contraindications

None.

Patient preparation

1. Transabdominal – full bladder

    Transvaginal – empty bladder

2. Patient consent.[1]

    It is always advisable to have a chaperone.

Equipment

5–10-MHz transducers.
Colour Doppler is useful in the assessment of complex adnexal mass lesions helping to differentiate retracted clot from solid components with a blood supply.

Contrast medium

Galactose monosacharride microparticles (Echovist) are used as a specific contrast agent employed in the assessment of tubal patency; spillage of the microparticles into the peritoneal cavity infers patency.

Reference

1. General Medical Council (2008) *Consent: Patients and Doctors Making Decisions Together.* London: General Medical Council.

Further reading

Ascher, S.M. & Reinhold, C. (2002) Imaging of cancer of the endometrium. *Radiol. Clin. North Am.* **40(3)**, 563–576.

Bates, J. (2006) *Practical Gynaecological Ultrasound.* 2nd edn. Cambridge University Press, Cambridge.

Bhatt, S., Ghazale, H. & Dogra, V.S. (2007) Sonographic evaluation of ectopic pregnancy. *Radiol. Clin. North Am.* **45(3)**, 549–560.

Funt, S.A. & Hann, L.E. (2002) Detection and characterization of adnexal masses. *Radiol. Clin. North Am.* **40(3)**, 591–608.

6

ULTRASOUND OF THE SCROTUM

Indications

1. Suspected testicular tumour
2. Suspected epididymo-orchitis
3. Hydrocoele
4. Acute torsion. In boys or young men in whom this clinical diagnosis has been made and emergency surgical exploration is planned, US should not delay the operation. Although colour Doppler may show an absence of vessels in the ischaemic testis, it is possible that partial untwisting resulting in some blood flow could lead to a false-negative examination
5. Suspected varicocoele
6. Scrotal trauma.

Contraindications

None.

Patient preparation

Consent.

Equipment

7.5–15 MHz transducer. Linear array for optimum imaging. Stand-off may be helpful in some cases.

Technique

1. Patient supine with legs together. Some operators support the scrotum on a towel draped beneath it or in a gloved hand.
2. Both sides are examined with longitudinal and transverse scans enabling comparison to be made.
3. Real-time scanning enables the optimal oblique planes to be examined.
4. In comparing the 'normal' with the 'abnormal' side, the machine settings should be optimized for the normal side, especially for colour Doppler. They should not be changed until both sides have been compared.
5. Patient should also be scanned standing upright and a Valsalva manoeuvre can be performed if a varicocoele is suspected.

Further reading

Kim, W., Rosen, M.A., Langer, J.E., et al. (2007) US MR imaging correlation in pathologic conditions of the scrotum. *Radiographics* **27(5)**, 1239–1253.
Pearl, M.S. & Hill, M.C. (2007) Ultrasound of the scrotum. *Semin. Ultrasound CT MR.* **28(4)**, 225–248.

CT OF THE REPRODUCTIVE SYSTEM

Indications:

1. Staging ovarian cancer
2. Staging germ cell tumours

Technique:

See "routine staging scan" as described in chapter 5 (page 140).

MAGNETIC RESONANCE IMAGING OF THE REPRODUCTIVE SYSTEM

Indications

1. Staging of cervical and uterine cancer
2. Characterization of complex ovarian mass
3. Suspected Mullerian tract anomalies
4. Investigation of endometriosis
5. Staging of ovarian cancer, although CT is often preferred
6. Assessment of pelvic floor
7. Scrotal MR can be used, generally after US, to further characterize a mass as intra or extra testicular and to determine the location of intra-abdominal undescended testis
8. Localization and morphology of uterine fibroids prior to consideration for uterine artery embolization.

Artifacts

Artifact from small-bowel peristalsis and, to a lesser extent, colonic peristalsis can occasionally be a problem in the pelvis and glucagon may be used to minimize this. Respiratory artifact is less of a problem in the pelvis than in the upper and mid abdomen. Movement from anterior abdominal wall fat can be suppressed using a saturation band.

Pulse sequences

For midline structures (uterus, cervix and vagina) sagittal T1-weighted and T2-weighted spin-echo sequences can be augmented with further axial sequences angled to regions of interest as required. Inclined axial images perpendicular to the long axis of the uterus or the long axis of the cervix are helpful for uterine and cervical abnormalities respectively.

The ovaries may be assessed with axial and coronal T1-weighted and T2-weighted spin-echo sequences. T1-weighted fat saturated sequences are used to identify haemorrhage (e.g. within endometriomas) and to help characterize fat-containing masses.

Perfusion imaging of the uterus can be used to assess the effectiveness of uterine fibroid therapy.

MRI is also used to measure the pelvic outlet in pelvimetry in order to avoid radiation dose.

Scrotal MR is generally performed with the scrotum supported as in US, using a surface coil. High-resolution axial, sagittal and coronal T2-weighted spin echo scans are obtained with a T1-weighted scan to identify haemorrhage. Large field-of-view (FOV) scans should be performed to assess the inguinal canal for the presence of a hernia.

6

Gadolinium i.v. can be given if necessary to assess perfusion. Scans should include the pelvis and kidneys if an undescended testis is being investigated.

Further reading

Brown, M.A., Martin, D.R. & Semelka, R. (2006) Future directions in MR imaging of the female pelvis. *Magn. Reson. Imaging Clin. N. Am.* **14(4)**, 431–437.

Burn, P.R., McCall, J.M., Chinn, R.J., et al. (2000) Uterine fibroleiomyoma: MR imaging appearances before and after embolization of uterine arteries. *Radiology* **214(3)**, 729–734.

Coakley, F.V. (2002) Staging ovarian cancer: role of imaging. *Radiol. Clin. North Am.* **40(3)**, 609–636.

Hamm, B., Forstner, R. & Kim, E.S., et al. (2008) MRI and CT of the female pelvis. *J. Nucl. Med.* **49(5)**, 862.

Humphries, P.D., Simpson, J.C., Creighton, S.M., et al. (2008) MRI in the assessment of congenital vaginal anomalies. *Clin. Radiol.* **63(4)**, 442–448.

Martin, D.R., Salman, K., Wilmot, C.C., et al. (2006) MR imaging evaluation of the pelvic floor for the assessment of vaginal prolapse and urinary incontinence. *Magn. Reson. Imaging. Clin. N. Am.* **14(4)**, 523–535.

Scheidler, J. & Heuck, A.F. (2002) Imaging of cancer of the cervix. *Radiol. Clin. North Am.* **40(3)**, 577–590.

Respiratory system

Methods of imaging the respiratory system

1. Plain films
2. Computed tomography (CT)
3. Radionuclide imaging (V/Q scans)
4. Ultrasound (US) – for pleural disease
5. Magnetic resonance imaging (MRI)
6. Positron emission tomography (PET)

Further reading

Hansell, D.M., Armstrong, P., Lynch, D.A., et al. (2005) Technical considerations. In: *Imaging of Diseases of the Chest*. 4th edn. London: Elsevier/Mosby; 1–26.

Klein, J.S. (ed.) (2000) Interventional chest radiology. *Radiol. Clin. North Am.* **38(2)**.

Müller, N.L. (2002) Computed tomography and magnetic resonance imaging: past, present and future. *Eur. Resp. J.* **19(35, suppl)**, 3s–12s.

COMPUTED TOMOGRAPHY OF THE RESPIRATORY SYSTEM

Indications

1. In the assessment of pulmonary masses
2. To exclude metastatic disease
3. In the assessment of diffuse infiltrative lung disease (high-resolution CT)
4. Arterial assessment (pulmonary emboli, aortic dissection)
5. In the assessment of bronchiectasis and large airway stenosis. Planning for therapeutic procedures to the airways, e.g. bronchial stent insertion.[1]

Technique

1. **Volume scan** – usually performed with intravenous contrast enhancement at a rate of $3\,\mathrm{ml\,s^{-1}}$ with a delay of 25–$40\,\mathrm{ml\,s^{-1}}$ depending on the speed of the CT scanner. However, bolus tracking software can be used to specifically trigger the scan for the assessment of relevant vascular structures, e.g. aorta in suspected aortic dissection or pulmonary artery in suspected pulmonary embolism (see below).

2. **High-resolution scan** – usually performed without intravenous (i.v.) contrast:

   a. Patient lies supine but additional prone images[2] may be required to confirm reversible dependent change

   b. On full inspiration, either incremental 1-mm slices at 10-mm to 20-mm intervals OR using multidetector scanner, volume scan with high-resolution reconstruction of 1-mm thick slices at 5–10-mm interval. A volume scan has the potential benefit of post-processing capabilities. Three-dimensional reformatting can help to illustrate the cranio-caudal distribution of pulmonary fibrosis, e.g. distribution of disease on coronal reformats

   c. Additional expiratory images can be performed in suspected air-trapping and airways disease

   d. Image reconstruction using 'bone' algorithm, i.e. high-resolution algorithm which reduces standard CT image smoothing

   e. Maximize spatial resolution using smallest field of view possible.

References

1. Boiselle, P.M. & Ernst, A. (2002) Recent advances in central airway imaging. *Chest* **121(5)**, 1651–1660.
2. Kashiwabara, K. & Kohshi, S. (2006) Additional computed tomography scans in the prone position to distinguish early interstitial lung disease from dependent density on helical computed tomography screening patient characteristics. *Respirology* **11(4)**, 482–487.

Further reading

Beigelman-Aubry, C., Hill, C., Guibal, A., et al. (2005) Multi-detector row CT and postprocessing techniques in the assessment of diffuse lung disease. *RadioGraphics.* **25(6)**, 1639–1652.

COMPUTED TOMOGRAPHY-GUIDED LUNG BIOPSY

Indications

1. Investigation of a pulmonary opacity when other diagnostic techniques have failed to make a diagnosis
2. Investigation of a new chest lesion in a patient with a known malignancy
3. To obtain material for culture when other techniques have failed to identify the causative organism in a patient with persistent consolidation.

All biopsies should be planned after case discussion at a multidisciplinary meeting with a respiratory physician, radiologist and oncologist where the balance of benefit versus risk can best be assessed. Central lesions are preferably biopsied trans-bronchially either by standard bronchoscopy or transbronchial needle aspirate with endoscopic US guidance.

Contraindications

1. Vascular: bleeding diathesis, concurrent administration of anticoagulants, significant pulmonary arterial or venous hypertension. Vascular lesions such as aneurysms or arterio-venous malformations should have already been suspected at pre-biopsy discussion and should not be subjected to biopsy
2. Respiratory: contralateral pneumonectomy, presence of bullae or seriously impaired respiratory function, such that a pneumothorax could not be tolerated. The procedure should not be performed if the patient plans air travel within 6 weeks of the procedure
3. Suspected hydatid disease
4. Extremely uncooperative patient.

Equipment

1. Biopsy needle – fine needle aspirate can be performed if there is an on-site pathology service. Otherwise a cutting needle biopsy is used, of which there are several types available, e.g. Temno cutting needle or Cook Quick-Core. Coaxial needle biopsy systems can be used as these reduce the number of passes through the pleura. 18 or 20G needles are most often used
2. Full resuscitation equipment including a chest drain.

Patient preparation

1. Premedication with diazepam may be required. However, the patient must remain cooperative so that a consistent breathing pattern can be maintained during the procedure

2. The procedure may be performed on an outpatient basis with observation for 4–6 hours post procedure, but a bed should be available in case of complications
3. Clotting screen
4. Pulmonary function tests (spirometry).

Aftercare

1. Close observation post procedure for at least 1 h in a supervised ward or recovery area, preferentially with the patient lying in a position where the biopsy site is dependent, e.g. right lateral decubitus if right lateral biopsy
2. Chest X-ray in expiration at approximately 1 h post procedure. If a pneumothorax has developed then the further management will depend on the clinical condition of the patient. This may involve further close observation, aspiration or chest drain insertion, depending on the degree of patient dyspnoea and distress
3. High-risk patients such as those with pre-existing impairment of respiratory function are best admitted overnight.

Complications

1. Pneumothorax in 20%. However, a chest drain is necessary in only a small minority (about 3%). The incidence of pneumothorax is increased if:
   a. the operator is inexperienced
   b. larger bore needles are used
   c. there is an increased number of punctures
   d. small or central lesions are biopsied
   e. the needle traverses a fissure.
2. Local pulmonary haemorrhage (10%)
3. Haemoptysis (2–5%)
4. Other complications, such as implantation of malignant cells along the needle track, spread of infection and air embolism, are all extremely rare
5. The current documented death rate is 0.15%.

Further reading

Anderson, J.M., Murchison, J. & Patel, D. (2003) CT-guided lung biopsy: factors influencing diagnostic yield and complication rate. *Clin. Radiol.* **58 (10)**, 791–797.

Aviram, G., Schwartz, D.S., Meirsdorf, S., et al. (2005) Transthoracic needle biopsy of lung masses: a survey of techniques. *Clin. Radiol.* **60(3)**, 370–374.

Manhire, A., Charig, M., Clelland, C., et al. (2003) BTS Guidelines: Guidelines for radiologically guided lung biopsy. *Thorax* **58(11)**, 920–936.

Richardson, C.M., Pointon, K.S., Manhire, A.R., et al. (2002) Percutaneous lung biopsies: a survey of UK practice based on 5444 biopsies. *Br. J. Radiol.* **75(897)**, 731–735.

METHODS OF IMAGING PULMONARY EMBOLISM

1. *Plain film chest radiograph.* The initial chest radiograph is often normal. Numerous signs have been described in association with pulmonary embolism but, overall, the chest radiograph is neither specific nor sensitive.
2. *Ventilation/perfusion (V/Q) radionuclide scanning.* The technique is described later in this chapter. Interpretation of V/Q images is not clear-cut and there are a number of causes for the typical V/Q mismatch. Diagnostic criteria developed divide results into normal, low-probability, intermediate (or indeterminate) and high-risk groups. Specificity and sensitivity are such that, if the criteria place the images in the normal group, pulmonary embolism is virtually excluded and if the images fit the criteria for high risk it is very likely (85–90%). In the intermediate risk group specificity is poor and further imaging may be required.
3. *Doppler ultrasound* of leg veins to confirm deep vein thromboses.
4. *Multidetector CT pulmonary angiography* (CTPA) of the chest to diagnose pulmonary emboli down to subsegmental level. Can be complemented with a CT venography sequence performed at the same examination as CTPA (see Chapter 10).
5. *Pulmonary arteriography* was traditionally the 'gold standard' and will detect most pulmonary emboli but has now largely been replaced by multidetector CT.

Diagnostic pathways can be planned using an algorithm of clinical probability of pulmonary embolus together with the result of D-dimer assay.

Further reading

Roy, P.M., Colombet, I., Durieux, P. et al. (2005) Systematic review and meta-analysis of strategies for the diagnosis of suspected pulmonary embolism. *BMJ* **331(7511)**, 259.

Stein, P.D., Woodard, P.K., Weg, J.G. et al. (2007) Diagnostic pathways in acute pulmonary embolism: recommendations of the PIOPED II investigators. *Radiology* **242(1)**, 15–21.

RADIONUCLIDE LUNG VENTILATION/PERFUSION (V/Q) IMAGING

Indications

1. Suspected pulmonary embolism
2. Assessment of perfusion and ventilation abnormalities, e.g. in congenital cardiac or pulmonary disease
3. Quantitative assessment of right-to-left shunting (perfusion only)
4. Quantitative assessment of differential perfusion and ventilation before lung cancer, lung transplant or lung volume reduction surgery.[1,2]

Contraindications (to perfusion imaging)

1. Right-to-left shunt – because of the risk of cerebral emboli
2. Severe pulmonary hypertension.

Neither of these are absolute contraindications (indeed, perfusion imaging can be used for assessment of shunts), and it may be considered acceptable to reduce the number of particles administered in these cases.

Radiopharmaceuticals

Perfusion

^{99m}Tc labelled macroaggregated albumin particles (MAA), 100 MBq max (1 mSv ED), 10–40 μm in diameter which occlude small lung vessels (<0.5% of total capillary bed).

Ventilation

1. ^{81m}Kr (krypton) gas, 6000 MBq max (0.2 mSv ED). Ideal generator-produced agent with a short $T_{1/2}$ of 13 s and a γ-energy of 190 keV. Simultaneous dual isotope ventilation and perfusion imaging is possible because of different γ-energy to ^{99m}Tc. Wash-in and wash-out studies are not possible. Expensive and limited availability
2. ^{99m}Tc-Technegas, 40 MBq max (0.6 mSv ED).[3] Ultrafine Tc labelled carbon particles, 5–20 nm in size. No simultaneous ventilation and perfusion imaging. Longer residence time in lungs than aerosols, so SPECT and respiration-gated studies possible. Similar diagnostic efficacy to krypton. Expensive dispensing system
3. ^{99m}Tc-DTPA, aerosol, 80 MBq max (0.4 mSv ED). Simultaneous ventilation and perfusion imaging not possible. Cheap and readily available alternative to krypton, but less suitable in patients with chronic obstructive airways disease or chronic asthma because clumping of aerosol particles is likely
4. ^{133}Xe (xenon) gas, 400 MBq max (0.4 mSv ED) diluted in 10 l and re-breathed for 5 min. Long $T_{1/2}$ of 5.25 days and a γ-energy of 81 keV. Ventilation must precede perfusion study because low

γ-energy would be swamped by scatter from ^{99m}Tc. Wash-in and wash-out studies are possible. Poor-quality images and rarely used.

Equipment

1. Gamma-camera, preferably multi-headed for SPECT
2. Low-energy general purpose collimator
3. Gas dispensing system and breathing circuit for ventilation.

Patient preparation

1. For ventilation, familiarization with breathing equipment
2. A current chest X-ray is required to assist with interpretation.

Technique

Perfusion

1. The injection may be given in the supine, semi recumbent or sitting position (N.B. MAA particle uptake is affected by gravity)
2. The syringe is shaken to prevent particles settling
3. A slow i.v. injection is given directly into a vein (particles will stick to a plastic cannula) over about 10 s. Avoid drawing blood into the syringe as this can cause clumping
4. The patient must remain in position for 2–3 min while the particles become fixed in the lungs
5. Imaging may begin immediately, preferably in the sitting position.

Ventilation

^{81m}Kr gas

This is performed at the same time as the perfusion study, either by dual isotope acquisition or swapping energy windows at each patient position:

1. The patient is positioned to obtain identical views to the perfusion images and asked to breathe normally through the mouthpiece.
2. The air supply attached to the generator is turned on and imaging commenced.

^{99m}Tc-DTPA aerosol

This scan is performed before the perfusion study, which may follow immediately unless there is clumping of aerosol particles in the lungs, in which case it is delayed for 1–2 h:

1. A DTPA kit is made up with approx. 600 MBq ^{99m}Tc per ml
2. ^{99m}Tc-DTPA is drawn into a 5 ml syringe with 2 ml air, then injected into the nebulizer and flushed through with air
3. The patient is positioned initially with their back to the camera, sitting if possible
4. The nose-clip is placed on the patient who is asked to breathe normally through the mouthpiece. The air supply is turned on to deliver a rate of 10 L min^{-1}

5. After reaching a sufficient count rate the air supply is turned off. The patient should continue to breathe through the mouthpiece for a further 15 s
6. The nose-clip is removed and the patient is given a mouth wash, then imaging is commenced.

Images

Anterior, posterior, left and right posterior obliques.

Since perfusion and ventilation images are directly compared, it is important to have identical views for each. Foam wedges between the patient's back and the camera assist accurate oblique positioning.

Additional techniques

1. SPECT imaging appears to significantly improve the specificity of the technique by reducing the number of intermediate probability scans.
2. Standardized interpretation of images can improve the clinical effectiveness of V/Q scans, and criteria have been published which are widely used.[4]

Aftercare

None.

Complications

Care should be taken when injecting MAA not to induce respiratory failure in patients with severe pulmonary hypertension. In these cases, inject very slowly.

References

1. Wang, S.C., Fischer, K.C., Slone, R.M., et al. (1997) Perfusion scintigraphy in the evaluation for lung volume reduction surgery: correlation with clinical outcome. *Radiology* **205(1)**: 243–248.
2. Win, T., Tasker, A.D., Groves, A.M., et al. (2006) Ventilation-perfusion scintigraphy to predict postoperative pulmonary function in lung cancer patients undergoing pneumonectomy. *Am. J. Roentgenol.* **187(5)**, 1260–1265.
3. Howarth, D.M., Lan, L., Thomas, P.A., et al. (1999) ^{99m}Tc Technegas ventilation and perfusion lung scintigraphy for the diagnosis of pulmonary embolus. *J. Nucl. Med.* **40(4)**, 579–584.
4. Freitas, J.E., Sarosi, M.G., Nagle, C.C., et al. (1995) Modified PIOPED criteria used in clinical practice. *J. Nucl. Med.* **36(9)**, 1573–1578.

Further reading

Gray, H.W. (2005) The lung. In: Sharp, P.F., Gemmell, H.G. & Murray A.D. (eds) *Practical Nuclear Medicine*. 3rd edn. London: Springer-Verlag; 179–204.
Riedel, M. (2004) Diagnosing pulmonary embolism. *Postgrad. Med. J.* **80(944)**, 309–319.

COMPUTED TOMOGRAPHY IN THE DIAGNOSIS OF PULMONARY EMBOLI

Technique

The technique will depend on individual CT scanner technology. Single-slice scanners require a longer scanning time than multi-detector scanners. Individual CT manufacturers will advise specific scanning protocols tailored to the scanner technology and speed. The volume of i.v. contrast and the scan delay may need to be increased for larger build patients.

Computed tomography pulmonary angiography – enhanced scan of pulmonary arterial system[1]

1. Volume of contrast medium – 110–150 ml or when dual phase injector available, 80–100 ml of contrast medium followed by saline chase of 30–50 ml
2. Delay:
   a. Preset delay of approximately 15 s for single slice; 22 s for 16 slice scanner; 26 s for 64 slice scanner
   OR
   b. Bolus tracking using software supplied with most multidetector scanners. A ROI (region of interest) is positioned over the pulmonary artery at the level of the carina. After commencing the injection a 'tracker scan' monitors the hounsfield level at the ROI and the scan is then triggered when the density at the ROI reaches a preset value
3. Rate of injection – $4 \, \mathrm{ml \, s^{-1}}$
4. Detector width/reconstruction (mm) – 0.625/1.25
5. Scan direction and extent – caudocranial direction helps reduce respiratory motion artifact at the lung bases. Less important with faster multislice scanners. Scan from lowest hemidiaphragm to lung apex
6. Image review and post-processing[2] – images should be reviewed at three settings:
   a. Mediastinal window (window width/window level 400/40 HU)
   b. Pulmonary embolism-specific window (700/100 HU)
   c. Lung window (1500/−600 HU).

Multiplanar reformatted images through the longitudinal axis of a vessel can be helpful to overcome difficulties encountered on axial sections of obliquely oriented arteries, aiding confidence in diagnosis or exclusion of thrombus.

7

References
1. Wittram, C. (2007) How I do it: CT pulmonary angiography. *Am. J. Roentgenol.* **188(5)**, 1255–1261.
2. Wittram, C., Maher, M.M., Yoo, A.J., et al. (2004) CT angiography of pulmonary embolism: diagnostic criteria and causes of misdiagnosis. *Radiographics* **24(5)**, 1219–1238.

Further reading
Remy-Jardin, M., Pistolesi, M., Goodman, L.R., et al. (2007) Management of suspected acute pulmonary embolism in the era of CT angiography: a statement from the Fleischner Society. *Radiology* **245(2)**, 315–329.
Schoepf, U.J & Costello, P. (2004) CT angiography for diagnosis of pulmonary embolism: state of the art. *Radiology* **230(2)**, 329–337.

PULMONARY ARTERIOGRAPHY

Indications

1. Demonstration of pulmonary emboli and other peripheral abnormalities, e.g. arteriovenous malformations, when less invasive investigations have been non-diagnostic.
2. Planning and performing therapeutic procedures such as catheter-directed thrombolysis or catheter embolectomy (in patients who cannot receive systemic thrombolysis due to bleeding risk and where surgical embolectomy is contraindicated).

Contraindications[1]

These include the general contraindications to any form of arteriography such as contrast allergy, renal failure and bleeding diatheses. There are more specific relative contraindications to diagnostic pulmonary arteriography:

1. Elevated right ventricular end-diastolic pressure (>20 mmHg) and/or elevated pulmonary artery pressure (>70 mmHg) – where the mortality rate is increased to 2–3%, instead of a standard documented mortality rate of 0.2–0.5%. Selective arteriography is advised if arteriography is still essential to patient management.
2. Left bundle branch block – right heart catheterization may induce complete heart block. A temporary pacemaker may need to be placed prior to the procedure.

Contrast medium

Low osmolar contrast material (LOCM) 370; $0.75 \, \text{ml} \, \text{kg}^{-1}$ at $20–25 \, \text{ml} \, \text{s}^{-1}$ (max. 40 ml).

Equipment

1. Fluoroscopy unit on a C- or U-arm, with digital subtraction facilities
2. Pump injector
3. Catheter: pigtail (coiled end, end hole and 12 side holes; see Fig. 8.3).

Technique

The Seldinger technique is used via the right femoral vein. The catheter is introduced via an introducer sheath. The catheter tip is sited, under fluoroscopic control, to lie 1–3 cm above the pulmonary valve. Pulmonary pressures should routinely be measured during the procedure. Lower injection rates are advised if the pressures are raised.

Additional techniques

1. If the entire chest cannot be accommodated on one field of view, the examination can be repeated by examining each lung. The catheter is advanced to lie in each main pulmonary artery in turn. For the right lung the patient, or the tube, is turned 10° LPO and for the left lung 10° RPO.
2. 40° caudal-cranial view: this view is optimal for the visualization of the bifurcation of the right and left pulmonary arteries, the pulmonary valve, annulus and trunk. With this manoeuvre the pulmonary trunk is no longer foreshortened and is not superimposed over its bifurcation.

Complications

The rate of minor complications is 1–3%. These include respiratory distress, major dysrhythmias, contrast reactions and renal failure. The current documented mortality rate is 0.2–0.5%.

For further details regarding general complications related to catheter techniques see page 216.

References

1. Gotway, M.B., Reddy, G.P. & Dawn, S.K. (2005) Pulmonary thromboembolic disease. In: Webb, W.R. & Higgins, C.B. (eds) *Thoracic Imaging: Pulmonary and Cardiovascular Radiology*. Philadelphia: Lippincott Williams & Wilkins; 609–629.

Further reading

Kucher, N. (2007) Catheter embolectomy for acute pulmonary embolism. *Chest* **132(2)**, 657–663.
Uflacker, R. (2001) Interventional therapy for pulmonary embolism. *J. Vasc. Interv. Radiol.* **12(2)**, 147–164.

7

BRONCHIAL STENTING

Indications

1. Compression or stricture secondary to malignant disease
2. Tracheal or bronchial stricture – either congenital or acquired, e.g. post lung transplant
3. Fistulae/dehiscence with the oesophagus or pleural cavity
4. Tracheobronchomalacia (relative indication).

Stents

1. Silicone polymers, e.g. Dumon (Novatech)
2. Metallic, e.g. Palmaz (Johnston & Johnston), Gianturco (Cook)
3. Covered – metallic mesh with polyurethane coating, e.g. covered Wallstent (Boston Scientific)
4. Hybrid – e.g. polyester/silicone or nitinol/silicone
5. Retrievable – e.g. either covered or uncovered nitinol stents, which allow retrieval or repositioning.

For malignant disease, polymer or covered stents should be used to prevent tumour in-growth.

Complications

1. Migration
2. Mucostasis
3. Obstruction, e.g. due to exuberant granulation tissue or tumour in-growth
4. Mechanical failure, e.g. stent fracture
5. Perforation.

Further reading

Dineen, K.M., Jantz, M.A. & Silvestri, G.A. (2002) Tracheobronchial stents. Review. *J. Bronchol.* **9(2)**, 127–137.
Lee, K.S., Lunn, W., Feller-Kopman, D., et al. (2005) Multislice CT evaluation of airway stents. *J. Thorac. Imaging* **20(2)**, 81–88.

MAGNETIC RESONANCE IMAGING OF THE RESPIRATORY SYSTEM

MRI only has a limited role in assessing the respiratory system as the susceptibility artifact from the large volume of air makes imaging the lungs difficult. The mediastinum and chest wall are well assessed by MRI due to the ability to image in the coronal and sagittal plane. MRI is particularly useful in the assessment of superior sulcus and neurogenic tumours as it can give information on the nature and extent of any intraspinal extension. Fast sequences and cardiac gating may be used to minimize motion artifacts. However, CT is quicker and more widely available. Multidetector CT technology can now give excellent multiplanar and three-dimensional reconstruction.

In the future MR pulmonary angiography may have a role to play in the diagnosis of pulmonary emboli, but it will probably be limited to a small cohort of patients in whom there is a relative contraindication to radiographic contrast or ionizing radiation.[1] At present, multi-detector CT scanning is the preferred method of investigation owing to its availability and ease of performance.

Reference

1. Fink, C., Ley, S., Schoenberg, S.O., et al. (2007) Magnetic resonance imaging of acute pulmonary embolism. *Eur. Radiol.* **17(10)**, 2546–2553.

Further reading

van Beek, E.J., Wild, J.M., Fink, C., et al. (2003) MRI for the diagnosis of pulmonary embolism. *J. Magn. Reson. Imaging* **18(6)**, 627–640.

7

PET AND PET-CT OF THE RESPIRATORY SYSTEM

In recent years, FDG-PET has become an essential lung-cancer imaging tool. A PET scan is currently recommended for the investigation of lung cancer where the lesion is greater than 1 cm in size. It also plays an important role in loco-regional and distant staging of non-small cell lung cancer (NSCLC). Patient preparation and the technique are fully described in Chapter 11. The scan can be performed either on an isolated PET scanner or a hybrid PET-CT scanner.

Recent studies suggest that PET is more sensitive than CT in measuring the biological effects of anti-cancer therapy. In the future PET-CT may have an additional role in predicting the response to anti-cancer treatment when patients have a scan performed to assess the early response after induction therapy.

Further reading

Devaraj, A., Cook, G.J., Hansell, D.M. (2007) PET/CT in non-small cell lung cancer staging – promises and problems. *Clin. Radiol.* **62(2)**, 97–108.

Vansteenkiste, J.F. & Stroobants, S.S. (2006) PET scan in lung cancer: current recommendations and innovation. *J. Thorac. Oncol.* **1(1)**, 71–73.

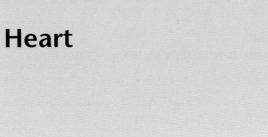

8

Heart

Methods of imaging the heart

1. Chest radiography
2. Fluoroscopy and angiocardiography
3. Echocardiography, including the transoesophageal technique
4. Computed tomography (CT)
5. Radionuclide imaging:
   a. Ventriculography
   b. Myocardial perfusion imaging
6. Magnetic resonance imaging (MRI).

ANGIOCARDIOGRAPHY

Diagnostic catheterization has predominantly been replaced by echocardiography (including transoesophageal echocardiography), radionuclide ventriculography and MRI. Angiocardiography is usually used as part of an interventional therapeutic procedure and can be performed simultaneously with cardiac catheterization during which pressures and oximetry are measured in the cardiac chambers and vessels that are under investigations. The right heart, left heart and great vessels are examined together or alone, depending on the clinical problem.

Indications

1. Congenital heart disease and anomalies of the great vessels – mostly in the paediatric population. Either for diagnosis or therapeutic procedures such as transcatheter closure of patent foramen ovale, atrial septal defect (ASD), ventricular septal defect (VSD) and patent ductus arteriosus

2. Valve disease, myocardial disease and ventricular function. Balloon valvuloplasty can be performed during the procedure to treat stenotic valvular disease if necessary.

Contrast medium

Low osmolar contrast material (LOCM) 370 (see Table 8.1).

Equipment

1. Biplane digital fluoroscopy and cine radiography with C-arms to facilitate axial projections
2. Pressure recording device
3. Electrocardiogram (ECG) monitor
4. Blood oxygen analyser
5. Catheter:
   a. For pressure measurements and blood sampling: Cournand (Fig. 8.1), 4–7-F
   b. For angiocardiography: National Institutes of Health (NIH) (Fig. 8.2) or pigtail (Fig. 8.3), 4–8-F.

Table 8.1 Volumes of contrast media in angiocardiography

	Injection site			
	Ventricle			Aorta or pulmonary artery
Adult	1 ml kg^{-1} at 18–20 ml s^{-1}			0.75 ml kg^{-1} at 18–20 ml s^{-1} (max. 40 ml)
Child				
First year	1.5 ml kg^{-1}	injected over 1–2 s	75% of the ventricular volume	
2–4 years	1.2 ml kg^{-1}			
5 years	1.0 ml kg^{-1}			

In general, hypoplastic or obstructed chambers require smaller volumes and flow rates and large shunts require greater volumes and flow rates of contrast medium.

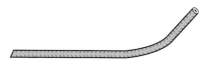

Figure 8.1 Cournand catheter. End holes: 1 Side holes: 0.

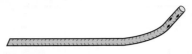

Figure 8.2 National Institutes of Health (NIH) catheter. End holes: 0 Side holes: 4 or 6.

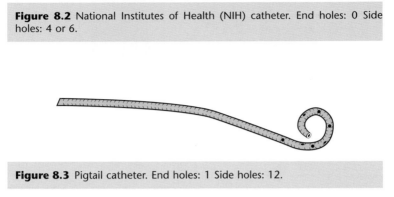

Figure 8.3 Pigtail catheter. End holes: 1 Side holes: 12.

Technique

1. Right-sided cardiac structures and pulmonary arteries are examined by introducing a catheter into a peripheral vein. In babies the femoral vein may be the only vein large enough to take the catheter. If an atrial septal defect is suspected, the femoral vein approach offers the best chance of passing the catheter into the left atrium through the defect. In adults the right antecubital or basilic vein may be used. The cephalic vein should not be used because it can be difficult to pass the catheter past the site where the vein pierces the clavipectoral fascia to join the axillary vein. The catheter, or introducer, is introduced using the Seldinger technique. (The NIH catheter must be introduced via an introducer as there is no end hole for a guidewire.)
2. In children it is usually possible to examine the left heart and occasionally the aorta by manipulating a venous catheter through a patent foramen ovale. In adults the aorta and left ventricle are studied via a catheter passed retrogradely from the femoral artery.
3. The catheter is manipulated into the appropriate positions for recording pressures and sampling blood for oxygen saturation. Following this, angiography is performed.

Image acquisition

Using digital angiography at 30 frames s^{-1} with axial alignment of the heart, i.e. the X-ray beam is aligned perpendicular to the long axis of the heart (Fig. 8.4). The long axis of the heart is usually oblique to

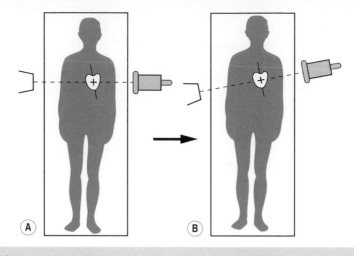

Figure 8.4 Principles of axial angiography. Alignment of the heart perpendicular to the X-ray beam.

the long axis of the patient's body and cardiac angiography suites have movable C-arms which allow correct positioning by movement of the equipment alone without disturbing the patient (Fig. 8.4b). Further rotation of the direction of the X-ray beam is used to profile those areas of the heart under examination. Useful views are:

1. *40° cranial/40° left anterior oblique (LAO) (hepatoclavicular or four-chamber) view* – the beam is perpendicular to the long axis of the heart and aligns the atrial septum and posterior interventricular septum parallel to the beam
2. *Long axial 20° right anterior oblique (RAO) (long axial oblique) view* – the lateral tube and image intensifier are angled 25–30° cranially, to align with the long axis of the heart, and 20° RAO.

CORONARY ARTERIOGRAPHY

Indications
1. Diagnosis of the presence and extent of ischaemic heart disease
2. After revascularization procedures
3. Congenital heart lesions
4. Therapeutic percutaneous coronary intervention – balloon angioplasty and stenting.

Diagnostic arteriography can be supplemented by intravascular ultrasound (US) to determine the nature and extent of plaque within the vessel wall or angioscopy in some centres.

Contrast medium

LOCM 370, 8–10 ml given as a hand injection for each projection.

Equipment

1. Digital angiography with C-arm
2. Pressure recording device and ECG monitor
3. Judkins (Fig. 8.5) or Amplatz (Fig. 8.6) catheters – the left and right coronary artery catheters are of different shape.

Patient preparation

As for routine arteriography.

Preliminary image

Chest X-ray.

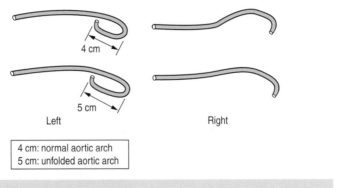

4 cm

5 cm

Left   Right

4 cm: normal aortic arch
5 cm: unfolded aortic arch

Figure 8.5 Judkins coronary artery catheters. End holes: 1 Side holes: 0

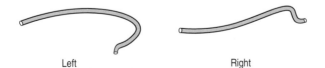

Left   Right

Figure 8.6 Amplatz coronary artery catheters. End holes: 1 Side holes: 0

Technique

The catheter is introduced using the Seldinger technique via the radial, brachial or femoral artery and advanced until its tip lies in the ostium of the coronary artery.

Image acquisition

Angiography (30 frames s^{-1}) is performed in the following positions:

Right coronary artery
1. With radial puncture: 30° RAO, 45° LAO, 45° LAO/20° cranial
2. With femoral puncture: as above.

Left coronary artery
1. With radial puncture: 30° RAO, 10° RAO, 60° LAO, hepatoclavicular view (see above)
2. With femoral puncture: additional lateral projection possible.

Complications

In addition to the general complications discussed in Chapter 9, patients undergoing coronary arteriography may be liable to:

1. Arrhythmias – such as non-sustained atrial fibrillation with right heart catheterization or non-sustained ventricular arrhythmia with left ventriculography
2. Ostial dissection by the catheter
3. Access site complications – local haematoma, femoral artery pseudoaneurysm or arterio-venous fistula. Mostly with femoral route.

CARDIAC COMPUTED TOMOGRAPHY (INCLUDING CORONARY COMPUTED TOMOGRAPHIC ANGIOGRAPHY)

As a result of advances in CT technology, non-invasive cardiac imaging is becoming central to the diagnosis and management of patients with cardiac disease. This is the result of fast scan times and cardiac gating facilities available with multidetector CT scanners. Whilst the examination is tailored to assessment of the cardiac structures, CT imaging gives the benefit over conventional cardiac and coronary angiography of demonstrating clinically significant non-cardiac findings within the adjacent mediastinum, lungs or upper abdomen,[1] and can give additional information regarding plaque characterization.

Cardiac CT may be performed as:

1. Unenhanced CT scan for coronary artery calcium scoring
2. Contrast enhanced CT coronary angiography (CTA)
3. Contrast enhanced CT for myocardial assessment or cardiac valve imaging (specialist centres only).

The coronary artery calcium (CAC) score is calculated from the volume of calcium present in the coronary arteries. A high score indicates an increased risk of adverse coronary events and CAC scoring has been used as a screening tool for subclinical cardiac disease. Absence of coronary artery calcification does not exclude atheroma but is associated with a low risk of adverse coronary event. Evidence shows that scores will probably need to be matched to age, sex and ethnic background.[2]

Coronary computed tomographic angiography

Documented mean effective radiation dose for coronary CTA ranges from 6 to 25 mSv[3] and reported mean effective dose for conventional catheter angiography is 5.6 mSv.[4] Further improvements in CT technology continue to reduce effective dose but there must be constant awareness with attempt to minimize dose wherever possible. Tailored coronary CTA is well-documented to have a high negative predictive value for coronary artery stenosis.[5,6]

Indications

1. Patients with known or suspected chronic coronary artery disease.
2. As a screening test in asymptomatic high-risk patients or patients with atypical chest pain.
3. As an alternative to diagnostic coronary angiography when planning percutaneous angiographic intervention or as post-procedure follow-up.
4. Visualization of coronary artery grafts, including the entire course of the left internal mammary artery (LIMA) graft to its distal anastomosis on the coronary artery.

Technique

The exact technique will depend on individual CT scanner technology and requires a multidetector CT which is 16 slice or above. Each CT manufacturer will advise scan protocols tailored to their specific scanners; however, general parameters useful for coronary artery assessment cardiac CT are as follows:[7]

1. For optimal imaging, the patient should have a regular heart rate of 50–65 beats per minute during the scan. Either oral or intravenous (i.v.) beta-blockers are often given to slow the heart rate before scanning. ECG monitoring with clear QRS complex is required. Radiation dose can be reduced by cardiac gating with prospective ECG triggering and radiation dose

8

modulation by decreasing X-ray tube output during systole – only data acquired during diastole are used for evaluation of coronary arteries.[8]

2. Volume of contrast medium – 95–100 ml LOCM 350–400 mgI/ml followed by saline chase of 50 ml through cannula in right antecubital vein. (The saline chase reduces streak artifact from dense contrast in the right side of the heart, whilst the right-sided cannulation reduces streak artifact from the left subclavian artery or internal mammary coronary graft.) An initial unenhanced scan is sometimes used to assess the coronary artery calcium score, provide landmarks for planning of the contrast run and allow the patient to become accustomed to the scan.

3. Delay:
   a. Preset delay of 18–20 s
   OR, preferably,
   b. Bolus tracking using software supplied with the multidetector scanner. A ROI (region of interest) is positioned over the ascending aorta. After commencing the injection a 'tracker scan' monitors the hounsfield level at the ROI and the scan is then triggered when the density at the ROI reaches a preset value, e.g.150 HU

4. Rate of injection – LOCM 400 at $5\,\mathrm{ml\,s^{-1}}$ or LOCM 350 at $6\,\mathrm{ml\,s^{-1}}$

5. Collimator/reconstruction width (mm) – 0.6 to 0.75/0.75 to 1 as per available CT technology[9]

6. Rotation time/tube voltage – fastest possible with available scanner technology/120 kV

7. Scan direction and extent – cranio-caudal from tracheal bifurcation to 1 cm below heart

8. Image reconstruction, review and post-processing – images can be reconstructed at various times through the cardiac cycle from the R–R peak, usually expressed as percentage through the length of the cycle. Image review using axial scans, multiplanar reconstructions (MPR), curved MPRs, volume rendering and surface shaded display all useful to analyse the vessel pathway, wall and caliber.

References

1. Weinreb, J.C., Larson, P.A., Woodard, P.K., et al. (2005) American College of Radiology clinical statement on noninvasive cardiac imaging. *Radiology* **235**, 723–727.
2. Preis, S.R. & O'Donnell, C.J. (2007) Coronary heart disease risk assessment by traditional risk factors and newer subclinical disease imaging: is a 'one-size-fits-all' approach the best option? Editorial. *Arch. Intern. Med.* **167(22)**, 2399–2401.

3. Mahesh, M. & Cody, D.D. (2007) AAPM/RSNA physics tutorial for residents: physics of cardiac imaging with multiple-row detector CT. *RadioGraphics* **27**, 1495–1509.
4. Coles, D.R., Smail, M.A., Negus, I.S., et al. (2006) Comparison of radiation doses from multislice computed tomography coronary angiography and conventional diagnostic angiography. *J. Am. Coll. Cardiol.* **47**, 1840–1845.
5. Abdulla, J., Abildstrom, S.Z., Gotzsche, O., et al. (2007) 64-multislice detector computed tomography coronary angiography as potential alternative to conventional coronary angiography: a systematic review and meta-analysis. *Eur. Heart J.* **28(24)**, 3042–3050.
6. Nieman, K. Cademartiri, F., Lemos, P.A., et al. (2002) Reliable noninvasive coronary angiography with fast submillimeter multislice spiral computed tomography. *Circulation* **106**, 2051–2054.
7. Schoepf, U.J., Zwerner, P.L., Savino, G., et al. (2007) Coronary CT angiography: how I do it. *Radiology* **244**, 48–63.
8. Earls, J.P., Berman, E.L., Urban, B.A., et al. (2008) Prospectively gated transverse coronary CT angiography versus retrospectively gated helical technique: improved image quality and reduced radiation dose. *Radiology* **246**, 742–753.
9. Pugliese, F., Mollet, N.R., Hunink, M.G., et al. (2008) Diagnostic performance of coronary CT angiography by using different generations of multisection scanners: single center experience. *Radiology* **246**, 384–393.

Further reading

Gershlick, A.H., de Belder, M., Chambers, J., et al. (2007) Role of non-invasive imaging in the management of coronary artery disease: an assessment of likely change over the next 10 years. A report from the British Cardiovascular Society Working Group. *Heart* **93**, 423–431.
Vanhoenacker, P.K., Heijenbrok-Kal, M.H., Van Heste, R., et al. (2007) Diagnostic performance of multidetector CT angiography for assessment of coronary artery disease: meta-analysis. *Radiology* **244**, 419–428.

8

RADIONUCLIDE VENTRICULOGRAPHY

Indications

Gated blood-pool study[1]

1. Evaluation of ventricular function; particularly left ventricular ejection fraction (LVEF)
2. Assessment of myocardial reserve in coronary artery disease
3. Cardiomyopathy, including the effects of cardio-toxic drugs.

First pass radionuclide angiography[2,3]

1. Evaluation of right ventricular ejection fraction (RVEF)
2. Detection and quantification of intra-cardiac shunts.

Contraindications

Significant arrhythmias may make gated blood-pool imaging impossible.

Radiopharmaceuticals

^{99m}Technetium-in-vivo-labelled red blood cells, 800 MBq max (8 mSv ED).

Before radiolabelling with ^{99m}Technetium (^{99m}Tc)-pertechnetate, the red blood cells are 'primed' with an injection of stannous pyrophosphate. The stannous ions reduce the pertechnetate and allow it to bind to the pyrophosphate which adsorbs on to the red blood cells.

Equipment

1. Gamma-camera: equipped with low-energy general purpose collimator
2. Imaging computer: list-mode or multi-gated acquisition (MUGA)
3. ECG monitor with gating pulse output.

Patient preparation

1. An i.v. injection of 'cold' stannous pyrophosphate ($20\,\mu g\ kg^{-1}$) is given directly into a vein 20–30 min before the pertechnetate injection. (Avoid injection via long plastic Teflon coated cannula which may result in a poor label.)
2. Three ECG electrodes are placed in standard positions to give a gating signal.

Technique

Gated blood-pool study

1. Patient supine
2. The ECG trigger signal is connected
3. I.v. injection of ^{99m}Tc pertechnetate
4. One minute is allowed for the bolus to equilibrate before computer acquisition is commenced (see 'Films' below).

List mode is best, where individual events are stored as their x, y coordinates along with timing and gating pulses. This allows maximum flexibility for later manipulation and framing of data. Around 5 million counts should be acquired. However, MUGA mode is adequate, and is still the most commonly used. In this, the start of an acquisition cycle is usually triggered by the R wave of the patient's ECG. A series of 16–32 fast frames are recorded before the next R wave occurs. Each of these has very few counts in from a single cycle, so every time the R wave trigger arrives another set of frames is recorded and summed with the first. The sequence continues until 100–200 kilo-counts per frame have been acquired in about 10 min. Some degree of arrhythmia can be tolerated using the technique of 'buffered bad beat rejection', where cardiac cycles of irregular length are rejected and the data not included in the images. The length of time to acquire an image set increases as the proportion of rejected beats rises.

First-pass radionuclide angiography

This provides information on right ventricular function and intra-cardiac shunts, although only from one view unless a multi-headed camera or bi-planar collimator is available:

1. Positioning depends upon the clinical question. For ventricular function evaluation, the patient lies supine with the camera against the chest in the RAO 30° position for best visualization of the right atrium and ventricle, or the LAO 35–45° position for best visualization of the left ventricle. A caudal tilt of 15–30° may improve separation of the ventricles. For assessment of shunting, the camera is positioned anteriorly.
2. The ECG trigger signal is connected.
3. The validity of the first-pass study is dependent on the quality of the bolus injection. For RVEF assessment, the ^{99m}Tc-pertechnetate is injected over approximately 3 s (too tight a bolus will not provide sufficient cardiac cycles for evaluation; too slow an injection will result in poor image statistics before circulation through the lung capillary bed and left side of the heart). However, for shunt quantification, ^{99m}Tc-pertechnetate is injected in as tight a bolus as possible by using the Oldendorf or similar technique (see Chapter 1).
4. Gated list-mode computer acquisition is started as the bolus is released. Although the first pass usually takes a maximum of 10–15 s, it is advisable to continue data acquisition for up to 50 s in case of slow bolus arrival. (If list mode is not available, a short-frame dynamic study with 20 frames s^{-1} or faster on a 64×64 matrix may be used, although it is unlikely that gating information will be able to be stored, so calculation of RVEF will be sub-optimal. For shunt assessment, a rate of 2 frames s^{-1} is reasonable.)
5. A gated blood-pool study follows, as above.

Images

Gated blood-pool study

A number of views may be recorded, depending on the clinical problem:

1. LAO 35–45° with a 15–30° caudal tilt, chosen to give best separation between left and right ventricles. Patient supine. This view is sufficient if only LVEF is required

8

2. Anterior, patient supine
3. LPO, chosen to give best separation between atria and ventricles. Patient in right lateral decubitus position.

Analysis

Gated blood-pool study
1. The LVEF is calculated
2. Systolic, diastolic, phase and amplitude images are generated
3. The frames can be displayed in cine mode to give good visualization of wall motion.

First-pass study
1. The RVEF can be calculated
2. Serial images can be produced showing the sequence of chamber filling
3. A time-activity curve from the pulmonary region can be used for quantitative assessment of a shunt
4. Chamber transit times may be calculated.

Additional techniques

1. Gated blood-pool imaging can be carried out during controlled exercise with appropriate precautions to assess ventricular functional reserve. Leg exercise using a bed-mounted bicycle ergometer is the method of choice. Shoulder restraints and hand grips help to reduce upper body movement during imaging. For patients unable to exercise effectively, stress with dobutamine infusion is used.[4] Under continuous monitoring, the dose is incrementally increased from 5 to $20 \mu g \, kg^{-1} \, min^{-1}$, infusing each dose for 3 min. The infusion is stopped when S-T segment depression of >3 mm, any ventricular arrhythmia, systolic blood pressure >220 mmHg, attainment of maximum heart rate, or any side-effects occur
2. Gated single photon emission computed tomography (SPECT) blood pool acquisition can be used for measurement of left as well as the right ventricular function using special software (Autoquant+) which calculates the left and right ventricular volumes
3. With gated SPECT using the myocardial perfusion imaging agents $^{99}Tc^m$-MIBI and $^{99}Tc^m$-tetrofosmin (see 'Radionuclide myocardial perfusion imaging'), it is possible to combine ventriculography and perfusion scans in a single study.[5,6]

When acquiring gated SPECT studies ventricular parameters are usually measured during rest study only because of the length of the examination (20 min).

Aftercare

1. Monitor recovery from exercise
2. Normal radiation safety precautions (see Chapter 1).

Complications

Complications are related to the exercise test and include induction of angina, cardiac arrhythmias and cardiac arrest.

References

1. Metcalfe, M.J. (2005) Radionuclide ventriculography. In: Sharp, P.F., Gemmell, H.G. & Murray, A.D. (eds) *Practical Nuclear Medicine*. London: Springer.
2. Friedman, J.D., Berman, D.S., Borges-Neto, S., et al. (2006) First-pass radionuclide angiography. *J. Nucl. Cardiol.* **13(6)**, e42–55.
3. Williams, K.A. (2005) Measurement of ventricular function with scintigraphic techniques: part 1 – imaging hardware, radiopharmaceuticals, and first-pass radionuclide angiography. *J. Nucl. Cardiol.* **12(1)**, 86–95.
4. Konishi, T., Koyama, T., Aoki, T., et al. (1990) Radionuclide assessment of left ventricular function during dobutamine infusion in patients with coronary artery disease: comparison with ergometer exercise. *Clin. Cardiol.* **13**, 183–188.
5. Fukuoka, S., Maeno, M., Nakagawa, S., et al. (2002) Feasibility of myocardial dual-isotope perfusion imaging combined with gated single photon emission tomography for assessing coronary artery disease. *Nucl. Med. Commun.* **23(1)**, 19–29.
6. Anagnostopoulos, C. & Underwood, S.R. (1998) Simultaneous assessment of myocardial perfusion and function: how and when? *Eur. J. Nucl. Med.* **25**, 555–558.

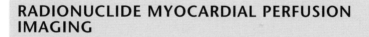

RADIONUCLIDE MYOCARDIAL PERFUSION IMAGING

Indications

1. Diagnosis and assessment of extent and severity of myocardial ischaemia or infarction
2. Assessment of myocardial viability
3. Evaluation of prognosis
4. Evaluation of effects of angioplasty and bypass surgery on myocardial perfusion with pre- and post-intervention imaging.

Contraindications

1. Unstable angina
2. Frequent ventricular arrhythmias at rest
3. Contraindications to pharmacological stress agent
4. Second-degree heart block
5. Severe valvular disease, especially aortic valve stenosis.

Radiopharmaceuticals[1,2]

1. *99mTc-methoxyisobutylisonitrile (MIBI or sestamibi)*, up to 800 MBq (8 mSv ED) for planar imaging, 800 MBq (8 mSv ED) for SPECT (or 1600 MBq max. for the total of two injections in single day rest/exercise protocols). Cationic complex with myocardial uptake in near proportion to coronary blood flow but minimal redistribution. There is also, normally, liver uptake and biliary excretion, which can cause inferior wall artifacts on SPECT if care is not taken. Separate injections are required for stress/rest studies, but image timing is flexible due to minimal redistribution

2. *99mTc-tetrofosmin (Myoview)* (activity and radiation dose as for MIBI). Similar uptake characteristics and diagnostic efficacy to MIBI, but with easier preparation

3. *201Tl-thallous chloride*, 80 MBq max. (18 mSv ED). Thallium is a potassium analogue with initial rapid myocardial uptake in near proportion to coronary blood flow, and subsequent washout and redistribution. Hence, unlike the ^{99}Tc^m agents, same-day stress/rest redistribution studies can be performed with a single injection. With principal photon energies of 68–72 and 167 keV and $T_{1/2}$ of 73 h, it is not ideal for imaging and gives a higher radiation dose than the newer ^{99m}Tc alternatives. It is increasingly being replaced by ^{99m}Tc agents. However, many still consider ^{201}Tl for assessment of myocardial viability and hibernation, with either re-injection at rest or a separate day rest-redistribution study giving the greatest sensitivity.

4. *18FDG + blood flow PET*. The radio-isotope gold standard for viability assessment, but not widely available[3]

5. *Rubidium-82 PET*. This study can be used to assess myocardial perfusion. Not widely available.

Equipment

1. SPECT-capable gamma-camera, preferably dual-headed
2. Low-energy, high-resolution, general purpose or specialized cardiac collimators
3. Pharmacological stressing agent (adenosine, dipyridamole or dobutamine) or exercise (bicycle ergometer or treadmill)
4. Nitroglycerin (tablets or sublingual spray) to enhance resting uptake of ischaemic, but viable segments
5. ECG monitor
6. Resuscitation facilities including defibrillator
7. Aminophylline to reverse possible severe bronchospasm after dipyridamole infusion
8. Lidocaine to reverse serious arrhythmias caused by dobutamine infusion

Patient preparation

1. Nil by mouth or light breakfast 4–6 h prior to test
2. Cessation of cardiac medication on the day of the test if possible. ß-blockers can be continued and adenosine stress used. Avoid caffeine for 24 h if using dipyridamole or adenosine.

Technique

The principal of the technique is to compare myocardial perfusion under conditions of pharmacological stress or physical exercise, with perfusion at rest. Diseased but patent arterial territories will show lower perfusion under stress conditions than healthy arteries, but will show relatively improved perfusion at rest. Infarcted tissue will show no improvement at rest. Hence, prognostic information on the likelihood of adverse cardiac events and the benefits of revascularization can be gained.[4]

Stress regime

Pharmacological stress has become increasingly widely used instead of physical exercise.[5] The optimal stress technique aims to maximize coronary arterial flow. The preferred pharmacological stressing agent is adenosine infusion ($0.14 \, mg \, kg^{-1} \, min^{-1}$ for 6 min).[6] Adenosine is a potent coronary vasodilator. It reproducibly increases coronary artery flow by more than maximal physical exercise (which often cannot be achieved in this group of patients). It has a short biological half-life of 8–10 s, so most side-effects are reversed simply by discontinuing infusion. Stressing with adenosine has now largely replaced dipyridamole, which will not be discussed here.

There are circumstances where adenosine is contraindicated, e.g. asthma, second-degree heart block or systolic blood pressure $<100 \, mmHg$. Dobutamine stress may be employed in these circumstances.[7] Dobutamine acts as a $ß_1$ receptor agonist, increasing contractility and heart rate. Under continuous monitoring, the dose is incrementally increased from 5 to $20 \, \mu g \, kg^{-1} \, min^{-1}$, infusing each dose for 3 min. The infusion is terminated when S-T segment depression of $>3 \, mm$, any ventricular arrhythmia, systolic blood pressure $>220 \, mmHg$, attainment of maximum heart rate, or any side-effects occur. Dobutamine is contraindicated in patients with aortic aneurysm. New, more specific targeted agents such as regadenoson (A_{2A} adenosine receptor agonist) are being developed which could be used in asthmatic patients rather than dobutamine.[8]

^{99m}Tc-MIBI or tetrofosmin rest/stress test

Because MIBI and tetrofosmin have minimal redistribution, separate injections are needed for stress and rest studies. Two-day protocols are optimal, but it is often more convenient to perform both studies on the same day. A number of groups have shown that this is possible without significantly degrading the results, most effectively when the resting study is performed first.[9]

2-Day protocol (stress/rest)

1. Initiate pharmacological stress or exercise
2. Up to 800 MBq MIBI or tetrofosmin is administered i.v. at maximal stress, continuing the stress protocol for 2 min post injection to allow uptake in the myocardium
3. 10–30 min post injection, a milky drink or similar is given to promote biliary clearance; high fluid intake will dilute bowel contents
4. Images are acquired 15–30 min after tetrofosmin or 60–120 min after sestamibi injection. If there is excessive liver uptake or activity in small bowel close to the heart, imaging should be delayed by a further 60 min
5. Depending on the clinical situation, if the stress scan is completely normal the patient may not need to return for the rest scan[10]
6. Preferably 2–7 days later, the patient returns for a resting scan
7. Glyceryl trinitrate (GTN) (two 0.3 mg tablets) or equivalent sublingual spray may be given to improve blood flow to ischaemic, but viable segments[11]
8. Immediately, up to 800 MBq MIBI or tetrofosmin i.v. is administered and proceed as for stress imaging.

1-Day protocol (stress/rest)

1. Initiate pharmacological stress or exercise; up to 400 MBq MIBI or tetrofosmin i.v. is administered at maximum stress
2. Image as per 2-day protocol
3. A minimum of 2 h after first tetrofosmin injection and minimum of 4 h after sestamibi injection, GTN is administered as above, followed by up to 1200 MBq MIBI or tetrofosmin (with longer period between injections, the activity of the second injection may be reduced)
4. Image as per 2-day protocol.

^{201}Tl stress/rest test

Since ^{201}Tl redistributes after injection, stress/rest studies can be performed with a single injection. However, stress image timing is more critical:

1. Initiate pharmacological stress or exercise
2. Administer 80 MBq ^{201}Tl i.v. at maximal stress, continuing the stress protocol for 1 min post injection to allow uptake in the myocardium
3. Image immediately (<5 min)
4. Image at rest 3–4 h after redistribution period, during which time patients should not eat

5. If fixed defects are present in exercise and rest images and assessment of viability and hibernation is required, either:
   a. administer a second smaller dose of 40 MBq ^{201}Tl, giving GTN pre injection, and image 20–30 min later. If defects still persist, image again at 18–24 h
   OR
   b. perform a separate day rest-redistribution study with 80 MBq ^{201}Tl after GTN, and image at 20–30 min and 3–4 h.

Images

Spect

1. Position patient as comfortably as possible with their arms above their head (or at least the left arm) if possible. SPECT images may be severely degraded by patient movement, so attention should be paid to keeping the patient very still
2. For the ^{99}Tc^m agents, check for activity in bowel loops close to the inferior wall of the heart. This can cause artifacts in the reconstructed images, so if significant activity is seen, delay the imaging to give greater time for clearance
3. 180° orbit from RAO 45° to LPO 45°, elliptical if possible. With modern dual-headed systems, this can be achieved with the heads at 90° to each other to minimize the amount of camera rotation required
4. Matrix size and zoom to give a pixel size of 6 mm
5. 60 projections, with a total imaging time of about 30–40 min for single and 15–25 min for dual-head systems
6. View the projections as a cine before the patient leaves the department. If available, perform software motion correction. If there is significant movement that cannot be corrected, repeat imaging. Beware 'diaphragmatic creep', particularly on ^{201}Tl patients breathless after exercise, where the average position of the diaphragm changes as they recover.

Analysis

1. Short, vertical long and horizontal long axis views are reconstructed, taking care to use the same orientation for stress and rest image data sets (modern systems have automatic alignment software).
2. Two-dimensional circumferential profile or 'bull's-eye' polar maps may be generated.

Additional techniques

1. Gated SPECT is now recommended,[12] and with special software (e.g. Cedars Sinai QGS package, Emory cardiac tool box) can provide additional information on ventricular wall motion, ejection fraction and chamber volume. It can also improve

specificity by reducing artifactual defects caused by regional myocardial motion and wall thickening.

2. Bull's-eye maps can be compared to normal databases and displayed quantitatively in terms of severity and extent of relative underperfusion.[13]

3. Attenuation and scatter correction using scanning transmission line sources or CT are now available on most modern dual-headed systems. This technique can improve diagnostic specificity by correcting attenuation artifacts and thereby increasing the normalcy rate. However, algorithms are still being improved, so at present it is wise to view the attenuation-corrected and uncorrected images together to identify possible introduced artifacts.[14]

4. The combination of rest ^{201}Tl and exercise ^{99m}Tc MIBI or tetrofosmin can be used to assess both ischaemia and viability.[15]

Aftercare
1. Monitoring of patient post-exercise
2. Normal radiation safety precautions (see Chapter 1).

Complications
Complications are related to stress and exercise and include: induction of angina, cardiac arrhythmias, cardiac arrest and bronchospasm after adenosine.

References
1. Reyes, E., Loong, C.Y., Harbinson, M., et al. (2006) A comparison of Tl-201, Tc-99m sestamibi, and Tc-99m tetrofosmin myocardial perfusion scinitgraphy in patients with mild to moderate coronary stenosis. *J. Nucl. Cardiol.* **13(4)**, 488–494.
2. Kapur, A., Latus, K.A., Davies, G., et al. (2002) A comparison of three radionuclide myocardial perfusion tracers in clinical practice: the ROBUST study. *Eur. J. Nucl. Med. Mol. Imaging* **29(12)**, 1608–1616.
3. Nandalur, K.R., Dwamena, B.A., Choudhri, A.F., et al. (2008) Diagnostic performance of positron emission tomography in the detection of coronary artery disease: a meta-analysis. *Acad. Radiol.* **15(4)**, 444–451.
4. Travin, M.I. & Bergmann, S.R. (2005) Assessment of myocardial viability. *Semin. Nucl. Med.* **35(1)**, 2–16.
5. Travain, M.I. & Wexler, J.P. (1999) Pharmacological stress testing. *Semin. Nucl. Med.* **29**, 298–318.
6. Takeishi, Y., Takahashi, N., Fujiwara, S., et al. (1998) Myocardial tomography with technetium-99m-tetrofosmin during intravenous infusion of adenosine triphosphate. *J. Nucl. Med.* **39**, 582–586.
7. Verani, M.S. (1994) Dobutamine myocardial perfusion imaging. *J. Nucl. Med.* **35**, 737–739.
8. Iskandrian, A.E., Bateman, T.M., Belardinelli, L., et al. (2007) Adenosine versus regadenoson comparative evaluation in myocardial perfusion

imaging: results of the ADVANCE phase 3 multicenter international trial. *J. Nucl. Cardiol.* **14(5)**, 645–658.

9. Tadehara, F., Yamamoto, H., Tsujiyama, S., et al. (2008) Feasibility of a rapid protocol of 1-day single-isotope rest/adenosine stress Tc-99m sestamibi ECG-gated myocardial perfusion imaging. *J. Nucl. Cardiol.* **15(1)**, 35–41.

10. Lavalaye, J.M., Shroeder-Tanka, J.M., Tiel-van Buul, M.M., et al. (1997) Implementation of technetium-99m MIBI SPECT imaging guidelines: optimizing the two-day stress-rest protocol. *Int. J. Card. Imaging* **13**, 331–335.

11. Thorley, P.J., Sheard, K.L., Wright, D.J. et al. (1998) The routine use of sublingual GTN with resting ^{99}Tc^m-tetrofosmin myocardial perfusion imaging. *Nucl. Med. Commun.* **19**, 937–942.

12. Travin, M.I., Heller, G.V., Johnson, L.L., et al. (2004) The prognostic value of ECG-gated SPECT imaging in patients undergoing stress Tc-99m sestamibi myocardial perfusion imaging. *J. Nucl. Cardiol.* **11(3)**, 253–262.

13. Schwaiger, M. & Melin, J. (1999) Cardiological applications of nuclear medicine. *Lancet* **354**, 661–666.

14. Banzo, I., Pena, F.J., Allende, R.H., et al. (2003) Prospective clinical comparison of non-corrected and attenuation- and scatter-corrected myocardial perfusion SPECT in patients with suspicion of coronary artery disease. *Nucl. Med. Commun.* **24(9)**, 995–1002.

15. Kim, Y., Goto, H., Kobayshi, K., et al. (1999) A new method to evaluate ischemic heart disease: combined use of rest thallium-201 myocardial SPECT and Tc-99m exercise tetrofosmin first pass and myocardial SPECT. *Ann. Nucl. Med.* **13**, 147–153.

MAGNETIC RESONANCE IMAGING OF THE CARDIAC SYSTEM

One of the earliest applications of cardiac MRI was the anatomical delineation of congenital heart disease when the pathology could not be completely evaluated by echocardiography. More recently cardiac MRI has been found to be a very effective method of functional assessment of the heart. Not only has it an important role in the assessment of ventricular function, myocardial mass and myocardial viability,[1,2] but it is also increasingly used for clinical rest and stress perfusion measurements. It is particularly valuable in distinguishing ischaemic from non-ischaemic cardiomyopathy.[3]

References

1. Berman, D.S., Hachamovitch, R., Shaw, L.J., et al. (2006) Roles of nuclear cardiology, cardiac computed tomography, and cardiac magnetic

resonance: assessment of patients with suspected coronary artery disease. *J. Nucl. Med.* **47(1)**, 74–82.

2. Weinreb, J.C., Larson, P.A., Woodard, P.K., et al. (2005) American College of Radiology clinical statement on noninvasive cardiac imaging. *Radiology* **235**, 723–727.

3. Jackson, E., Bellenger, N., Seddon, M., et al. (2007) Ischaemic and non-ischaemic cardiomyopathies - cardiac MRI appearances with delayed enhancement. *Clin. Radiol.* **62**, 395–403.

Further reading

Bhatnagar, P., Mankad, K., Hoey, E., et al. (2008) Cardiac radiology: subspecialty web review. *Clin. Radiol.* **63**, 370–372.

Finn, J.P, Nael, K., Deshpande, V., et al. (2006) Cardiac MR imaging: state of the technology. *Radiology* **241**, 338–354.

Arterial system

Methods of imaging the arterial system
1. Catheter angiography
2. Ultrasound (US)
3. Computed tomography (CT)
4. Magnetic resonance imaging (MRI)

Further reading
Collins, R., Cranny, G., Burch, J., et al. (2007) A systematic review of duplex ultrasound, magnetic resonance angiography and computed tomography angiography for the diagnosis and assessment of symptomatic, lower limb peripheral arterial disease. *Health Technol. Assess.* **11(20),** iii–iv, xi–xiii, 1–184.
Kaufman, J.A. & Lee, M.J. (eds) (2004) *Vascular and Interventional Radiology: The Requisites.* Philadelphia: Elsevier-Mosby.

INTRODUCTION TO CATHETER TECHNIQUES

The basic technique of arterial catheterization is also applicable to veins.

Patient preparation
1. The patient will need admission to hospital. Careful preparation before the procedure and observation after are required. With the introduction of smaller diameter catheters, day case admission may be appropriate for routine peripheral angiography and some angioplasty cases.
2. If the patient is on anticoagulant treatment, blood clotting should be within an acceptable therapeutic 'window'.

3. The radiologist or a suitably trained person should see the patient preferably several days prior to the procedure in order to:
   a. explain the procedure
   b. obtain informed consent
   c. assess the patient, with special reference to renal function, blood pressure and peripheral pulses as a baseline for post-arteriographic problems.

Puncture sites

1. Femoral artery – most frequently used
2. Brachial artery – a high approach is preferable
3. Axillary artery
4. Radial artery.

Equipment for the Seldinger technique

Needles

The technique of catheter insertion via double-wall needle puncture and guidewire is known as the Seldinger technique. The original Seldinger needle consisted of three parts:

1. An outer thin-walled blunt cannula
2. An inner needle
3. A stilette.

Many radiologists now prefer to use modified needles:

1. Double-wall puncture with a two-piece needle consisting of a bevelled central stilette and an outer tube
2. Single-wall puncture with a simple sharp needle (without a stilette) with a bore just wide enough to accommodate the guidewire.

Guidewires

Basic guidewires consist of two central cores of straight wire around which is a tightly wound coiled wire spring (Fig. 9.1). The ends are sealed with solder. One of the central core wires is secured at both ends – a safety feature in case of fracturing. The other is anchored in solder at one end, but terminates 5 cm from the other end, leaving a soft flexible tip. Some guidewires have a movable central core so the tip can be flexible or stiff. Others have a J-shaped tip which is useful for negotiating vessels with irregular walls. The size of the J-curve is denoted by its radius in mm. Guidewires are polyethylene coated but may be coated with a thin film of Teflon to reduce friction. Teflon, however, also increases the thrombogenicity, which can be countered by using heparin-bonded Teflon. The most common sizes are 0.035 and 0.038 inch diameter. A more recent development is hydrophilic guidewires. These frequently have a metal

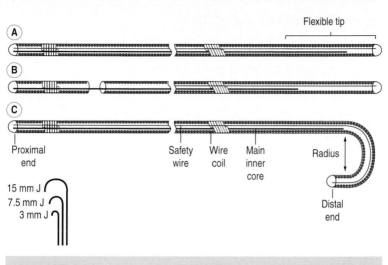

Figure 9.1 Guidewire construction. (a) Fixed core, straight. (b) Movable core, straight. (c) Fixed core, J-curve.

mandrel as their core. They are very slippery with excellent torque and are useful in negotiating narrow tortuous vessels. They require constant lubrication with saline.

Catheters

Most catheters are manufactured commercially, complete with end hole, side holes, preformed curves and Luer lock connection. They are made of polyurethane or polyethylene. Details of the specific catheter types are given with the appropriate technique.

Some straight catheters may be shaped by immersion in hot sterile water until they become malleable, forming the desired shape and then fixing the shape by cooling in cold sterile water. For the average adult a 100-cm catheter with a 145-cm guidewire is suitable for reaching the aortic branches from a femoral puncture.

The introduction of a catheter over a guidewire is facilitated by dilation of the track with a dilator (short length of graded diameter tubing). If the patient has a large amount of subcutaneous fat in the puncture area, catheter control will be better if it is manipulated through an introducer sheath. This is also indicated where it is anticipated that frequent catheter exchanges may be required.

Taps and connectors

These should have a large internal diameter that will not increase resistance to flow. Luer locks stop the tap detaching during high-pressure injections.

FEMORAL ARTERY PUNCTURE

This is the most frequently used puncture site providing access to the left ventricle, aorta and its branches and has the lowest complication rate of the peripheral sites.

Relative contraindications

1. Blood dyscrasias
2. Femoral artery aneurysm or pseudoaneurysm
3. Local soft-tissue infection
4. Severe hypertension
5. Ehlers–Danlos syndrome (due to the vessel wall being easily torn).

Technique (Fig. 9.2)

1. The patient lies supine on the X-ray table. Both femoral arteries are palpated and if pulsations are of similar strength the side opposite the symptomatic leg may be chosen. This leaves the symptomatic side untouched and free from groin puncture complications if future vascular surgery is undertaken. If all else

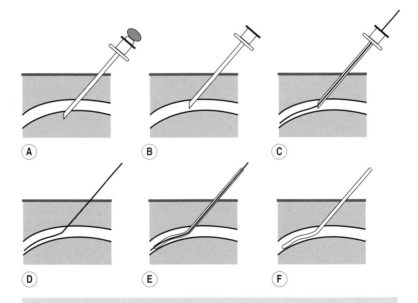

Figure 9.2 Seldinger technique. (a) Both walls of vessel punctured. (b) Stilette removed. Needle withdrawn so that bevel is within the lumen of the vessel and blood flows from the hub. (c) Guidewire inserted through needle. (d) Needle withdrawn, leaving guidewire in situ. (e) Catheter threaded over wire. (f) Guidewire withdrawn.

is equal, then the right side is technically easier (for right-handed operators).

2. The appropriate catheter and guidewire are selected and their compatibility checked by passing the guidewire through the catheter and needle.

3. The location and point of puncture of the femoral artery must be considered. The external iliac artery arches anteriorly and laterally as it passes under the inguinal ligament and continues as the femoral artery. Attempts to puncture the artery cephalad to the ligament may result in a puncture deep in the pelvis at a point where haemostasis is difficult to secure by manual compression and where peri-catheter and post-procedure bleeding may be obscured by preferential passage of blood into the retroperitoneum. Brief preliminary fluoroscopy of the groin can identify the centre of the femoral head with the intention of puncturing the artery at this point. This increases the likelihood of hitting the common femoral artery and facilitates haemostasis post-procedure by allowing the artery to be compressed against bone. The inguinal skin fold does not reliably correlate with the position of the inguinal ligament. The entire common femoral artery lies above the skin fold in more than 75% of western European subjects.[1] Direct US guidance is increasingly routinely used for vascular puncture.

4. Using aseptic technique, local anaesthetic is infiltrated either side of the artery down to the periosteum. A 3–5-mm stab incision is made over the artery to reduce binding of soft tissues on the catheter. In thin patients the artery may be very superficial and the skin may need to be pinched-up or deflected laterally, to avoid cutting the artery.

5. The artery is immobilized by placing the index and middle fingers of the left hand on either side of the artery, and the needle is held in the right hand. The needle is advanced through the soft tissues until transmitted pulsations are felt. Both walls of the artery are punctured through-and-through (single-wall puncture increases the risk of intimal dissection). The stilette is removed, and the needle hub is depressed so that it runs more parallel to the skin and is then withdrawn until pulsatile blood flow indicates a satisfactory puncture. Poor flow may be due to:

   a. the end of the needle lying in or against the vessel wall or within plaque
   b. aorto-iliac stenosis giving low femoral artery pressure
   c. hypotension – due to vasovagal reaction during the puncture
   d. femoral vein puncture.

9

6. When good flow is obtained the guidewire is introduced through the needle and advanced gently along the artery using intermittent fluoroscopy to avoid engaging the vessel wall. When the wire is in the descending thoracic aorta the needle is withdrawn over the guidewire, keeping firm pressure on the puncture site to reduce bleeding. The free portion of guidewire is then wiped clean with a wet sponge and the catheter threaded over it. For 5-F or greater diameter catheters, particularly those which are curved, a dilator is recommended matched to catheter size. The catheter is advanced up the descending aorta, under fluoroscopic control, and when in a satisfactory position the guidewire is withdrawn.

7. Catheter patency can be maintained by continuous flushing from a pressurized bag of heparinized saline (2500 units in 500 ml of 0.9% saline) attached through a three-way tap, or by intermittent manual flushing throughout the procedure. Flushing should be done rapidly otherwise the more distal catheter holes will remain unflushed.

8. At the end of the procedure the catheter is withdrawn and manual compression of the puncture site should be maintained for 5–10 min.

Aftercare

1. Bed rest – typically for 4 h, but longer at the discretion of the operator. Larger catheters, antiplatelet therapy and anticoagulation require longer observation

2. Careful observation of the puncture site for hemorrhage

3. Pulse and blood pressure observation, e.g. half-hourly for 4 h and then 4-hourly for the remainder of 24 h, if the larger catheter systems are used.

Reference

1. Lechner, G., Jantsch, H., Waneck, R., et al. (1988) The relationship between the common femoral artery, the inguinal crease, and the inguinal ligament: a guide to accurate angiographic puncture. *Cardiovasc. Intervent. Radiol.* **11**, 165–169.

HIGH BRACHIAL ARTERY PUNCTURE

Indications

As for femoral artery puncture, but as this approach is associated with a higher incidence of complications, it should only be used if femoral artery puncture is not possible.

Contraindications

1. Atherosclerosis of the axillary or subclavian arteries
2. Subclavian artery aneurysm.

Technique

1. The patient lies on the X-ray table with his arm in supination. The peripheral pulses are palpated and the brachial artery localized approximately 10 cm above the elbow.
2. A small incision is made in the skin, 1–2 cm distal to the selected point of arterial puncture.
3. A single-wall puncture needle is used, with an acute angle of entry into the artery.
4. A straight, soft-tipped guidewire is introduced when good pulsatile flow is obtained.
5. A 5-F pigtail catheter is introduced over the guidewire and its pigtail formed in the aorta.
6. At the end of the procedure the catheter tip is straightened using the guidewire and then removed. This reduces the risk of intimal damage and flap formation during withdrawal of the catheter.

AXILLARY ARTERY PUNCTURE

Indications

As for femoral artery puncture, but this approach is associated with a higher incidence of complications than femoral or high brachial artery puncture and should only be used if these techniques are not possible.

9

Contraindications

1. Atherosclerosis of the axillary or subclavian arteries
2. Subclavian artery aneurysm.

Technique

1. The patient lies supine on the X-ray table with his arm fully abducted. The puncture point is just distal to the axillary fold. It is infiltrated with local anaesthetic.
2. A small incision is made in the skin 1–2 cm distal to the point of the arterial puncture.
3. The needle is directed more horizontally than the femoral approach and along the line of the humerus.
4. Following satisfactory puncture the remainder of the technique is as for femoral artery catheterization.

GENERAL COMPLICATIONS OF CATHETER TECHNIQUES

Due to the anaesthetic
See Chapter 18.

Due to the contrast medium
See Chapter 2.

Due to the technique
Diagnostic angiography is an invasive procedure and complications are expected. The majority of these are minor, e.g. groin haematoma. Recommended upper limits for complication rates have been produced by the Society of Cardiovascular and Interventional Radiology (SCVIR):[1] these rates are included in the following discussion.

Local

The most frequent complications occur at the puncture site. Complication rate is lowest with a femoral puncture site:

1. *Haemorrhage/haematoma* – the commonest complication. Small haematomas occur in up to 20% of examinations and large haematomas in up to 4%. The SCVIR threshold for haematomas requiring transfusion, surgery or delayed discharge after diagnostic angiography is 0.5%. Haematoma formation is greater with larger catheters, more frequent catheter exchanges and heparin, antiplatelet or thrombolytic agents. Haematoma formation is also greater when the femoral artery is punctured high because of inadequate compression of the artery following catheter removal.

2. *Arterial thrombus* may be due to:
   a. stripping of thrombus from the catheter wall as it is withdrawn
   b. trauma to the vessel wall.
   Factors implicated in increased thrombus formation are:
   a. large catheters
   b. excessive time in the artery
   c. many catheter changes
   d. inexperience of the radiologist
   e. polyurethane catheters, because of their rough surface.
   The incidence is decreased by the use of:
   a. heparin-bonded catheters
   b. heparin-bonded guidewires
   c. flushing with heparinized saline.

3. *Infection at the puncture site.*

4. *Damage to local structures*. Especially the brachial plexus during axillary artery puncture. Femoral nerve palsy can result from inadvertent infiltration of the nerve with local anaesthetic. It is short-lived but should prompt very cautious subsequent mobilization of the patient in case the leg 'gives way'. More protracted femoral nerve damage can be due to excessive haematoma or pseudoaneurysm formation in the groin.

5. *Pseudoaneurysm*. The SCVIR threshold for diagnostic angiography is 0.2%. It presents as a pulsatile mass at the puncture site any time after arteriography and is due to communication between the lumen of the artery and a cavity within semi-solid or organized haematoma. Arterial puncture below the common femoral artery bifurcation increases the risk of this complication. Some may require surgical or interventional radiological repair.

6. *Arteriovenous fistula* – rare. SCVIR threshold is 0.1%. More common when puncture is below the common femoral artery bifurcation, because at this level the vein lies posterior to the artery and both are punctured in the standard double-wall technique.

Distant

1. *Peripheral embolus* – from stripped catheter thrombus. Emboli to small digital arteries will resolve spontaneously; emboli to large arteries may need aspiration thrombectomy through a catheter or surgical embolectomy. The SCVIR threshold is 0.5%.

2. *Atheroembolism* – more likely in older subjects. J-shaped guidewires are less likely to dislodge atheromatous plaques.

3. *Air embolus*. May be fatal in coronary or cerebral arteries. It is prevented by:
   a. ensuring that all taps and connectors are tight
   b. always sucking back when a new syringe is connected
   c. ensuring that all bubbles are excluded from the syringe before injecting
   d. keeping the syringe vertical, plunger up, when injecting.

4. *Cotton fibre embolus*. Occurs when syringes are filled from a bowl containing swabs or when a guidewire is wiped with a dry gauze pad. This very bad practice is prevented by:
   a. separate bowls of saline for flushing and wet swabs
   OR, preferably,
   b. a closed system of perfusion.

5. *Artery dissection* – due to entry of the catheter, guidewire or contrast medium into the subintimal space. It is recognized by resistance to passage of the guidewire or catheter, poor back-bleeding from the catheter hub, increased resistance to injection of contrast medium or subintimal contrast medium on fluoroscopy. The risk of serious dissection is reduced by:

9

    a. not using a single-wall needle with a long bevel
    b. using floppy J-shaped guidewires
    c. using catheters with multiple side holes
    d. employing a small volume manual test injection prior to a pump injection
    e. careful and gentle manipulation of catheters.

6. *Catheter knotting* – more likely during the investigation of complex congenital heart disease. Non-surgical reduction of catheter knots is discussed by Thomas and Sievers.[2] Surgical removal after withdrawal of the knotted end to the groin may be the only solution in some cases.

7. *Catheter impaction*:
    a. in a coronary artery produces cardiac ischaemic pain
    b. in a mesenteric artery produces abdominal pain.
    There should be rapid wash-out of contrast medium after a selective injection. A sound of sucking air on removing the guidewire and poor back-bleeding from the catheter indicate an impacted (wedged) catheter tip.

8. *Guidewire breakage* – more common in the past and tended to occur 5 cm from the tip, where a single central core terminates.

9. *Bacteraemia* – rarely of clinical significance.

References

1. Singh, H., Cardella, J.F., Cole, P.E., et al. (2003) Quality improvement guidelines for diagnostic arteriography. *J. Vasc. Interv. Radiol.* **14,** S283–S288.
2. Thomas, H.A. & Sievers, R.E. (1979) Nonsurgical reduction of arterial catheter knots. *Am. J. Roentgenol.* **132,** 1018–1019.

ASCENDING AORTOGRAPHY

Echocardiography, multislice CT, and MRI are preferable initial imaging modalities for assessment of the ascending aorta.

Indications

1. Aortic aneurysm, trauma or dissection
2. Atheroma at the origin of the major vessels
3. Aortic regurgitation (echocardiography is more sensitive and less invasive if available)
4. Congenital heart disease – particularly the demonstration of congenital or iatrogenic aorto-pulmonary shunts and coarctation
5. As a preliminary to endovascular intervention, e.g. aneurysm repair.

Contrast medium

Low osmolar contrast material (LOCM) 370, $0.75\,ml\,kg^{-1}$ (max. 40 ml). Inject at 18–$20\,ml\,s^{-1}$.

Equipment

1. Digital fluoroscopy unit with C-arm capable of 20–30 frames s^{-1}
2. Pump injector
3. Catheter:
   a. pigtail (Fig. 8.3)
   OR
   b. Gensini (Fig. 9.3)
   OR
   c. National Institutes of Health (NIH) (Fig. 8.2).

Technique

1. The catheter is introduced using the Seldinger technique via the femoral artery, and its tip sited 1–3 cm above the aortic valve.
2. The patient is positioned 45° RPO to open out the aortic arch, and to show the aortic valve and the left ventricle to best advantage.
3. A test injection is performed to ensure that:
   a. the catheter is correctly placed in relation to the aortic valve (which is particularly important in the hyperkinetic heart)
   b. the catheter tip is not in a coronary artery.

Films

20–30 frames s^{-1}.

Additional films

If, on the original run, the right common carotid artery overlies the right innominate artery or an aneurysm is present on the anterior aspect of the ascending aorta, the injection is repeated with the patient positioned left posterior oblique (LPO).

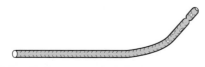

Figure 9.3 Gensini catheter. Note tapered end. End holes: 1 Side holes: 6.

ARTERIOGRAPHY OF THE LOWER LIMB

Indications
1. Arterial ischaemia
2. Trauma
3. Arteriovenous malformation.

Methods
Both lower limbs
1. Catheter angiography – using a pigtail catheter introduced via the femoral artery and sited proximal to the aortic bifurcation
2. Brachial or axillary puncture.

One lower limb
1. Using a femoral artery catheter:
   a. introduced retrogradely and sited in the ipsilateral common iliac artery
   b. introduced retrogradely from the contralateral side and sited in the common iliac, external iliac or femoral artery (sidewinder catheter)
   c. introduced antegradely.

   If thin 4-F catheters are used, only day-case admission is necessary.

Contrast medium
All of these techniques can be performed under local anaesthesia with LOCM. 10–20 ml of 300 mg I ml^{-1} concentration is suitable for the examination of one limb. 50 ml of 350 mg I ml^{-1}, at a rate of 12–15 ml s^{-1}, is suitable for a catheter aortogram.

BALLOON ANGIOPLASTY

Also known as percutaneous transluminal angioplasty or balloon dilation.

Indications
1. Dilation of localized vascular stenoses, mainly of the renal, iliac, lower limb and coronary arteries.
2. Recanalization of occluded segments of vessels in selected cases. Dilation procedures are often combined with preparatory diagnostic angiography in the same session; the majority are done under local anaesthetic. The procedure is often needed after lysis of arterial thrombus: this is outlined below.

Equipment

1. Digital fluoroscopy unit with C-arm capable of angiography and preferably with 'road mapping' facilities
2. Arterial pressure measuring equipment (optional)
3. Catheters:
   a. Gruntzig double-lumen balloon dilation catheters. Various manufacturers offer a wide range of balloon length and diameter combinations as well as catheter-shaft lengths, depending on the site and size of the vessel to be angioplastied
   b. Van Andel dilation catheter (a tapered, straight Teflon catheter, occasionally useful)
   c. straight Teflon or polyethylene catheters.
4. Guidewires:
   a. 0.035 or 0.038-inch diameter wires, typically 145 cm long; a slippery hydrophilic guidewire may be helpful for crossing tight stenoses
   b. 250 cm exchange guidewire.
5. Thrombolytic agents may be infused into recently thrombosed vessels, prior to angioplasty.

Technique

Principles

1. Adequate angiograms must be obtained before proceeding to angioplasty.
2. Angioplasty is always performed with the guidewire remaining across the stenosis or occlusion until the procedure is completed.
3. Adequate vascular surgical assistance must be readily available before attempting angioplasty.
4. If the history suggests that a thrombosis has occurred within the previous 3 weeks, thrombolysis may be helpful.
5. The patient should be anticoagulated during the procedure, using 3000–5000 units of heparin.
6. The balloon diameter is selected by reference to the measured size of the normal artery on the preceding angiogram, allowing for magnification.

Renal arteries

1. The tip of a suitable guidewire is negotiated through and beyond the stenosis in the renal artery, from either the femoral or high brachial artery approach.
2. A balloon catheter of appropriate diameter is positioned across the stenosis and distended (approx. 7 atmospheres for 1 min) after injecting 3000 units of heparin. A post-dilation angiogram is then taken. If a residual stenosis remains, further dilations or implantation of a metallic stent may be necessary.

Iliac arteries

1. These are preferably dilated from a retrograde femoral puncture on the side of the lesion.
2. If the femoral pulse is absent or difficult to feel, it may be located using US guidance or road mapping from a contralateral femoral approach. Alternatively a sidewinder catheter can be introduced from the opposite groin and a guidewire directed over the aortic bifurcation and across the lesion.
3. If possible, a femoral artery pressure should be measured immediately after introducing the catheter, and before a guidewire is passed through the lesion. This is to assess the severity of the pressure gradient before and after angioplasty.
4. A suitable guidewire is then advanced carefully through the stenosis. If the lesion is eccentrically situated, it may be preferable to advance using a pre-shaped catheter, to inject contrast medium to position the catheter, and then to advance through the patent lumen, avoiding possible intimal dissection from below. If the lesion is particularly tight, a hydrophilic wire may be useful.
5. A catheter is passed over the guidewire and into the distal aorta.
6. Some operators do not give heparin for straightforward iliac angioplasties.
7. The guidewire is removed, to allow a pressure measurement in the aorta. It is then replaced and the catheter exchanged for a balloon catheter. After dilating the lesion, an angiogram is performed and pressures checked to ensure that a significant gradient no longer exists. A wire or catheter remains across the stenosis until this is confirmed.

Femoral arteries (common, and origins of superficial femoral and profunda arteries)

1. These cannot easily be approached by an antegrade puncture on the side of the lesion since there is little room to manoeuvre and exchange catheters.
2. The contralateral femoral artery is catheterized using a sidewinder catheter. The tip is positioned in the iliac artery ipsilateral to the lesion and a guidewire advanced down through the lesion. The catheter is then exchanged for a balloon catheter and, after injecting heparin 3000 units, the lesion is dilated and a check angiogram performed before the guidewire is withdrawn. A long introducer sheath across the bifurcation facilitates smooth tracking of catheters and permits check arteriography throughout the procedure whilst still maintaining the wire across the lesion.

Superficial femoral and popliteal arteries

1. An antegrade puncture is performed (pointing in the direction of arterial flow) aiming to hit the femoral artery as it passes over the femoral head. The skin puncture site is correspondingly higher than a retrograde puncture. US is invaluable in antegrade punctures and most experienced operators use it wherever possible.
2. A 15-mm J-guidewire can be used to select the required branch; usually the superficial femoral artery.
3. The guidewire is advanced almost down to the lesion, and a straight Teflon or polyethylene catheter is inserted over the guidewire to the same point. The wire is then gently passed across the lesion with the catheter following. Digital road mapping guidance is helpful in many instances. A van Andel dilation catheter may be useful once the lesion has been traversed by the guidewire.
4. If gentle injection of contrast medium outlines a channel parallel to the expected lumen, dissection has occurred. The catheter should be withdrawn and attempts made to regain the lumen.
5. When the lesion has been passed the catheter is exchanged for a balloon catheter (usually 5 mm in diameter), 3000 units of heparin are injected and dilation is performed. The distal 'run-off' should be carefully assessed on the post-angioplasty films; success is related to the adequacy of 'run-off' and it is necessary to ensure that there has been no distal embolization of thrombus or atheroma.

Catheter-directed arterial thrombolysis

1. Chemical thrombolysis plays a role in the treatment of acute ischaemia of the leg due to:
   a. in-situ thrombosis of a stenosed vessel
   b. occluded lower-limb arterial bypass graft
   c. thrombosed popliteal aneurysm with no demonstrable distal run-off
   d. infra-inguinal embolus (sometimes iatrogenic post-angioplasty).
2. Thrombolysis should be undertaken in consultation with a vascular surgeon and should not compromise the leg unnecessarily by delaying surgical treatment. An acute episode less than 24-h old is more likely to respond to thrombolysis. After 14 days surgery is preferable to thrombolysis.[1]
3. Irreversible limb ischaemia requires amputation to avoid reperfusion syndrome.
4. Absolute contraindications to thrombolysis include stroke within the preceding 2 months, a recent gastrointestinal bleed

and neurosurgery or head trauma. Relative contraindications are major trauma or surgery, severe hypertension, brain tumour and recent eye surgery.

5. Recombinant tissue plasminogen activator (rt-PA) is the most widely used agent in the United Kingdom. It can be used as local boluses of, for example, 5 mg at 5–10-min intervals or as a low dose infusion at $0.5–2\,mg\,hour^{-1}$.

6. Catheter placement for thrombolysis is typically achieved by passing a guidewire alongside or through the thrombus and advancing a catheter into the proximal end. The catheter is firmly fixed to the skin to prevent dislodgement. A bolus of rt-PA followed by infusion is then administered through the catheter and the patient returned to a high-dependency ward for observation of signs of haemorrhage. Monitoring of clotting factors such as fibrinogen levels does not influence the likelihood of haemorrhagic complications.

7. Depending on the initial progress and discretion of the operator the patient returns after several hours for check angiography through the catheter. If necessary the catheter is advanced and infusion continued until satisfactory lysis, or the procedure is discontinued if progress is poor. Successful thrombolysis often reveals underlying stenoses as the cause of the occlusion. These are angioplastied at completion.

8. There are catheters manufactured for delivering fibrinolytics as a high pressure spray through multiple side holes over several centimeters of occluded vessel. These may be used manually or connected to a dedicated pump that measures and times the 'pulse sprays'. This method has an added mechanical lytic effect and allows faster lysis. Other devices used in thrombolysis include hydrolyzing and mechanical thrombectomy catheters.

9. Bleeding complications are frequent, including haemorrhagic stroke in up to 2%.[2]

10. Thrombolysis is used widely wherever arterial and venous thrombosis occurs in the body. Many applications are not universally accepted and are off-license uses of the thrombolytic agent.

It is an important tool in the management of thrombosed hae-modialysis access.

Aftercare

1. The pulses distal to the artery that has been dilated and the colour of the toes should be observed half-hourly for 4 h
2. Aspirin 150 mg daily (for life, unless there is a contraindication)
3. Reinforcement of the need to stop smoking.

Complications

Due to technique

1. Perforation of iliac artery leading to retroperitoneal haemorrhage
2. Embolization of clot or atheroma distally down either leg. This may be removed by suction thrombo-embolectomy or surgical embolectomy
3. Occlusion of main artery
4. Occlusion of collateral artery
5. Major groin haematoma formation, which may suddenly develop several hours after the procedure is completed
6. False aneurysm formation at the puncture site
7. Cholesterol embolization. Catheter manipulation disrupts atheroma and releases cholesterol crystals into the arterial circulation causing occlusion at arteriolar level. Pulses may be present and arteries patent angiographically but patients are restless and develop severe tissue ischaemia in the affected vascular territory with skin mottling, limb loss, stroke, bowel infarction and renal failure.

References

1. Ouriel, K., Shortell, C.K., DeWeese, J.A., et al. (1994) A comparison of thrombolytic therapy with operative revascularization in the initial treatment of acute peripheral arterial ischemia. *J. Vasc. Surg.* **19**, 1021–1030.
2. Dawson, K., Armon, A., Braithwaite, B.D., et al. (1996) Stroke during intra-arterial thrombolysis: a survey of experience in the UK (abstr). *Br. J. Surg.* **83**, 568.

Further reading

Working Party on Thrombolysis in the Management of Limb Ischemia. (2003) Thrombolysis in the management of lower limb peripheral arterial occlusion – a consensus document. *J. Vasc. Interv. Radiol.* **14(9 Pt 2)**, S337–S349.

9

VASCULAR EMBOLIZATION

Indications

1. To control bleeding – from the gastrointestinal and genitourinary tracts, from the lungs and after trauma.
2. To infarct or reduce the blood supply to tumours or organs.
3. To reduce or stop blood flow through arteriovenous malformations, aneurysms, fistulae or varicoceles.

4. To reduce the blood flow in priapism.
5. As treatment for uterine fibroids.

Equipment
1. Digital fluoroscopy unit with C-arm capable of angiography and preferably with 'road mapping' facilities.
2. Pre-shaped femoro-visceral catheters. These should not have side holes since their presence promotes clumping of particles and fibres at the catheter tip leading to blockage of the lumen. Size and shape will depend on the particular problem. Balloon occlusion catheters and co-axial catheters may also be useful.
3. Embolic materials:
    a. Liquid – 50% dextrose, alcohol, quick-setting glues and polymers
    b. Particulate – gel-foam, polyvinyl alcohol, autologous clot
    c. Solid – Gianturco steel coils, detachable balloons.

The material used depends on the lesion, its site and the duration of the occlusion required. Use of materials other than those listed has been reported.

Patient preparation
1. As for arteriography
2. Some procedures are painful and sedo-analgaesia may be needed.

Technique
Principles
1. All therapeutic occlusions are potentially dangerous: the expected gain must justify the risk.
2. Adequate knowledge of the vascular anatomy must be available before commencing.
3. The operator must be an experienced angiographer.
4. The lesion must be selectively catheterized. When permanent occlusion is required, the centre of the lesion should be filled with non-absorbable material (e.g. silicone spheres, polyvinyl-alcohol, polymer) before the supplying blood vessels are occluded.
5. Reflux of embolic material is likely to occur as the blood flow slows down; injection of emboli should be done slowly with intermittent gentle injections of contrast medium to assess flow and progress.
6. It is safer to come back another day than to continue for too long.

Aftercare

1. Observation of temperature pulse and blood pressure for signs of sepsis or bleeding
2. Observation of the tissues distal to the occluded vessel should be maintained for 24 h
3. Analgesia as required (patient controlled administration).

Complications

1. Misplacement of emboli: this may occur without the operator being aware that it has happened.
2. There may be propagation of thrombus, with embolization to the lungs or elsewhere.
3. Post-embolization syndrome results from infarcted tissue releasing toxins into the circulation. It comprises pain, fever, malaise, raised white cell count and inflammatory indices and transient impairment of renal function. Infarcted tissue can cause fever for up to 10 days. However, this tissue can become infected, and antibiotics may be required.

VASCULAR ULTRASOUND

US is a reliable, non-invasive, inexpensive test which is well tolerated by patients and widely used for assessment of the arterial system. Intra-abdominal or pelvic arteries are examined with US, but it is best suited to relatively superficial vessels such as those of the neck or lower limb. Chest arteries cannot be assessed by US because the sound will not adequately penetrate air or bone. The main disadvantages of US are the marked operator dependant nature of the technique and lengthy examination times for some studies.

The main components of arterial vascular US studies are:

1. Grey-scale US: gives anatomical information and detailed assessment of vessel wall including areas of intimal thickening or calcification
2. Pulsed-wave Doppler: measures changes in frequency of US waves reflected by moving blood within the vessel (Doppler shift). These data are used to calculate a detailed graph of direction and velocity of flow in the vessel. The normal pattern of flow differs between various arteries and flow patterns change at sites of disease such as narrowing (i.e. velocity of flow increases)

9

3. Colour Doppler: uses the same information as pulsed-wave Doppler but displays flow as colour superimposed in the arterial lumen on grey-scale imaging. Colour represents the direction and velocity of flow with red conventionally indicating flow towards the US transducer and blue representing flow away from the transducer. Rapid flow is displayed as white or yellow. This is helpful in selection of regions for detailed assessment with pulsed-wave Doppler or detection of A-V fistulae or pseudo-aneurysm
4. Power Doppler: a modification of colour Doppler which is more sensitive to slow flow or flow in small structures. However, it does not give information on direction or velocity of flow.

Further reading
Pellerito, J.S. (2001) Current approach to peripheral arterial sonography. *Radiol. Clin. North Am.* **39(3)**, 553–567.

COMPUTED TOMOGRAPHIC ANGIOGRAPHY

As CT technology has developed during the past few years, particularly with the introduction of 16 and 64 slice multidetector CT (MDCT) scanners, the quality and diagnostic usefulness of CT angiography (CTA) has improved dramatically.

CTA is performed as a block of very thin axial MDCT images obtained during the rapid peripheral intravenous (i.v.) infusion of iodinated contrast. The acquisition is timed to coincide with the peak density of contrast in arteries and the images subsequently re-constructed using post-processing techniques such as multi-planar reconstruction (MPR) or maximum intensity projections (MIP).

Although CTA involves administration of iodinated contrast (see Chapter 2) and significant radiation dose, there are many advantages: imaging is very rapid – usually less than 30 s to acquire the main dataset even for extended scans including lower limbs, scanners are readily available, unstable patients can be monitored with standard equipment, and valuable information is obtained about the blood vessel wall and surrounding structures.

PERIPHERAL (LOWER LIMB) COMPUTED TOMOGRAPHIC ANGIOGRAPHY

Description of other specific CTA methods are found in appropriate chapters.

Indications

1. Lower-limb ischaemia
2. Arterio-venous malformation
3. Trauma.

Patient preparation

General precautions for use of ionizing radiation (Chapter 1) and iodinated contrast (Chapter 2). The nature and purpose of the examination is explained to the patient.

Technique

For optimum images a MDCT scanner with at least a 16 slice detector is used:

1. Contrast: 100–150 ml LOCM 300
2. Contrast injection rate: $4\,ml\,s^{-1}$ via a peripheral vein
3. Range: lower abdominal aorta to heel, or extended as upper abdominal aorta to heel.
4. Slice thickness: 3 mm
5. Reconstruction increment: 1.5 mm
6. Delay:
   a. Preset empirical delay, using manufacturer's guidelines for individual scanner
   OR
   b. Bolus tracking technique, choosing a region of interest (ROI) in the aorta just above the upper range of the scan and monitoring contrast density in ROI during injection until it reaches a predetermined value (usually 100 hounsfield units), which triggers the CT acquisition. This is the preferred technique.

Aftercare and complications

For iodinated contrast see Chapter 2.

Further reading

Chow, L.C. & Rubin, G.D. (2002) CT angiography of the arterial system. *Radiol. Clin. North Am.* **40(4)**, 729–749.
Duddalwar, V.A. (2004) Multislice CT angiography: a practical guide to CT angiography in vascular imaging and intervention. *Br. J. Radiol.* **77 (Spec no. 1)**, S27–S38.

MAGNETIC RESONANCE ANGIOGRAPHY

Guidelines on MR safety and selection of patients must be followed (see Chapter 1).

MR angiography (MRA) is now in widespread clinical use and is a highly sensitive and specific tool for assessment of the arterial system. For most examinations contrast-enhanced MRA with i.v. gadolinium (see Chapter 2) is now the preferred method. Gadolinium i.v. shortens the T1 relaxation time of blood so blood appears bright when imaged with a very short TR (repetition time) and other structures on the image appear dark. Timing of the contrast injection is critical. Imaging without contrast is used infrequently, but may be either a 'bright blood' cine technique, to demonstrate both anatomical and functional data, or 'black blood' imaging, which gives useful morphological information.

The thoracic and abdominal aorta, carotid arterial system and major branches of the aorta including subclavian, celiac, superior mesenteric and renal arteries are routinely imaged with MRA. The pulmonary arteries are harder to image at MRA. Images are most often obtained as a block of thin coronal images (three-dimensional imaging) with contrast enhancement. Images are post-processed, including maximum intensity projection (MIP) series.

Previously, the arteries of the pelvis and peripheral arteries of the lower limb were difficult to image due to limited longitudinal field of view in MR scanners. More recent developments including elongated MR coils and 'moving-table' multi-station MRA have made high-quality examination of these vessels possible with a single injection of contrast and short imaging time. In some centres peripheral MRA is now routine and has replaced diagnostic catheter angiography.

Further reading

Earls, J.P. & Edelman, R.R. (2006) Magnetic resonance angiography: body applications. In: Edelman, R.R., Hesselink, J.R., Zlatkin, M.B., et al. (eds), *Clinical Magnetic Resonance Imaging*. Philadelphia: Saunders-Elsevier.

Ho, V.B. & Corse, W.R. (2003) MR angiography of the abdominal aorta and peripheral vessels. *Radiol. Clin. North Am.* **41(1)**, 115–144.

Venous system

Methods of imaging the venous system
1. Contrast venography
2. Ultrasound (US)
3. Impedance plethysmography
4. Radionuclide imaging
5. Computed tomography (CT)
6. Magnetic resonance imaging (MRI).

Further reading
Kaufman, J.A. & Lee, M.J. (eds) (2004) *Vascular and Interventional Radiology: The Requisites.* Philadelphia: Elsevier-Mosby.
Scarvelis, D. & Wells , P.S. (2006) Diagnosis and treatment of deep-vein thrombosis. *CMAJ* **175**, 1087–1092.

PERIPHERAL VENOGRAPHY

Intravenous (i.v.) peripheral venography is an invasive procedure requiring i.v. injection of contrast medium and the use of ionizing radiation. Marked limb swelling can result in failure to cannulate a vein which precludes use of the technique. False-negative results do occur. It is still considered the gold standard for diagnosis of deep venous thrombosis, but is now only rarely performed.

LOWER LIMB
Method
Intravenous venography.

Indications

1. Deep venous thrombosis
2. To demonstrate incompetent perforating veins (Doppler ultrasound is preferable)
3. Oedema of unknown cause
4. Congenital abnormality of the venous system.

Contraindications

Local sepsis.

Contrast medium

Low osmolar contrast material (LOCM) 240.

Equipment

1. Fluoroscopy unit with spot film device
2. Tilting radiography table.

Patient preparation

The leg should be elevated overnight to lessen oedema if leg swelling is severe.

Technique

1. The patient is supine and tilted 40° head up, to delay the transit time of the contrast medium.
2. A tourniquet is applied tightly just above the ankle to occlude the superficial venous system. This may also occlude the anterior tibial veins, and so their absence should not automatically be interpreted as due to venous thrombosis.
3. A 19G butterfly needle (smaller if necessary) is inserted into a vein on the dorsum of the foot. If the needle is too near the ankle, the contrast medium may bypass the deep veins and so give the impression of deep venous occlusion.
4. 40 ml of contrast medium is injected by hand. The first series of spot films is then taken.
5. A further 20 ml bolus is injected quickly whilst the patient performs a Valsalva manoeuvre to delay the transit of contrast medium into the upper thigh and pelvic veins. The patient is tilted quickly into a slightly head down position and the Valsalva manoeuvre is relaxed. Alternatively, if the patient is unable to comply, direct manual pressure over the femoral vein whilst the table is being tilted into the head-down position will achieve the same effect. Films are taken 2–3 s after releasing pressure.
6. At the end of the procedure the needle should be flushed with 0.9% saline to lessen the chance of phlebitis due to contrast medium.

Films

Collimated to include all veins:

1. Anterior posterior (AP) of calf
2. Both obliques of calf (foot internally and externally rotated)
3. AP of popliteal, common femoral and iliac veins.

Aftercare

The limb should be exercised.

Complications

Due to the contrast medium

1. As for the general complications of intravascular contrast media (Chapter 2)
2. Thrombophlebitis
3. Tissue necrosis due to extravasation of contrast medium. This is rare, but may occur in patients with peripheral ischaemia
4. Cardiac arrhythmia – more likely if the patient has pulmonary hypertension.

Due to the technique

1. Haematoma
2. Pulmonary embolus – due to dislodged clot or injection of excessive air.

UPPER LIMB

Method

I.v. venography.

Indications

1. Oedema
2. To demonstrate the site of venous occlusion or stenosis
3. Superior vena cava obstruction

Contrast medium

LOCM 300.

Equipment

Fluoroscopy unit with spot film device.

Patient preparation

None.

Technique

For i.v. venography:

10

1. The patient is supine
2. An 18G butterfly needle is inserted into the median cubital vein at the elbow. The cephalic vein is not used, as this bypasses the axillary vein
3. Spot films are taken of the region of interest during a hand injection of 30 ml of contrast medium. Alternatively a digital subtraction angiographic run can be performed at 1 frame per s.

Aftercare

None.

Complications

Due to the contrast medium
See Chapter 2.

CENTRAL VENOGRAPHY

SUPERIOR VENA CAVOGRAPHY

Indications

1. To demonstrate occlusion or stenosis of the central veins
2. As a preliminary examination in transvenous interventional techniques
3. Congenital abnormality of the venous system, e.g. left-sided superior vena cava.

Contrast medium

LOCM 370, 60 ml.

Equipment

Rapid serial radiography unit, or preferably a C-arm with digital subtraction angiography.

Patient preparation

None.

Technique

1. The patient is supine
2. 18G butterfly needles are inserted into the median antecubital vein of both arms
3. Hand injections of contrast medium 30 ml per side, are made simultaneously, as rapidly as possible by two operators.

The injection is recorded by rapid serial radiography (see 'Films' below). The film sequence is commenced after about two-thirds of the contrast medium has been injected.

N.B. If the study is to demonstrate a congenital abnormality, or on the rare occasion that the opacification obtained by the above method is too poor, a 5-F catheter with side holes, introduced by the Seldinger technique, may be used.

Films/images

Images are obtained at a rate of one per second for 10 s.

Aftercare

None, unless a catheter is used.

Complications

Due to the contrast medium
See Chapter 2.

INFERIOR VENA CAVOGRAPHY

Indications

1. To demonstrate the site of venous obstruction, displacement or infiltration
2. As a preliminary examination in transvenous interventional techniques
3. Congenital abnormality of the venous system.

Contrast medium

LOCM 370, 40 ml.

Technique

1. With the patient supine, the catheter is inserted into the femoral vein using the Seldinger technique (see Chapter 9). A Valsalva manoeuvre may facilitate venepuncture by distending the vein. The vein can be punctured blindly by palpating the femoral artery pulsation and aiming to its medial side, but it is preferable to puncture the vein under direct US guidance.
2. Any obstruction to the passage of the catheter may indicate thrombus in the iliac veins or that the catheter and wire have entered an ascending lumbar vein. Fluoroscopy and gentle hand injection of contrast will clarify.
3. An injection of 40 ml of contrast medium is made at 20 ml s by a pump injector, and recorded by rapid serial radiography or as a digital subtraction run at 2 frames s^{-1}.

10

Aftercare

1. Pressure at venepuncture site
2. Routine observations for 2 h.

Complications

Due to the contrast medium
See Chapter 2.

Due to the technique
See Chapter 9 – complications of catheter technique.

PORTAL VENOGRAPHY

Methods

1. Late-phase superior mesenteric angiography (see p. 80)
2. Trans-splenic approach (discussed below)
3. Paraumbilical vein catheterization
4. Transjugular transhepatic approach.[1]

Indications

1. To demonstrate prior to operation the anatomy of the portal system in patients with portal hypertension.
2. To check the patency of a portosystemic anastomosis.

Contrast medium

LOCM 370, 50 ml.

Equipment

1. Rapid serial radiography unit
2. Arterial catheter (SMA approach)
3. 10-cm needle (20G) with stilette and outer plastic sheath, e.g. Longdwell (trans-splenic approach).

Patient preparation

1. Admission to hospital. A surgeon should be informed in case complications of procedure arise (for the trans-splenic approach)
2. Clotting factors are checked
3. Severe ascites is drained
4. Nil orally for 5 h prior to the procedure
5. Premedication, e.g. diazepam 10 mg orally.

Technique

Superior mesenteric angiography
See page 80.

For trans-splenic approach

1. With the patient supine, the position of the spleen is percussed or identified with US. The access point is as low as possible in the midaxillary line, usually at the level of the tenth or eleventh intercostal space.
2. The region is anaesthetized using a sterile procedure.
3. The patient is asked to hold their breath in mid-inspiration, and the needle is then inserted inwards and upwards into the spleen (about three-quarters of the length of the needle is inserted, i.e. 7.5 cm). The needle and stilette are then withdrawn, leaving the plastic cannula in situ. Blood will flow back easily if the cannula is correctly sited. The patient is then asked to breathe as shallowly as possible to avoid trauma to the spleen from excessive movement of the cannula.
4. A test injection of a small volume of contrast medium under screening control can be made to ensure correct siting of the cannula. If it has transfixed the spleen, simple withdrawal into the body of the spleen is not acceptable, as any contrast medium subsequently injected would follow the track created by the withdrawal. A new puncture is necessary.
5. When the cannula is in a satisfactory position, the splenic pulp pressure may be measured with a sterile manometer. (It is normally 10–15 cm H_2O.)
6. A hand injection of 50 ml of contrast medium is made in 5 s and recorded by rapid serial radiography/digital subtraction angiography. The cannula should be removed as soon as possible after the injection to minimize trauma to the spleen.
7. Occasionally a patent portal vein will fail to opacify, owing to major portosystemic collaterals causing reversed flow in the portal vein. The final arbiter of portal vein patency is direct mesenteric venography performed at operation. The maximum width of a normal portal vein is said to be 2 cm.

Films

Rapid serial radiography or digital subtraction runs: one film per second for 10 s.

Aftercare

1. Blood pressure and pulse; initially quarter-hourly, subsequently 4-hourly.
2. The patient must remain in hospital overnight.

10

Complications

Due to the contrast medium
See Chapter 2.

Due to the technique
1. Haemorrhage
2. Subcapsular injection
3. Perforation of adjacent structures (e.g. pleura, colon)
4. Splenic rupture
5. Infection
6. Pain (especially with an extra-capsular injection).

Due to the catheter
See Chapter 9.

Reference
1. Rosch, J., Antonovic, R. & Dotter, C.T. (1975) Transjugular approach to the liver, biliary system, and portal circulation. *Am. J. Roentgenol.* **125**, 602–608.

Further reading
Tamura, S., Kodama, T., Kihara, Y., et al. (1992) Right anterior caudocranial oblique projection for portal venography; its indications and advantages. *Eur. J. Radiol.* **15**, 215–219.

TRANSHEPATIC PORTAL VENOUS CATHETERIZATION

Indications
To localize pancreatic hormone-secreting tumours before operation.

Contraindications
There are none specific to the technique. Ascites and hepatic cirrhosis make the procedure more difficult.

Contrast medium
LOCM 370, to demonstrate anatomy and position of catheter.

Technique
1. 5-ml samples of blood are taken at points along the splenic vein, superior mesenteric vein and first part of the portal vein. The samples are numbered sequentially, and the site from which

each was taken is marked on a sketch map of the portal drainage system. Simultaneous peripheral blood samples should be obtained at the same time as each portal sample to assess changing blood levels.

2. The accuracy of sampling can be improved by selective catheterization of pancreatic veins using varying shapes of catheter.[1]

Reference

1. Reichardt, W. & Ingemansson, S. (1980) Selective vein catheterization for hormone assay in endocrine tumours of the pancreas. Technique and results. *Acta. Radiol. Diagn.* **21**, 177–187.

ULTRASOUND

Ultrasound is the most widely used imaging method for the venous system; the advantages are that it is low cost and readily available. It can be used to assess the following:

1. Lower limb veins
2. Upper limb veins
3. Abdominal veins including renal veins, hepatic and portal veins, and inferior vena cava
4. Venous anatomy to assist in central venous line placement, e.g. for the internal jugular or subclavian vein.

10

US is most commonly used for assessment of patients with suspected venous thrombosis, particularly of the lower limb. It is also useful to assess arterio-venous fistulae; both therapeutic fistulae created for haemodialysis and those occurring as a complication of interventional vascular procedures, and for pre-surgical planning in patients with varicose veins. Both duplex and colour Doppler techniques are utilized.

Duplex

Duplex scanning involves a combination of pulsed Doppler and real-time US for direct visualization. Expansion and filling of the normal echo-free lumen can be identified but slow-moving blood may be misinterpreted as thrombus. Valsalva manoeuvre will cause expansion in the normal vein but is not a totally reliable sign. Pulsed Doppler assesses flow. Enhancement of flow due to respiratory excursion or manual calf compression suggests patency. The most reliable sign of patency is compressibility. Direct pressure with the US probe over the vein will cause the normal vein to collapse. If thrombus is present, this will not occur.

Colour Doppler

Colour Doppler examination gives a visual representation of flow over a segment of vein.

LOWER LIMB VENOUS ULTRASOUND

Indications

1. Suspected deep vein thrombosis
2. Follow-up of known deep vein thrombosis
3. To guide access for interventional venous procedures.

Equipment

5–7.5-MHz transducer with colour Doppler.

Technique

1. Patient supine with foot-down tilt. The popliteal and calf veins can easily be examined with the patient sitting with legs dependent or lying on a tilted couch with flexed knees and externally rotated hips. The femoral veins and external iliac veins are examined supine. The popliteal veins may be examined with the patient prone.
2. Longitudinal and transverse scans for external iliac, femoral and popliteal veins. For tibial and peroneal veins, these may be supplemented by oblique coronal scans.
3. Each vein may be identified by real-time scanning and colour Doppler. If in any doubt it may be confirmed as a vein by the spectral Doppler tracing. A normally patent vein should be completely occluded in real time by directly applied transducer pressure. This is not always possible for the superficial femoral vein at the adductor canal.
4. The normal venous signal is phasic and in the larger veins varies with respiration. Flow can be stopped by a Valsalva manoeuvre and is augmented by distal compression of the foot or calf. Acute thrombus may be non-echogenic but, in this case, the vein should not fill with colour Doppler and should not be completely compressible. The thrombus tends to become echogenic after a few days.
5. Although this technique is less well established for the exclusion of thrombus in the calf vessels, it has been shown

to have a sensitivity and specificity close to that of venography. Cannulation of a vein and injection of contrast medium can thus be avoided.

UPPER LIMB VENOUS ULTRASOUND

Indications
As for lower limb US, upper limb US is much less commonly performed.

Equipment
5–7.5-MHz transducer with colour Doppler.

Technique
1. The patient should be recumbent on a couch wide enough to support the upper limb and trunk comfortably.
2. With the arm in a neutral position at the patient's side, the subclavian vein is assessed either from above or below the clavicle. The image plane is parallel to the long axis of the vein. Diagnostic criteria for upper limb thrombosis are the same as those used for the lower limb, but the Doppler waveform in the upper limb venous system is more pulsatile because of proximity to the heart. The upper limb also has a much more extensive network of potential collateral venous pathways and care should be taken to avoid confusion of a patent collateral vein with the potentially occluded deep venous structure under examination.
3. The arm is then abducted and the axillary and brachial veins examined. The transducer should be placed high in the axilla to identify the proximal axillary vein and the Doppler characteristics of the axillary and brachial veins followed to assess for spontaneous and phasic flow, and appropriate response to augmentation and Valsalva manoeuvre. Both transverse and longitudinal imaging planes should be used, including assessment of response to compression.

The examination can be extended to include the cephalic, basilic and forearm veins.

Further reading
Hamper, U.M., DeJong, M.R. & Scoutt, L.M. (2007) Ultrasound evaluation of the lower extremity veins. *Radiol. Clin. North Am.* **45(3)**, 525–547.

Weber, T.M., Lockhart, M.E. & Robbin, M.L. (2007) Upper extremity venous Doppler ultrasound. *Radiol. Clin. North Am.* **45(3)**, 513–524.

IMPEDANCE PLETHYSMOGRAPHY

This technique depends on the principle of the capacity of the veins to fill and empty in response to temporary obstruction to venous outflow by occlusion of the thigh veins with a pneumatic cuff. Changes in calf volume produce changes in impedance measured by electrodes applied to the calf. The technique is demanding and requires skilled personnel. Clinical states that impair venous return, such as cardiac failure and pelvic pathology and also arterial insufficiency, produce abnormal results. Many centres use impedance plethysmography in conjunction with clinical pretest probability scoring and/or plasma D-dimer assay to identify patients who do not need to proceed to US or venography.[1]

Reference

1. Ginsberg, J.S., Kearon, C., Douketis, J., et al. (1997) The use of D-dimer testing and impedance plethysmographic examination in patients with clinical indications of deep vein thrombosis. *Arch. Intern. Med.* **157**, 1077–1081.

RADIOISOTOPES

Thrombus may be imaged with ^{111}In- or ^{99m}Tc-in vitro-labelled platelets. These are of limited routine clinical application.

COMPUTED TOMOGRAPHY

Multidetector CT (MDCT) with standard i.v. contrast and scan delay protocols for the chest or abdomen/pelvis (see Chapter 1) is very effective for detection of compression or thrombosis of major veins including the superior and inferior vena cavae, iliac and renal veins.

Although it would be possible to perform direct lower-limb CT venography after infusion of contrast via a foot vein, this technique has found little application and is not used in clinical practice.

In a group of selected patients with suspected pulmonary embolus (PE), MDCT of the lower limbs from iliac crest to popliteal fossa,

2 min after completion of CT pulmonary angiography (indirect CT venography), may be used as an alternative to US for detection of lower limb deep venous thrombosis. However, there is a significant associated radiation dose and there is no diagnostic advantage over US.[1] Indirect CT venography is not recommended in patients with suspected deep vein thrombosis, but without suspected PE. It should only be used as an alternative to US in patients undergoing CT for suspected PE for whom identification of DVT is considered necessary[2] or those with a high probability of PE, including patients with history of previous venous thrombo-embolism and possible malignancy.[3]

References
1. Goodman, L.R., Stein, P.D., Matta, F., et al. (2007) CT venography and compression sonography are diagnostically equivalent: data from PIOPED II. *Am. J. Roentgenol.* **189(5)**, 1071–1076.
2. Thomas, S.M., Goodacre, S.W., Sampson, F.C., et al. (2008) Diagnostic value of CT for deep vein thrombosis; results of a systematic review and meta-analysis. *Clin. Rad.* **63**, 299–304.
3. Hunsaker, A.R., Zou, K.H., Poh, A.C., et al. (2008) Routine pelvic and lower extremity CT venography in patients undergoing pulmonary CT angiography. *Am. J. Roentgenol.* **190(2)**, 322–326.

MAGNETIC RESONANCE

10

Standard guidance applies on selection of patients suitable for MRI examination (see Chapter 1).

MRI is well suited to imaging the venous system, but because of cost and limited availability it is used infrequently. Peripheral MR venography (MRV)[1] is currently used in selected cases of venous thrombosis in pregnant subjects and where fractured limbs are immobilized in casts. It is useful in evaluation of congenital abnormalities of peripheral venous anatomy and venous malformations.

The multi-planar imaging capabilities allow demonstration of complex venous anatomy and cine sequences, including velocity-encoded phase mapping, can provide functional information regarding direction and velocity of venous blood flow. MRI can be used to 'age' thrombus and differentiate acute from chronic clot. MRV does not involve ionizing radiation and i.v. gadolinium has a wider safety profile than iodinated contrast used for CT. Imaging can be performed using slice-by-slice (two-dimensional) or volume (three-dimensional) acquisition. Post-processing techniques, including maximum intensity projection (MIP) images, are used.

MRV sequences can be performed without i.v. contrast, e.g. time-of-flight imaging or phase contrast imaging sequences. However, these techniques are susceptible to signal loss due to slow flow or turbulence, and have largely been replaced by faster and more accurate i.v. gadolinium contrast-enhanced MRV studies.

MR venography offers unique diagnostic possibilities for abdominal, pelvic and thoracic veins,[2] and development of blood pool contrast agents (see Chapter 2) will further improve clinical usefulness of these procedures.[3]

References

1. Sampson, F.C., Goodacre, S.W., Thomas, S.M., et al. (2007) The accuracy of MRI in diagnosis of suspected deep vein thrombosis: systematic review and meta-analysis. *Eur. Radiol.* **17**, 175–181.
2. Butty, S., Hagspiel, K.D., Leung, D.A., et al. (2002) Body MR venography. *Radiol. Clin. North Am.* **40(4)**, 899–919.
3. Prince, M.R. & Sostman, H.D. (2003) MR venography: unsung and underutilized. *Radiology* **226(3)**, 630–632.

Lymph glands, lymphatics and tumours

POSITRON EMISSION TOMOGRAPHY IMAGING

Positron emission tomography (PET) imaging is a technique used to detect and accurately stage malignant disease, to differentiate benign and malignant tissue, and to assess response to treatment. Until recently, PET imaging availability was restricted due to high capital cost and logistics of radiopharmaceutical supply. It uses short-lived cyclotron-produced radionuclides such as ^{18}Fluorine, ^{11}Carbon, ^{13}Nitrogen and ^{15}Oxygen with half-lives of 110, 20, 10 and 2 min respectively. ^{18}Fluorine is the only one of these that has a half-life long enough to allow it to be produced off-site. This does permit 2-[^{18}F] fluoro-2-deoxy-d-glucose (^{18}F-FDG), the single most important PET radiopharmaceutical, to be used by sites without their own cyclotron.

The widespread acceptance of PET as a major advance is due to two major factors:

1. There is increased recognition in the literature of the role of the main PET tracer ^{18}F-FDG, a glucose analogue that is taken up in tissue in proportion to cellular glucose metabolism. This is particularly useful for tumour imaging, since most tumours have increased glucose metabolism and will concentrate FDG. Malignant cells are characterized by increased glucose transporter molecules at the cell surface. FDG is phosphorylated by the enzyme hexokinase to a polar intermediate which does not cross cell membranes well and is, therefore, trapped in the cell. Hexokinase levels and activity are increased in malignant cells. The reverse reaction (glucose-6-phosphatase) is slow and the enzyme is commonly deficient in cancer cells.
2. Integrated PET CT scanners are now available. These units have separate PET and CT scanners installed in the same gantry.

The patient undergoes a conventional CT scan (usually performed with low exposure factors to reduce radiation dose) immediately followed by a PET scan without moving on the same table-top. This allows fusion of the anatomical information from CT with the functional data from the PET scan, and hence accurate anatomical localization of metabolically active disease. The density data from the CT scan is also used to correct the PET data for differential attenuation of the emitted photons within the patient.

Normal physiological uptake is seen in organs that are hypermetabolic and big glucose users especially the brain and the heart, or active or recently active skeletal muscle. Variable uptake is seen in the gut and there is normal excreted urinary activity in the urinary tract. One confounding factor for interpretation may be normal physiological uptake in brown fat – particularly in the neck and paraspinal regions. Differentiation of this normal activity from pathology is greatly aided by the co-registration afforded by combined PET CT scanners.

However, FDG is not specific for cancer cells as any hypermetabolic cell such as those in sites of inflammation or infection will show increased uptake of FDG, so interpretation with reference to full clinical details and other imaging is important to avoid false-positive scans.

As the only PET tracer likely to be widely available in the near future, this section is restricted to FDG imaging. Discussion is also limited to the role of PET in oncological patients.

2-[^{18}F]FLUORO-2-DEOXY-D-GLUCOSE (^{18}F-FDG) PET SCANNING

Indications (oncology)

General
1. Distinguishing benign from malignant disease, e.g. lung nodules, brain lesions, etc.
2. Establishing the grade of malignancy, e.g. brain tumours, soft-tissue masses
3. Establishing the stage of disease, e.g. lung cancer, lymphoma, etc.
4. Establishing whether there is recurrent or residual disease, e.g. lymphoma, teratoma, seminoma, etc.
5. Establishing the site of disease in the face of rising tumour markers, e.g. colorectal, germ cell tumours, etc.

6. Establishing the response to therapy – pre, during and post therapy imaging
7. Identifying occult malignancy, e.g. paraneoplastic syndrome or the unknown primary in the setting of proven metastatic disease.

Specific

The following tumour specific indications are supported by grade A or grade B evidence (A: randomized controlled clinical trials, meta-analyses and systematic reviews; B: robust experimental or observational studies; C: other evidence where the advice relies on expert opinion and has the endorsement of respected authorities):

1. Lung cancer:
   a. Characterization of solitary pulmonary nodule where biopsy is not possible
   b. Staging of non-small cell lung cancer prior to surgery or radical radiotherapy.
2. Lymphoma:
   a. Assessment of residual masses post chemotherapy for disease activity
3. Colorectal cancer:
   a. Differentiation of local recurrence from post surgical or post radiotherapy fibrosis
   b. Exclusion of distant metastases prior to resection
4. Oesophageal cancer:
   a. Primary staging
5. Melanoma:
   a. Detection of distant metastases (sentinel node mapping preferred for regional nodal disease)
6. Thyroid cancer:
   a. Raised thyroglobulin; negative I-131 scan
7. Seminoma/teratoma:
   a. Assessing recurrent disease from seminoma or teratoma
   b. Residual masses post treatment
8. Soft-tissue sarcoma:
   a. Staging and grading
9. Other indications; there are other scenarios where PET may well be useful, but either the numbers are smaller or the evidence is more limited or less robust.

Contraindications

1. Recent chemotherapy – minimum interval of 2–3 weeks recommended
2. Recent radiotherapy – minimum interval of 8–12 weeks recommended
3. Poorly controlled diabetes, i.e. serum glucose $>8.5\,\mathrm{mmol\,l^{-1}}$ at time of scanning.

11

Patient preparation

1. Fasting for 4–6 h, with plenty of non-sugary fluids
2. Monitor blood glucose before injection to ensure it is not elevated. Elevated blood glucose levels result in diversion of glucose to muscle. Consider rescheduling patient if blood glucose elevated. Administration of insulin is counter-productive as this diverts glucose uptake to muscle
3. A mild sedative such as diazepam may be given to reduce physiological muscle and brown fat uptake
4. Oral contrast may be administered to aid interpretation of the CT. Attenuation correction artifact on the PET images secondary to the high-density contrast has been shown not to be clinically significant.

Technique

1. Up to the UK limit of 400 MBq ^{18}FDG intravenously (i.v.) (10 mSv effective dose (ED)) is administered.
2. To reduce muscle uptake of FDG, patients should remain in a relaxed environment such as lying in a darkened room (without talking if head and neck area are being imaged) between injection and scan.
3. Image at 1 h post injection. Later imaging has been reported to enhance tumour conspicuity due to a higher tumour to background ratio.
4. Imaging is preferred with the arms above the head to reduce beam hardening artifact on the CT.
5. CT:
   a. Low dose
   b. No i.v. contrast medium
   c. Positive or negative oral contrast agents according to local protocol are increasingly being used.
6. PET:
   a. From the base of skull to upper thighs (occasionally extended if melanoma or limb or head and neck tumours)
   b. 3–4 min for each of 5–6 bed positions for the PET
7. In some instances a diagnostic standard dose CT with i.v. contrast may be acquired as well, but in routine practice a diagnostic scan will usually be already available.

Other applications

Coronary artery disease (Chapter 8)
Assessment of myocardial viability.

Neurology (Chapter 13)
1. Location of epileptic foci
2. Assessment of dementia.

Further reading

British Nuclear Medicine Society Web Site guidelines – *www.bnms.org.uk* 2008

Cook, G.J., Wegner, E.A. & Fogelman, I. (2004) Pitfalls and artifacts in [18]FDG PET and PET/CT oncologic imaging. *Semin. Nucl. Med.* **34(2)**, 122–133.

Kapoor, V., McCook, B.M. & Torok, F.S. (2004) An introduction to PET CT imaging. *RadioGraphics* **24(2)**, 523–543.

Rohren, E.M., Turkington, T.G. & Coleman, R.E. (2004) Clinical applications of PET in oncology. *Radiology* **231(2)**, 305–332.

von Schulthess, G.K., Steinert, H.C. & Hany, T.F. (2006) Integrated PET/CT: current applications and future directions. *Radiology* **238(2)**, 405–422.

GALLIUM RADIONUCLIDE TUMOUR IMAGING

This is rarely used, having almost entirely been superseded by cross-sectional techniques and PET scanning.[1] The main disadvantages are the high radiation dose, the extended nature of the investigation, its non-specific nature, and difficulties in interpretation in the abdomen due to normal bowel activity.

Indications

1. Hodgkin's and non-Hodgkin's lymphoma: assessment of residual masses after therapy and early diagnosis of recurrence[1]
2. Gallium imaging has been used with variable success in a variety of other tumours, e.g. hepatoma, bronchial carcinoma, multiple myeloma and sarcoma
3. It has also been used in benign conditions such as sarcoidosis and for localization of infection or in suspected orthopaedic infection

11

Contraindications

None.

Radiopharmaceutical

[67]Ga-Gallium citrate, 150 MBq maximum (17 mSv ED).

Normal accumulation is seen in the liver, bone marrow and nasal sinuses, and variably in the spleen, salivary and lacrimal glands. There is significant excretion via the gut and some via the kidneys. [67]Ga has a half-life of 78 h and principal γ-emissions at 93, 185 and 300 keV, so image quality is fairly poor.

Equipment

1. Gamma camera, preferably with whole-body and single-photon emission computed tomography (SPECT) facilities
2. Medium- or high-energy collimator.

Patient preparation

If the abdomen is being investigated, laxatives may be given (if not contraindicated) for 2 days after injection of ^{67}Ga-citrate to clear bowel activity. Additionally, an enema or suppository may be given on the day of imaging.

Technique

1. ^{67}Ga-citrate is administered i.v.
2. Delayed images are acquired as below with energy windows about the lower two or all three of the main photopeaks.

Images

1. 48 and 72 h. Whole-body, spot views and SPECT as appropriate. SPECT can increase the sensitivity and specificity of the investigation
2. Non-specific bowel activity can be discriminated by imaging on two separate occasions. Activity in bowel contents should move between scans and abnormal areas of accumulation will be stationary. If there is still any doubt at 72 h, later images at up to 7 days may prove helpful.

Additional techniques

1. A radionuclide bone scan may be performed prior to gallium imaging.
2. A radiocolloid scan may help to discriminate between lesions in the region of the liver or spleen and normal uptake in these organs. Image subtraction techniques may be used.

Aftercare

Normal radiation safety precautions.

Complications

None.

Reference

1. Seam, P., Juweid, M.E. & Cheson, B.D. (2007) The role of FDG-PET scans in patients with lymphoma. *Blood* **110(10)**, 3507–3516.

Further reading
Bombardieri, E., Aktolun, C., Baum, R.P., et al. (2003) ^{67}Ga scintigraphy:
    procedure guidelines for tumour imaging. *Eur. J. Nucl. Med. Mol. Imaging.*
    30(12), BP125–131.
Front, D., Bar-Shalom, R. & Israel, O. (1997) The continuing clinical role of
    gallium 67 scintigraphy in the age of receptor imaging. *Semin. Nucl. Med.*
    27(1), 68–74.

RADIOIODINE METAIODOBENZYLGUANIDINE SCAN

Metaiodobenzylguanidine (MIBG) is a noradrenaline (norepineph-rine) analogue. It is taken up actively across cell membranes of sympathetic and adrenal medullary tissue into intracellular storage vesicles. There is no further metabolism, and it remains sequestered and localized in the storage vesicles of catecholamine-secreting tumours and tumours of neuroendocrine origin.[1]

Indications

Localization and staging of the following tumours of neuroendocrine origin:

1. Neuroblastoma
2. Phaeochromocytoma
3. Carcinoid tumours
4. Medullary thyroid carcinoma
5. Other neuroendocrine tumours.

Contraindications

None.

Radiopharmaceuticals

1. [123]Iodine(I)-metaiodobenzylguanidine (MIBG), 250 MBq
   typical, 400 MBq max (6 mSv ED with thyroid blockade). The
   13-h half-life of ^{123}I allows imaging up to 48 h
2. ^{131}I-labelled MIBG is also available, and is still in common use
   outside Europe where ^{123}I-MIBG is not made commercially.
   However, the higher photon energy of the emitted gamma rays
   renders it an inferior imaging agent and results in a higher
   radiation dose to the patient. It should only be
   considered where ^{123}I-MIBG cannot be obtained.

11

Equipment

1. Gamma-camera, preferably with whole-body imaging and SPECT capabilities
2. Low-energy general purpose collimator for ^{123}I.

Patient preparation

1. Where possible, stop medications that interfere with MIBG uptake.[2] These include tricyclic antidepressants, antihypertensives, cocaine, sympathomimetics, decongestants containing pseudoephedrine, phenylpropanolamine and phenylephrine (many available over the counter) and others.
2. Thyroid blockade, to reduce radiation dose to the thyroid continuing for 24 h after ^{123}I-MIBG injection:
   a. Adults – either oral potassium perchlorate (400 mg, 1 h before MIBG injection, then 200 mg every 6 h) or oral potassium iodate (85 mg twice daily starting 24 h before MIBG injection)
   b. Children – Lugol's iodine 0.1–0.2 ml diluted with water or milk three times a day starting 48 h before MIBG injection. Potassium iodate is more palatable – the tablets need splitting for paediatric dosage.

Technique

1. MIBG is administered slowly i.v. over 1–2 min (a fast injection may cause adrenergic side-effects).
2. Imaging at 24 h (sometimes additionally at 4 or 48 h), emptying bladder before pelvic views.

Images

1. Anterior and posterior abdomen, 10–20 min per view
2. Whole-body imaging for comprehensive search for metastases
3. SPECT may help to localize lesions, particularly in thorax and abdomen. Hybrid CT-SPECT scanners will help anatomical localization.

Additional techniques

1. If therapy with ^{131}I-MIBG is being considered, quantitative assessment can be performed using geometric mean and attenuation correction to calculate percentage of administered dose residing in tumour at 24 h.
2. ^{111}In-octreotide, which binds to somatostatin receptors frequently expressed in neuroendocrine and other tumours, is an alternative imaging agent to MIBG. It appears to be more sensitive for carcinoids, and may be useful in cases where the MIBG scan is negative. It also has therapeutic analogues under development.

Aftercare

Normal radiation safety precautions (see Chapter 1).

Complications

None.

References

1. Ilias, I. & Pacak, K. (2004) Current approaches and recommended algorithm for the diagnostic localization of pheochromocytoma. *J. Clin. Endocrinol. Metab.* **89(2)**, 479–491.
2. Solanki, K.K., Bomanji, J., Moyes, J., et al. (1992) A pharmacological guide to medicines which interfere with the biodistribution of radiolabelled meta-iodobenzylguanidine (MIBG). *Nucl. Med. Commun.* **13(7)**, 513–521.

SOMATOSTATIN RECEPTOR IMAGING

Somatostatin is a physiological neuropeptide which has biological effects including inhibition of growth hormone release, and suppression of insulin and glucagon excretion. Octreotide (a long-acting analogue of the human hormone, somatostatin) can be used therapeutically to inhibit hormone production by carcinoids, gastrinomas and insulinoma, etc. A number of tumours, particularly those of neuroendocrine origin, express neuroendocrine receptors. Imaging after the administration of radionuclide-labelled somatostatin analogues such as octreotide, therefore, allows their localization.[1]

Indications

Localization and staging of the following tumours of neuroendocrine origin:

1. Carcinoid
2. Gastrinoma
3. Phaeochromocytoma
4. Medullary cell Ca thyroid
5. Small cell lung cancer
6. Pituitary.

Although sometimes used for the assessment of insulinomas, these latter tumours are more variably visible with octreotide (approx. 50%) than carcinoids, gastrinomas and phaeochromocytomas, which are seen in 80–100% of cases.

11

Contraindications

None.

Radiopharmaceuticals

[111]Indium (In) pentetreotide (a DTPA conjugate of octreotide) 220 MBq i.v. (ED 17 mSv).

Equipment

1. Gamma-camera, preferably with whole-body imaging and SPECT capabilities
2. Medium energy for [111]In.

Patient preparation

1. Some centres use bowel preparation
2. Oral hydration to help with renal clearance. There is usually high renal uptake
3. In patients with possible insulinoma i.v. glucose should be available because of a small risk of inducing hypoglycaemia
4. Discontinue oral somatostatin to avoid competitive inhibition.

Technique

Image at 24 h and 48 h if necessary:

1. Anterior and posterior abdomen, 10–20 min per view
2. Whole-body imaging for comprehensive search for metastases
3. SPECT may help to localize lesions, particularly in thorax and abdomen. Hybrid CT-SPECT scanners will help anatomical localization.

Additional techniques

MIBG may be positive in octreotide negative tumours and vice versa.

Aftercare

Normal radiation safety precautions (see Chapter 1).

Complications

None.

Reference

1. Krenning, E.P., Kwekkeboom, D.J., Bakker, W.H., et al. (1993) Somatostatin receptor scintigraphy with [^{111}In-DTPA-D-Phe1] – and [^{123}I-Tyr3]-octreotide: the Rotterdam experience with more than 1000 patients. *Eur. J. Nucl. Med.* **20(8)**, 716–731.

LYMPH NODE IMAGING

RADIOGRAPHY

On plain films lymph nodes may show:

1. Directly:
   a. as a soft tissue mass, e.g. hilar lymph glands on a chest X-ray
   b. calcified nodes, e.g. following tuberculosis or treatment of malignancy
2. Indirect evidence from displacement of normal structures, e.g. displacement of ureters seen during excretion urography.

ULTRASOUND

Advantages:

1. Non-invasive and without risk to the patient
2. Helpful in the neck and axilla in particular, especially with Doppler analysis and US-guided fine-needle aspiration or core biopsy

Disadvantages:

1. Highly operator-dependent
2. Intestinal gas is a major factor in poor visualization. Unsuitable for the mediastinum.

COMPUTED TOMOGRAPHY

Technique is dealt with in other chapters.

Advantages:

1. Can image all nodes
2. Technically easy to perform.

Disadvantages:

1. Internal structure is not seen
2. Gives no indication of nature, apart from on the basis of size, and possibly on basis of enhancement characteristics.

MAGNETIC RESONANCE IMAGING

Technique is dealt with in other chapters.

Advantages:

1. Can image all nodes
2. Technically easy to perform.

Disadvantages:

1. Internal structure is not seen
2. Gives no indication of nature, apart from on the basis of size.

11

MAGNETIC RESONANCE LYMPHANGIOGRAPHY

Currently under assessment is MR lymphangiography. High-resolution T2*-weighted MR scans are obtained prior to and post the injection of lymphotropic superparamagnetic nanoparticles. Normal nodes are high signal on the pre-contrast scan, but lose signal on the post contrast signal due the T2* effect from the iron content in the particles taken up by normal reticuloendothelial cells. Nodes containing malignant tissue retain their high signal intensity on the post contrast scans and small tumour deposits can be detected in even normal-sized nodes.[1]

RADIOGRAPHIC LYMPHANGIOGRAPHY

This is a technically difficult and invasive examination requiring limited operative exposure of lymphatic vessels for cannulation, usually in the feet. Lipiodol, the usual contrast material, is no longer available and operator expertise is also largely no longer available. It has been superseded by cross-sectional imaging techniques such as US, CT and MRI, and functional assessment with FDG PET and some other radionuclide imaging procedures.

RADIONUCLIDE LYMPHOSCINTIGRAPHY

Lymphoscintigraphy provides a less invasive alternative to conventional lymphography. High-resolution anatomical detail is not possible.

Indications

1. Localization of the 'sentinel' node in breast carcinoma[2] and malignant melanoma using a hand-held probe. In recent years, this has become the major indication for lymphoscintigraphy. The technique in itself does not diagnose nodes affected by malignancy; rather it identifies the node most likely to be involved and, therefore, to allow histological sampling. Although still awaiting completion of long-term clinical trials, the early indications are that if the first or 'sentinel' node in the lymphatic drainage chain from the primary site is shown to have negative histology (approx. 60% of cases in breast cancer), then more extensive nodal clearance and associated morbidity can be avoided
2. Differentiation of lymphoedema from venous oedema
3. Assessment of lymphatic flow in lymphoedema.[3]

Contraindications

Hypersensitivity to human albumin products.

Radiopharmaceuticals

1. ^{99m}Technetium (Tc)-nanocolloidal albumin (particle size <80 nm), 40 MBq maximum (0.4 mSv ED) total for all injections. The colloid is injected intradermally and cleared from the interstitial space by lymphatic drainage.
2. A number of other colloids are used around the world for sentinel node imaging, and other radiopharmaceuticals have been used for lymphoscintigraphy.

Equipment

1. Gamma-camera
2. High-resolution general purpose collimator.

Patient preparation

Clean injection sites.

Technique

1. Sentinel node imaging:
   Example protocols are:
   a. breast carcinoma: inject ^{99m}Tc-colloid in approximately 5 ml volume intradermally for palpable lesions and around the tumour under US guidance for non-palpable lesions
   b. melanoma: inject ^{99m}Tc-colloid intradermally in a ring of locations around the melanoma site, with a volume of about 0.1 ml for each injection.
   Static images are taken at intervals until the first node is seen. For breast cancer, take anterior and left or right lateral images with the arm raised as for surgery. Mark the skin over the node in both axes to guide surgical incision and intraoperative location with a gamma-detecting probe. With effectively no background activity in the body, anatomical localization on the images is needed. A ^{57}Cobalt flood source (usually available for routine camera quality assurance) can be placed for a short period under the imaging couch to produce a body outline on the image.
2. Other anatomical sites of investigation or for investigation of lymphatic drainage/lymphoedema:
   a. ^{99m}Tc-colloid in 0.1–0.3 ml volume is injected intradermally at sites depending upon the area to be studied, e.g. for nodes below diaphragm and lower limb drainage – injections in each foot in the first and second web spaces for drainage or over the lateral dorsum of the foot for lymphatics or for axillary nodes and upper limb drainage injections in each hand in the second and third web spaces.
   b. Static images are taken of the injection site(s) immediately, followed by injection site, drainage route and liver images at

11

intervals, e.g. 15, 30, 60 and 180 min, continuing up to 24 h or until the liver is seen. Visualization of the liver indicates patency of at least one lymphatic channel (except early liver activity within 15 min, which implies some colloid entry into blood vessels).

Analysis

If more frequent imaging or a long dynamic study is performed, time-activity curves for regions along the drainage route can be plotted and used to quantify flow impairment.

Aftercare

Normal radiation safety precautions.

Complications

Anaphylactic reaction – rare.

References

1. Harisinghani, M.G., Barentsz, J., Hahn, P.F., et al. (2003) Noninvasive detection of clinically occult lymph-node metastases in prostate cancer. *New Engl. J. Med.* **348(25)**, 2491–2499.
2. Krynyckyi, B.R., Kim, C.K., Goyenechea, M.R., et al. (2004) Clinical breast lymphoscintigraphy: optimal techniques for performing studies, image atlas, and analysis of images. *RadioGraphics* **24(1)**, 121–145
3. Witte, C.L., Witte, M.H., Unger, E.C., et al. (2000) Advances in imaging of lymph flow disorders. *RadioGraphics* **20(6)**, 1697–1719.

RADIONUCLIDE IMAGING OF INFECTION AND INFLAMMATION

A number of radionuclide techniques exist for this, the most commonly used of which is radionuclide-labelled leucocyte imaging.[1,2] The ready availability and sensitivity for collections and inflammation of anatomical imaging techniques such as US and CT has, however, reduced the demand for radionuclide procedures.

Indications

1. Diagnosis and localization of obscure infection and inflammation in soft tissue and bone
2. Assessment of inflammatory activity in disorders such as inflammatory bowel disease, e.g. Crohn's.

Contraindications

None.

Radiopharmaceuticals

1. ^{111}In-labelled leucocytes, 20 MBq maximum (9 mSv ED). ^{111}In-oxine, tropolonate and acetylacetonate are highly lipophilic complexes that will label leucocytes, erythrocytes and platelets. The leucocytes have to be labelled in vitro and the labelled cell suspension reinjected. ABO/Rh-matched donor leucocytes can be used with neutropenic patients or to reduce infection hazard in HIV-positive patients. ^{111}In has a half-life of 67 h and principal gamma emissions at 171 and 245 keV. There is no confounding uptake in bowel and this technique may be more suitable for chronic or more low-grade infections because of the longer imaging window (4–48 h).

2. ^{99m}Tc-hexamethylpropyleneamineoxime (HMPAO)-labelled leucocytes, 200 MBq max (3 mSv ED). HMPAO is also a highly lipophilic complex which preferentially labels granulocytes. The cell-labelling technique is similar to that for ^{111}In, but HMPAO has the advantage that kits can be stocked and used at short notice. There is more bowel uptake as a result of biliary excretion than with ^{111}In-labelled leucocytes, so images must be taken earlier than 4 h post injection for diagnosis of abdominal infection. The ^{99m}Tc label delivers a lower radiation dose than ^{111}In-labelled leucocytes and has better imaging resolution, which can, for example, help to identify inflammation in small bowel.

3. ^{67}Ga-gallium citrate, 150 MBq max (17 mSv ED). This localizes in inflammatory sites. Formerly the most commonly used agent, it has now largely been replaced by labelled leucocyte imaging. There is significant bowel activity up to 72 h, so delayed imaging may be necessary for suspected abdominal infection, and accuracy in the abdomen is less than elsewhere. ^{67}Ga, with a T1/2 of 78 h and principal γ-emissions at 93, 185 and 300 keV, delivers a significantly higher radiation dose than ^{99m}Tc-HMPAO- and 111In-labelled leucocytes, but it has the advantage of requiring no special preparation.

4. ^{99m}Tc- or ^{111}In-human immunoglobulin (HIG). This is a newer agent for which a commercial kit is available for ^{99m}Tc labelling. It has the advantage of not requiring a complex preparation procedure, but its place relative to labelled leucocytes is still a matter of debate.

5. ^{99m}Tc-sulesomab (Leukoscan). This is another more recent commercial agent comprising a labelled antigranulocyte monoclonal antibody fragment. It also has a simple preparation

11

procedure, and is finding a role in the diagnosis of orthopaedic infections.

6. ^{18}F-FDG PET has been used to evaluate obscure infection or suspected infection of orthopaedic hardware.

Equipment

1. Gamma camera, preferably with whole body imaging facility
2. Low-energy high-resolution collimator for ^{99m}Tc, medium-energy for ^{111}In, medium- or high-energy for ^{67}Ga.

Patient preparation

None.

Technique

1. The radiopharmaceutical is administered intravenously
2. Image timing depends upon the radiopharmaceutical used and the suspected source of infection. Whole-body imaging may be employed for all of the radiopharmaceuticals:
   a. ^{111}In-labelled white cells. Static images are acquired at 3 and 24 h post injection. Further imaging at 48 h may prove helpful.
   b. ^{99m}Tc-HMPAO-labelled white cells. For suspected abdominal infections, image at 0.5 and 2 h, i.e. before significant normal bowel activity is seen. For other sites, image at 1, 2 and 4 h. Additional 24-h images may be useful.
   c. ^{67}Ga-citrate. Images are acquired at 48 and 72 h for regions where normal bowel, urinary and blood pool activity may obscure abnormal collection sites. Later images may prove helpful in non-urgent cases. Extremities and urgent cases may be imaged from as early as 6 h. If not contraindicated, laxatives given for 48 h post injection will help to clear bowel activity.

Additional techniques

1. The diagnosis of bone infection may be improved by combination with three-phase radioisotope bone scanning or bone marrow imaging.
2. Comparison with a radiocolloid scan may help to discriminate between infection in the region of the liver or spleen and normal uptake in these organs.

Aftercare

Normal radiation safety precautions (see Chapter 1).

Complications

None.

References

1. Peters, A.M. & Lavender, J.P. (1991) Editorial. Imaging inflammation with radiolabelled white cells; ^{99m}Tc-HMPAO or ^{111}In? *Nucl. Med. Commun.* **12**, 923–925.
2. Love, C. & Palestro, C.J. (2004) Radionuclide imaging of infection. *J. Nucl. Med. Technol.* **32(2)**, 47–57.

11

Bones and joints

Imaging modalities

1. **Plain films.** These are cheap, widely available and valuable screening tools in the preliminary assessment of osteoarticular symptoms. Standard views require a minimum of two views perpendicular to each other, e.g. antero-posterior and lateral projections. The pathological processes underlying osteolysis and osteosclerosis, e.g. infection, tumours, articular erosions, etc., are well advanced before they become radiographically visible and radiographs may appear normal despite the presence of significant bone and joint disease. Although there are limitations, plain films are very useful in the characterization and differential diagnosis of disease, e.g. trauma, bone tumours, arthritis. Despite the recent advances in imaging techniques, the radiograph remains the single most important investigation in the characterization of bone tumours.

2. **Arthrography.** The injection of radiographically positive (iodinated) and negative (air) contrast medium directly into the joint allows radiographic assessment of articular structures in conventional arthrography. The examination can then be supplemented with CT (CT arthrography) which provides more detailed assessment of intra-articular status and structures using bone and soft-tissue window settings. For optimal evaluation, reformatted CT images in three planes with MDCT are obtained. Arthrography using a dilute gadolinium-DTPA solution and imaging with MRI (MR arthrography) is increasingly used in the study of large joint disease, e.g. shoulder, hip and to a lesser extent wrist, elbow and ankle.

3. **Radionuclide imaging.** Bone scintigraphy enjoys a high sensitivity but a low specificity. It is widely used in the detection and follow-up of metastatic disease, characterization of lesions shown by other imaging modalities, and as a sensitive test for the detection of pathology such as infection.

4. **Ultrasound (US).** Advances in US technology have increasingly been applied to musculoskeletal disorders in both adult and paediatric age groups. Peri-articular structures (capsule, ligaments, tendons) are optimally imaged. Under US-guidance, therapy to soft-tissue disease can be accurately targeted, joint fluid aspirated and arthrographic agents instilled into joints.

5. **Computed tomography (CT).** This is very useful in complex bone trauma for accurate surgical planning, also many applications in assessment of bone tumours and infection. Joint anatomy and pathology in joints which are difficult to image in two perpendicular planes and in which there is bone overlap, e.g. shoulder, hip, sternoclavicular, sacroiliac joints are best depicted using CT. When employed in CT arthrography, the intra-articular status of joints can be optimally assessed.

6. **Magnetic resonance imaging (MRI).** MRI is the best imaging modality for joint assessment. In many joints, e.g. knee, it can be employed as the first and only means of imaging. In other joints, e.g. shoulder, MRI alone is used to image the rotator cuff, but MR arthrography is required for optimal imaging of the ligaments, capsule and labrum in post-traumatic instability. Direct MR arthrography using intra-articular injection of dilute gadolinium solution is also employed, in the hip primarily to image the labrum and in the wrist to assess the interosseous ligaments of the proximal carpal row and the triangular fibrocartilage. Indirect MR arthrography following intravenous (i.v.) injection of gadolinium-DTPA, which quickly diffuses into the joint via the synovium, is used in the detection and quantification of active synovitis, e.g. rheumatoid arthritis. This is particularly of value in small joints and in the post-operative assessment of large joints. MRI is widely used in the assessment of bone pathology such as tumour or infection.

MUSCULOSKELETAL MAGNETIC RESONANCE IMAGING – GENERAL POINTS

1. The large variety of MR sequences provides an opportunity to tailor the sequences to the tissues that need to be optimally imaged. See Table 12.1.

2. I.v. gadolinium-DTPA is used in musculoskeletal (MSK) imaging for:
   a. infections – to differentiate abscess from phlegmon
   b. tumours – to differentiate viable tumour from necrosis –
      to differentiate solid from cystic components
   c. post-operative spine – to differentiate recurrent disc herniation from scar tissue

Table 12.1 Optimizing magnetic resonance imaging sequences for musculo-skeletal tissues

Tissue type	Optimal magnetic resonance (MR) imaging sequences		
Bone	T1	STIR	T2 fat sat
Cartilage	GRE + fat sat	T2 fat sat	PD fat sat
Labrum	T1 fat sat (MR arthrogram)	T1 spin echo (MR arthrogram)	GRE T2*
Meniscus	T1	GRE T2*	PD fat sat
Tendons/ ligaments	T2 fat sat	GRE T2*	T1
Muscle	T1	STIR	T1 fat sat
Marrow	T1	STIR	PD fat sat
Synovium	T1 fat sat (i.v. gadolinium)	T1 spin echo (i.v. gadolinium)	T1

STIR=short tau inversion recovery, GRE=gradient echo, PD=proton density

    d. synovial disease, e.g. rheumatoid arthritis – to determine activity/response to treatment
    e. avascular necrosis, e.g. Perthes' disease, scaphoid fracture – to show viable tissue
    f. indirect MR arthrography – to delineate articular cartilage status, meniscal repair.
3. MR arthrography. Direct MR arthrography involves joint puncture and the intra-articular injection of a dilute gadolinium solution (saline and local anaesthetic can also be used). The amount of gadolinium needed to produce contrast by shortening the T1 effect of fluid is very small – before injection gadolinium-DTPA is diluted in a ratio of 1:100 with sterile saline solution (see below). Too much gadolinium-DTPA results in signal loss of the fluid ('black out'). The joint is distended and the recesses filled, delineating the intra-articular structures and separating them from adjacent tissues. In the lower limb, it allows accurate visualization of the labrum of the hip, the operated meniscus in the knee, and the impingement ankle syndromes, demonstrating associated osteochondral defects, loose bodies and synovial pathology more reliably than conventional MRI. In the upper limb, it is mostly utilized in the unstable shoulder to assess the damaged osteoarticular structures, the elbow and wrist joints. T1 spin echo and T1 fat

12

saturated sequences are used routinely in MR arthrography along with a T2 sequence in at least one plane to detect cysts, bone and soft-tissue oedema. Traction applied to joints at MR arthrography improves visualization of certain structures, e.g. long head of biceps origin in the shoulder, articular cartilage in the hip. MR arthrography avoids the requirement for diagnostic arthroscopy and aids in the therapeutic plan.

Further reading

Bergin, D. & Schweitzer, M.E. (2003) Indirect MR arthrography. *Skeletal Radiol.* **32**, 551–558.

Peh, W.C. & Cassar-Pullicino, V.N. (1999) Magnetic resonance arthrography: current status. *Clin. Radiol.* **54**, 575–587.

ARTHROGRAPHY – GENERAL POINTS

1. The conventional radiographs should always be reviewed prior to the procedure.
2. Aspiration of an effusion should always be performed before contrast medium is injected. The aspirate should be sent, where appropriate, for microscopy, culture (aerobic and anaerobic) and sensitivity, crystal analysis, cytology and biochemistry.
3. Conventional arthrography has largely been replaced by MRI, e.g. knee. It is still the mainstay for diagnosing adhesive capsulitis, and in demonstrating the exact site of abnormal articular communications, e.g. wrist and foot. Most arthrograms are currently carried out as a prelude to either CT or MR arthrography.
4. If a needle is correctly sited within a joint space, a test injection of a small volume of contrast medium will stream away from the needle tip around the joint. However, if it is incorrectly sited, the contrast medium will remain in a diffuse cloud around the tip of the needle. For this reason, it is important that the fluoroscopy-guided needle approach should aim to visualize the needle tip at all times during its trajectory. In the knee, fluoroscopy in the AP plane is used as the needle is advanced from a lateral approach; fluoroscopy of the ankle in the lateral projection allows needle-tip visualization as it is advanced via an anterior approach.

5. Needle placement may be 'blind' or under image guidance, e.g. fluoroscopy, CT, CT fluoroscopy or US. Measured effective doses given by an experienced radiologist show significant differences; in shoulder arthrography – fluoroscopy (0.0015 mSv), single slice CT (0.18 mSv) and CT fluoroscopy (0.22 mSv).[1]

6. The positive contrast medium is absorbed from the joint and excreted from the body in a few hours. However, intra-articular air may take up to 4 days to be completely absorbed from the joint space. Every effort should be made to eliminate air bubbles at injection for MR arthrography as they create artifacts.

7. Arthrography is well tolerated by patients with discomfort rated less severe than general MRI-related patient discomfort.[2]

8. Arthrography is a very safe procedure, with low complication rates. In a major study [3] there were 3.8% minor complications (vasovagal reaction, pain, synovitis) and 0.02% major complications (anaphylactic reaction, infection, vascular). This included 13 300 MR arthrograms with only a 0.03% complication rate, all of which were minor.

9. In the scheduling of CT and MR arthrography it is important to ensure that the examination is carried out within 30 min of fluoroscopy guided contrast medium intra-articular instillation. After this time contrast medium absorption will result in a suboptimal examination with resultant difficulties in interpretation.

ARTHROGRAPHY

Indications

1. **Intra-articular structures** e.g. cartilage, labrum, and tendons. The exact status of cartilage overlying osteochondritis dissecans (knee, ankle), labral tears (shoulder and hip) and anchor point of the long head of biceps requires CT or MR arthrography for accurate diagnosis.

2. **Capsular, ligamentous and tendon injuries.** Information regarding the presence, type, extent, gap and edges of torn capsular and peri-capsular structures (glenohumeral ligaments, rotator cuff tendons, lateral ankle ligaments) requires CT/MR arthrography.

3. **Loose body.** Loose bodies can be solitary or multiple, radiolucent or radio-opaque. CT arthrography using dilute contrast medium solution best depicts radiolucent bodies.

12

Double-contrast CT arthrography using only a small amount of positive contrast medium is best to delineate radio-opaque loose bodies, determine true size, and assess articular status of the joint.

4. **Para-articular cyst.** Synovial cysts and ganglia within para-articular soft tissues and bones can present with space-occupying lesions, which may migrate some distance away from the joint source of origin (popliteal cysts, iliopsoas bursa). Arthrography can demonstrate the articular communication either immediately or on delayed imaging.

5. **Prosthesis assessment** e.g. loosening, infection. Arthrography demonstrates abnormal interposition of contrast medium indicating loosening at the cement /bone or metal/ bone interface depending on the type of arthroplasty procedure carried out, while joint irrigation and aspiration fluid specimens are needed to confirm associated infection. Subtraction radiographic techniques are employed to facilitate interpretation, as the metal prosthesis and the barium impregnated cement are subtracted out of the final image.

6. **Pain block** e.g. bupivacaine $\pm$ steroid therapy. For difficult therapeutic decisions, diagnostic tests to confirm the pain source origin are increasingly being employed by instilling 0.5% bupivacaine intra-articularly. The addition of a steroid preparation can also aid in a longer period of pain control. If required, the injectate may act as the arthrographic agent for MRI done immediately after the pain block.

7. **Confirm location of calcified para-articular soft-tissue masses.** Calcified or ossified soft-tissue lesions in a para-articular location may or may not be intra-articular (e.g. synovial osteochondromatosis, myositis ossificans) requiring CT arthrography to help in their accurate localization.

8. **Diagnosis and distension therapy in adhesive capsulitis.** Usually employed in the shoulder in the treatment of frozen shoulder, the combination of anaesthetic, steroid and saline can be used to distend and rupture the joint after arthrographic confirmation of the diagnosis.

9. **Intra-articular chemical therapy** e.g. hyaluronic acid, fibrinolysis, radioactive synovectomy. The intra-articular injection of hyaluronic acid in joints suffering from mild to moderate osteoarthritis produces viscosupplementation of joint fluid, reducing pain and increasing the articular cartilage thickness. In fibrin-laden effusions due to chronic rheumatoid arthritis, injected intra-articular fibrinolytic agents aid in the aspiration of the joint fluid.

Contraindications

1. Local sepsis
2. Allergy to iodine or gadolinium
3. Contraindication to MRI (see Chapter 2); consider CT arthrography.

Contrast medium

Conventional/CT arthrography

Low osmolar contrast material (LOCM) is used, the most common of which are iohexol and iopamidol. A higher concentration is needed in larger joints but for the purposes of CT arthrography, especially in tight joints, a dilute solution (100–150 mg iodine/ 100 ml) has distinct advantages. Volume of contrast medium needed is directly proportional to the capacity of the joint in question, e.g. 15 ml in the shoulder, 6 ml in the elbow and 3 ml in the wrist. Double-contrast examination of the knee for a CT arthrogram to assess the patellofemoral joint requires 4 ml iodinated contrast medium with 40 ml of air.

Magnetic resonance arthrography

The contrast used contains both dilute gadolinium-DTPA and iodinated contrast (which is needed to confirm correct needle placement during injection), e.g. a combination of:

1. 0.1 ml gadolinium-DTPA
2. 10 ml sterile saline solution, and
3. 2 ml LOCM 200 mg I ml^{-1}.

The volume required varies according to the joint being assessed.

Equipment

1. Fluoroscopy unit with spot film device and fine focal spot (0.3 mm^2)
2. Overcouch tube.

Patient preparation

None.

Preliminary radiographs

Routine acquisition and evaluation of joint radiographs is recommended.

Radiographic views

1. AP and lateral views are routinely obtained after arthrography
2. Additional axial (e.g. shoulder) and oblique (e.g. ankle) views may be helpful

12

3. Dynamic assessment under fluoroscopic imaging with stress views may be useful, e.g. inversion/eversion in the ankle; abduction/adduction, weight-bearing views of the shoulder
4. Erect posture with external and internal rotation views in double-contrast shoulder studies
5. Radial and ulnar deviation views in radio-carpal, midcarpal and inferior radio-ulnar joints.

Aftercare

Driving after the procedure is not advisable. The patient is warned that there may be some discomfort in the joint for 1–2 days after the procedure. It is also necessary to refrain from strenuous exercise during this time. The injected air for a double-contrast procedure precludes air travel.

Complications

Due to the contrast medium
1. Allergic reactions
2. Chemical synovitis.

Due to the technique
1. Pain
2. Infection
3. Capsular rupture
4. Trauma to adjacent structures, e.g. neural/vascular structures
5. Air embolus (rare).

Other
Vasovagal reaction.

References
1. Binkert, C.A., Verdun, F.R., Zanetti, M., et al. (2003) CT arthrography of the glenohumeral joint: CT fluoroscopy versus conventional CT and fluoroscopy – comparison of image guidance techniques. *Radiology* **229**, 153–158.
2. Binkert, C.A., Zanetti, M. & Hodler, J. (2001) Patient's assessment of discomfort during MR arthrography of the shoulder. *Radiology* **221**, 775–778.
3. Hugo, P.C., Newberg, A.H., Newman, J.S., et al. (1998) Complications of arthrography. *Sem. Musculoskelet. Radiol.* **2**, 345–348.

Further reading
Andreisek, G., Duc, S.R., Froehlich, J.M., et al. (2007) MR arthrography of the shoulder, hip, and wrist: evaluation of contrast dynamics and image quality with increasing injection-to-imaging time. *Am. J. Roentgenol.* **188**, 1081–1088.
Tehranzadeh, J., Mossop, E.P. & Golshan-Momeni, M. (2006) Therapeutic arthrography and bursography. *Orthop. Clin. North Am.* **37**, 393–408.

ARTHROGRAPHY – SITE SPECIFIC ISSUES

There are various needle approaches using image guidance and the most commonly used ones are described.

KNEE

Technique

1. The patient lies supine; either a medial or a lateral approach can be used and it is as well to be familiar with both.
2. Using a sterile technique, the skin and underlying soft tissue are anaesthetized at a point 1–2 cm posterior to the mid-point of the patella.
3. A 21G needle is advanced into the joint space from this point by angling it slightly anteriorly so the tip comes to lie against the posterior surface of the patella. By virtue of the anatomy, the tip of the needle must be within the joint space (Fig. 12.1). A more horizontal approach may result in the needle penetrating the infra-patellar fat pad, resulting in an extra-articular injection of contrast.
4. Any effusion is aspirated. A test injection of a small volume of contrast medium can be made under fluoroscopic control to ensure the needle is correctly positioned and, if so, the contrast medium should be seen to flow rapidly away from the needle

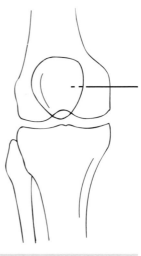

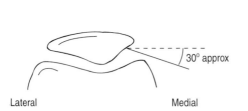

Lateral   Medial   30° approx

12

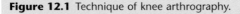

Figure 12.1 Technique of knee arthrography.

tip. If a satisfactory position is demonstrated, then the full volume of contrast medium (4 ml) and air (40 ml) may be injected for a double-contrast arthrogram.

5. The needle is then removed and the knee is manipulated to ensure even distribution of contrast medium within the joint; this is easily facilitated by asking the patient to walk around the room several times whilst bending the knee through as full a movement as possible.

6. The arthrogram is usually followed by CT to assess the patellofemoral articular status and its articular geometric relationship. Patellar tracking in different degrees of knee flexion can be done if needed. MDCT also assesses the medial and lateral articular and meniscal status optimally.

Further reading

Coumas, J.M. & Palmer, W.E. (1998) Knee arthrography. Evolution and current status. *Radiol. Clin. North Am.* **36(4)**, 703–728.

De Filippo, M., Bertellini, A., Pogliacomi, F., et al. (2008) Multidetector CT arthrography of the knee: diagnostic accuracy and indications. *Eur. J. Radiol.* March 6. Epub.

Mutschler, C., Vande Berg, B.C., Lecouvet, F.E., et al. (2003) Postoperative meniscus: assessment at dual–detector row spiral CT arthrography of the knee. *Radiology* **228**, 635–641.

HIP

Technique

1. The patient lies supine on the X-ray table, the leg is extended, internally rotated and the position maintained with sandbags so that the entire length of the femoral neck is visualized.

2. The position of the femoral vessels is marked to avoid inadvertent puncture.

3. The skin is prepared in a standard aseptic manner.

4. A metal marker (sterile needle) or a point on the skin is made to show the position of entry (Fig. 12.2) which should correspond to the midpoint of the inter-trochanteric line. After local anaesthetic infiltration a spinal needle (7.5 cm, 20 or 22G, short bevel) is then advanced vertically with mild forward angulation. The needle tip advances forward towards the femoral neck target under fluoroscopic control, aiming supero-laterally onto the femoral neck immediately below the junction of the femoral head with the neck laterally. The capsule may be thick and a definite 'give' felt when the needle enters the joint.

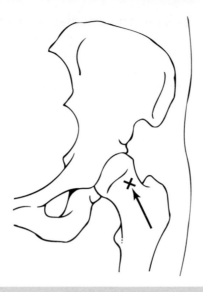

Figure 12.2 Technique of hip arthrography. x = site of entry into joint.

5. A test injection of contrast medium will demonstrate correct placement of the needle, as it flows away from the needle tip. Any fluid in the joint should be aspirated at this stage and sent for analysis.

6. Approximately 6–8 ml (1–2 ml in children) of contrast medium is injected. The exact amount depends on the capacity of the joint capsule. In MR arthrography, dilute gadolinium solution is used for contrast. Alternatively in a pain block procedure, 6–8 ml of 0.5% bupivacaine are injected intra-articularly and this can also act as the contrast medium for a limited MR arthrogram relying on T2 sequences. If examining a prosthetic joint, larger volumes of contrast medium may be required (15–20 ml). By adding a radioactive tracer to the infusate (^{99m}Tc-colloid) and subsequent imaging with a gamma-camera, a more accurate assessment of loosening can be made, perhaps because the tracer is less viscous than the contrast medium and extends to a greater extent along the prosthesis.

7. After injection of the contrast medium, the needle is removed and the joint is passively exercised to distribute the contrast medium evenly. Radiographic views are taken immediately and the patient sent to CT or MR scanning suites accordingly.

Radiographic views in the paediatric hip arthrogram

In children under the age of 10 years the procedure is usually done under general anaesthesia. A fuller conventional radiographic series is needed to assess the joint dynamics to help in the evaluation of treatment options particularly in developmental dysplasia of the hip:

1. AP hip
2. Frog lateral
3. Abduction and internal rotation
4. Maximum abduction
5. Maximum adduction
6. Push/pull views to demonstrate instability.

Further reading

Aliabadi, P., Baker, N.D. & Jaramillo, D. (1998) Hip arthrography, aspiration, block, and bursography. *Radiol. Clin. North Am.* **36(4)**, 673–690.

Devalia, K.L., Wright, D., Sathyamurthy, P., et al. (2007) Role of preoperative arthrography in early Perthes disease as a decision making tool. Is it really necessary? *J. Pediatr. Orthop. B* **16**, 196–200.

Grissom, L., Harcke, H.T. & Thacker, M. (2008) Imaging in the surgical management of developmental dislocation of the hip. *Clin. Orthop. Relat. Res.* **466**, 791–801.

Llopis, E. & Cerezal, L. (2008) Direct MR arthrography of the hip with leg traction: feasibility for assessing articular cartilage. *Am. J. Roentgenol.* **190**, 1124–1128.

Temmerman, O.P., Raijmakers, P.G., Deville, W., et al. (2007) The use of plain radiography, subtraction arthrography, nuclear arthrography, and bone scintigraphy in the diagnosis of a loose acetabular component of a total hip prosthesis: a systematic review. *J. Arthroplasty* **22**, 818–827.

SHOULDER

Technique

1. There are various approaches to needle placement, e.g. anterior (superior or inferior), modified anterior, and posterior to the glenohumeral joint. In the commonly used anterior approach the patient lies supine, with the arm of the side under investigation close to the body and in external rotation. This is to rotate the long head of the biceps out of the path of the needle. The articular surface of the glenoid will face slightly forwards, which is important as it allows a vertically placed needle to enter the joint space without damaging the glenoid labrum.

2. The coracoid process is an important landmark. Using a sterile technique, the skin and soft tissues are anaesthetized at a point 1 cm inferior and 1 cm lateral to the coracoid process. Position of needle entry point is optimized by fluoroscopy which also helps to ensure that the chosen needle trajectory is not impeded by an elongated coracoid process.

3. A spinal needle 21G needle is inserted vertically down into the joint space (Fig. 12.3). The vertical direction should intersect the junction of the middle and lower thirds of the cranio-caudal plane of the glenohumeral joint. This also allows precise control of the medio-lateral course of the needle. The position of the needle should be checked by intermittent screening. When it meets the resistance of the articular surface of the humeral head, it is withdrawn by 1–2 mm to free the tip. In the modified anterior approach where the needle traverses the rotator cuff interval, the needle is aimed towards the upper medial quadrant of the humeral head close to the articular joint line.

4. The intra-articular position of the needle is then confirmed by the injection of a small amount of the contrast medium under fluoroscopic control.

5. Then either the remainder of the iodinated contrast medium (15 ml in total) is injected for a single contrast examination, or sufficient air to distend the synovial sac (12 ml) is injected for a double-contrast examination. CT arthrography can be done after either type. In MR arthrography a dilute solution of gadolinium needs to be injected into the joint and this can be done by combining 1 ml of lidocaine, 2 ml of iodinated contrast medium ($200 \, \text{mg ml}^{-1}$) and 12 ml of dilute gadolinium solution ($2–2.5 \, \text{mmol l}^{-1}$). Sterile, premixed gadolinium-DTPA solutions are available for use in MR arthrography. Patients with an adhesive capsulitis may experience pain after much smaller amounts. If this is severe, then injection should be stopped.

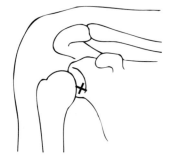

12

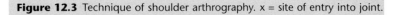

Figure 12.3 Technique of shoulder arthrography. x = site of entry into joint.

Resistance to injection is common, unlike injection into the knee, and more force is often required.

6. The needle is removed and the joint is gently manipulated to distribute the contrast medium.

7. CT arthrography examination is performed with the patient supine and positioned slightly eccentrically within the scanner to ensure that the shoulder is as close to the centre of the scanner as possible. The contralateral arm can be elevated above the head to minimize image artifacts. Scanning should be undertaken during arrested respiration to minimize motion artifact.

8. The area of interest in both CT/MR arthrography should include the acromion to the axillary recess. MDCT provides high-quality reformatted images in the three planes and MR images should also examine the joint in three planes. In addition when the arm is placed in the ABER position (abduction and external rotation), elegant MR views of the inferior capsule-labral complex and supraspinatus optimally study these structures.

Further reading

Chung, C.B., Dwek, J.R., Feng, S., et al. (2001) MR arthrography of the glenohumeral joint: a tailored approach. *Am. J. Roentgenol.* **177(1)**, 217–219.

Dépelteau, H., Bureau, N.J., Cardinal, E., et al. (2004) Arthrography of the shoulder: a simple fluoroscopically guided approach for targeting the rotator cuff interval. *Am. J. Roentgenol.* **182(2)**, 329–332.

Farmer, K.D. & Hughes, P.M. (2002) MR arthrography of the shoulder: fluoroscopically guided technique using a posterior approach. *Am. J. Roentgenol.* **178(2)**, 433–434.

Schneider, R., Ghelman, B. & Kaye, J.J. (1975) A simplified injection technique for shoulder arthrography. *Radiology* **114(3)**, 738–739.

ELBOW

Technique

Single contrast

1. The patient sits next to the table with the elbow flexed and resting on the table, the lateral aspect uppermost.

2. The radial head is located by palpation during gentle pronation and supination of the forearm. Using a sterile technique the skin and soft tissues are anaesthetized at a point just proximal to the radial head.

3. A 23G needle is then inserted vertically down into the joint space between the radial head and the capitellum (Fig. 12.4).

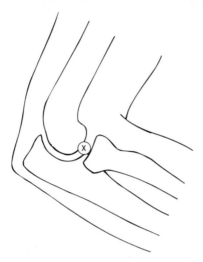

Figure 12.4 Technique of elbow arthrography. x = site of entry into joint.

4. An injection of a small volume of local anaesthetic will flow easily if the needle is correctly sited. This can be confirmed by the injection of a few drops of contrast medium under fluoroscopic control.
5. The remainder of the contrast medium (6–8 ml) is injected and the joint gently manipulated to distribute it evenly.

Double contrast
1. Position the patient as for single contrast technique and follow steps 1–4 above.
2. Inject 0.5 ml of contrast medium followed by 6–12 ml of air until the olecranon fossa is distended.

Further reading

Dubberley, J.H., Faber, K.J., Patterson, S.D., et al. (2005) The detection of loose bodies in the elbow: the value of MRI and CT arthrography. *J. Bone Joint. Surg. Br.* **87**, 684–686.

Steinbach, L.S. & Schwartz, M. (1998) Elbow arthrography. *Radiol. Clin. North Am.* **36(4)**, 635–649.

Waldt, S. & Bruegel, M. (2005) Comparison of multislice CT arthrography and MR arthrography for the detection of articular cartilage lesions of the elbow. *Eur. Radiol.* **15**, 784–791.

12

WRIST

Technique

Radiocarpal joint

1. The patient is seated next to the screening table with the forearm resting in a neutral prone position. The wrist should be supported over a wedge with about 10–15° of flexion.
2. Using a sterile technique, the skin and soft tissues are anaesthetized at a point over the midpoint of the scapho-capitate joint (Fig. 12.5).
3. A 23G needle is inserted into the joint by advancing it downwards and at an angle of about 15° proximally.
4. Contrast medium (2–4 ml) is injected under fluoroscopic control; if any leakage occurs into the midcarpal joint or distal radio-ulnar joints, then spot views should be taken. If this is not done, it is possible to miss small tears that later become obscured by the anterior and posterior extensions of the radiocarpal joint.

Midcarpal joint

1. The wrist is positioned as for radiocarpal injection, but with ulnar deviation, as this widens the joint space.
2. The skin and soft tissues are anaesthetized at point over the mid-point of the scapho-capitate joint (Fig. 12.5).
3. A 23G needle is inserted vertically into the joint space under fluoroscopic control.
4. Contrast medium (2 ml) is injected under fluoroscopic control, ideally with video-recording facility, until the joint space is full. Without continuous monitoring it may not be possible

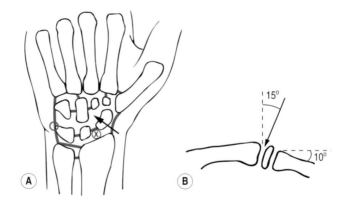

Figure 12.5 Technique of wrist arthrography. (a) AP view, x = point of entry to radiocarpal joint, arrow = point of entry to midcarpal joint. (b) Lateral view, arrow indicates cranial angulation required for needle with dorsal approach to radiocarpal joint.

to tell which of the ligaments separating the midcarpal from the radiocarpal joint are torn allowing interarticular communication.

Further reading

Joshy, S., Ghosh, S., Lee, K., et al. (2008) Accuracy of direct MR arthrography in the diagnosis of triangular fibrocartilage complex tears of the wrist. *Int. Orthop.* **32**, 251–253.

Linkous, M.D. & Gilula, L.A. (1998) Wrist arthrography today. *Radiol. Clin. North Am.* **36(4)**, 651–672.

Moser, T., Dosch, J.C., Moussaoui, A., et al. (2007) Wrist ligament tears: evaluation with MRI and combined MDCT and MR arthrography. *Am. J. Roentgenol.* **188**, 1278–1286.

Ruegger, C., Schmid, M.R., Pfirrmann, C.W., et al. (2007) Peripheral tear of the triangular fibrocartilage: depiction with MR arthrography of the distal radioulnar joint. *Am. J. Roentgenol.* **188**, 187–192.

Tirman, R.M., Weber, E.R., Snyder, L.L., et al. (1985) Midcarpal wrist arthrography for the detection of tears of the scapholunate and lunotriquetral ligaments. *Am. J. Roentgenol.* **144**, 107–108.

ANKLE

Technique

1. The patient lies in the lateral decubitus position with the ankle plantar-flexed. An anterior approach is used with fluoroscopic guidance of the needle with the ankle in the true lateral projection (Fig. 12.6).

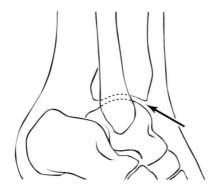

12

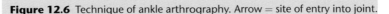

Figure 12.6 Technique of ankle arthrography. Arrow = site of entry into joint.

2. Using a sterile technique, the skin is anaesthetized at a point midway to the bimalleolar distance which places the needle lateral to the dorsalis pedis artery.
3. A 21G needle is inserted and advanced into the anterior joint space and contrast medium injected to confirm correct needle position, and then to distend the joint (4–6 ml).
3. The availability of volume acquisition with MDCT allows reformatted images in the three planes, which can detect small cartilage defects.
4. If MDCT is not available the CT scanner gantry is tilted to obtain, as closely as is possible, true coronal sections through the ankle.

Further reading

Cerezal, L., Abascal, F., García-Valtuille, R., et al. (2005) Ankle MR arthrography: how, why and when? *Radiol. Clin. North Am.* **43**, 693–707.

Davies, A.M. & Cassar-Pullicino, V.N. (1989) Demonstration of osteochondritis dissecans of the talus by coronal computed tomographic arthrography. *Br. J. Radiol.* **62(744)**, 1050–1055.

Schmid, M.R., Pfirrmann, C.W., Hodler, J., et al. (2003) Cartilage lesions in the ankle joint: comparison of MR arthrography and CT arthrography. *Skeletal Radiol.* **32**, 259–265.

TENDON IMAGING

Methods of imaging tendons

1. Tenography
2. US
3. CT
4. MRI.

General points

With the advent of CT, US and MRI, the indications for tenograghy (direct injection of contrast into the tendon sheath) are exceptionally rare. Although CT does show tendons and their relationship to joints and peri-articular structures, US and MRI also show the intrinsic tendon structure and differentiate fluid within the sheath from the tendon. The higher resolution of US enables better depiction of internal architecture of superficial tendons. In addition, dynamic assessment to exclude subluxing tendons can be done sonographically.

ULTRASOUND OF THE PAEDIATRIC HIP

Indications
1. Developmental dysplasia of the hip
2. Hip effusion
3. Slipped femoral capital epiphysis.

Technique
Developmental dysplasia of the hip
With US the unossified elements of the hip – femoral head, greater trochanter, labrum, triradiate cartilage – as well as the bony acetabular roof, can be identified in the first 6 months of life.[1] After 9–12 months, the degree of ossification precludes adequate imaging by US and plain film radiography becomes superior. There are two main methods, static and dynamic, and both may be used during one examination.

Static (Graf) method
This assesses the morphology and geometry of the acetabulum. Although independent of the position of the infant, it is recommended that the infant be placed in the decubitus position. A single longitudinal image is obtained with the transducer placed over the greater trochanter and held at right angles to all the anatomical planes. The following landmarks are identified in the following sequence: chondro-osseous boundary between femoral shaft and head, joint capsule, labrum, cartilaginous roof and superior bony rim of acetabulum. Although most images can be 'eyeballed', angles can be measured from the image and form the basis for the Graf classification.

Dynamic method
This assesses the stability of the hip when stressed. The hip is studied in the coronal and axial planes with the infant supine. With the hip flexed and adducted, the femur is pushed and pulled with a piston-like action.[2]

Hip-joint effusion
Approximately 50% of children with acute hip pain have intra-articular fluid[3] and the sensitivity of US for detecting effusion approaches 100%. With the child supine, the hip is scanned anteriorly with the transducer parallel to the femoral neck. Bulging of the anterior portion of the joint capsule can be readily identified.[4] The normal distance between the bony femoral neck and the joint capsule is always less than 3 mm, and the difference between the affected and unaffected sides should not be greater than 2 mm.

Slipped femoral capital epiphysis

Although plain radiographs constitute the usual means of diagnosis, a mild posterior slip can be identified in the acute situation by longitudinal scanning along the femoral neck.

References

1. Yousefzadeh, D.K. & Ramilo, J.L. (1987) Normal hip in children: correlation of US with anatomic and cryomicrotome sections. *Radiology* **165**, 647–655.
2. Clarke, N.M., Harcke, H.T., McHugh, P., et al. (1985) Real time ultrasound in the diagnosis of congenital dislocation and dysplasia of the hip. *J. Bone Joint Surg. Br.* **67**, 406–412.
3. Dörr, U., Zieger, M. & Hauke, H. (1988) Ultrasonography of the painful hip. Prospective studies in 204 patients. *Pediatr. Radiol.* **19**, 36–40.
4. Miralles, M., Gonzalez, G., Pulpeiro, J.R., et al. (1989) Sonography of the painful hip in children: 500 consecutive cases. *Am. J. Roentgenol.* **152**, 579–582.

RADIONUCLIDE BONE SCAN

Indications

1. Staging of cancer and response to therapy, especially breast and prostate
2. Assessment and staging of primary bone tumours
3. Painful orthopaedic prostheses to differentiate infection from loosening
4. Bone or joint infection
5. Trauma not obvious on X-ray, e.g. stress fractures
6. Bone pain
7. Avascular necrosis and bone infarction
8. Assessment of non-accidental injury in children
9. Metabolic bone disease for complications such as fractures
10. Arthropathies, e.g. rheumatoid
11. Reflex sympathetic dystrophy
12. Assessment of extent multifocal disorders such as Paget's disease and fibrous dysplasia.

Contraindications

None.

Radiopharmaceuticals

^{99m}Tc-methylene diphosphonate (MDP) or other ^{99m}Tc-labelled dipho-sphonate, 500 MBq typical, 600 MBq max (3 mSv ED). For single pho-ton emission computed tomography (SPECT) 800 MBq (5 mSv ED).

These compounds are phosphate analogues which are stable in vivo and rapidly excreted by the kidneys, providing a good con-trast between bone and soft tissue.

Equipment

1. Gamma-camera, preferably with SPECT and whole body imaging
2. Low-energy high-resolution collimator.

Patient preparation

The patient must be well hydrated.

Technique

1. ^{99m}Tc-diphosphonate is injected i.v. When infection is suspected or blood flow to bone or primary bone tumour is to be assessed, a bolus injection is given with the patient in position on the camera. A three-phase study is then performed with arterial, blood-pool and delayed static imaging.
2. The patient should be encouraged to drink plenty and empty the bladder frequently to minimize radiation dose.
3. The bladder is emptied immediately prior to imaging to prevent obscuring the sacrum and bony pelvis.
4. Delayed static imaging is performed ≥2 h after injection: up to 4 h for imaging of extremities and up to 6 h for those patients on dialysis or in renal failure.

Images

Standard

High-resolution images are acquired with a pixel size of 1–2 mm:

1. The whole skeleton. The number of views will depend upon the field of view of the camera and whether a whole-body imaging facility is available. A point to consider is that whole-body images will have lower resolution than spot views over parts of the skeleton where the camera is some distance from the patient (unless a body-contour tracking facility is available), since resolution falls off with distance. Spot views should be overlapping.
2. Anterior oblique views of the thorax are useful to separate sternum and spine uptake.
3. For examination of the posterior ribs, scapula or shoulder, an extra posterior thorax view with arms above the head should be taken to move the scapula away from the ribs.

4. For imaging small bones and joints, magnified views should be taken, with a pinhole collimator if necessary.
5. SPECT can be useful for lesion localization, e.g. in vertebrae and joints, and to detect avascular necrosis.[1] CT-SPECT fusion is likely to be even more helpful, analogous to the improved specificity and diagnostic confidence seen with PET-CT as opposed to PET alone.[2]

Three-phase

1. *Arterial phase 1*: 1–2 s frames of the area of interest for 1 min post-injection
2. *Blood pool phase 2*: 3-min image of the same area 5 min post injection
3. *Delayed phase 3*: views ≥2 h post injection, as for standard imaging.

Analysis

1. For the arterial phase, time-activity curves are created for regions of interest symmetrical about the mid-line.
2. For SPECT, reconstruction of transaxial, coronal, sagittal and possibly oblique slices to demonstrate the lesion.

Additional techniques

SPECT and CT-SPECT can be useful for improved lesion detection and localization in complex bony structures, e.g. spine and knees.[1,2]

Aftercare

Normal radiation safety precautions (see Chapter 1).

Complications

None.

Competing modalities

FDG-PET (see Chapter 11) and whole body MRI (e.g. with diffusion-weighted techniques) may be competitive for oncological purposes. MRI is often preferred for localized orthopaedic applications, but has limited applicability in the presence of a prosthesis.

References

1. Murray, I.P. & Dixon, J. (1989) The role of single photon emission computed tomography in bone scintigraphy. *Skeletal Radiol.* **18**, 493–505.
2. Utsunomiya, D., Shiraishi, S., Imuta, M., et al. (2006) Added value of SPECT/CT fusion in assessing suspected bone metastasis: comparison with scintigraphy alone and nonfused scintigraphy and CT. *Radiology* **238**, 264–271.

Further reading

Brooks, M. (2005) The skeletal system. In: Sharp, P.F., Gemmell, H.G. & Murray, A.D. (eds) *Practical Nuclear Medicine*. 3rd edn. London: Springer-Verlag; 143–161.

Love, C., Din, A.S., Tomas, M.B., et al. (2003) Radionuclide bone imaging: an illustrative review. *RadioGraphics* **23**, 341–358.

12

Brain

Methods of imaging the brain

Imaging the brain's structure and examining its physiology, both in the acute and elective setting, is now the domain of multiplanar, computer-assisted imaging. The imaging modalities in use today include the following:

1. **Computed tomography (CT).** This is the technique of choice for the investigation of serious head injury; for suspected intracranial haemorrhage, stroke, infection and other acute neurological emergencies. CT is quick, efficient and safer to use in the emergency situation than MRI.

2. **Magnetic resonance imaging (MRI).** This is the best and most versatile imaging modality for the brain, constrained only by availability, patient acceptability, and the logistics and safety of patient handling in emergency situations. New protocols and higher field strength magnets have raised the sensitivity of MRI in epilepsy imaging, acute stroke, aneurysm detection and follow-up post treatment of neoplastic and vascular disorders. It is the only effective way of diagnosing multiple sclerosis.

3. **Angiography.** This is very important in intracranial haemorrhage (ICH), especially subarachnoid haemorrhage (SAH). However, with the widespread availability of multi-detector CT scanners, CT angiography (CTA) is now preferentially used in ischaemic stroke, SAH and ICH. Angiography is still requested for pre-operative assessment of tumours and angiographic expertise is vital for the performance of many neurointerventional procedures.

4. **Radionuclide imaging.** There are two principal methods. The first is regional cerebral blood flow scanning, still more used in research than in clinical management, especially in the dementias and in movement disorders such as Parkinsonism; second is positron emission tomography (PET). By this method focal hyper-metabolism may be shown using F-18-fluorodeoxyglucose, for

example in epilepsy, and cell turnover may be shown using[11] C-methionine, for example in tumour studies.

5. **Ultrasound (US).** This is particularly helpful in neonates and during the first year of life to image haemorrhagic and ischaemic syndromes, developmental malformations, and hydrocephalus using the fontanelles as acoustic windows. In adults, transcranial Doppler may be used for intracerebral arterial velocity studies to assess the severity of vasospasm.

6. **Plain films of the skull.** These are of little value except in head injury.

COMPUTED TOMOGRAPHY OF THE BRAIN

Indications

CT is the imaging modality most commonly used in triaging acute neurological disease. For non-emergency indications CT is second best, but is still widely used, often because it is more broadly available and simpler to interpret. The indications include the following:

1. Following major head injury (if the patient has lost consciousness, has impaired consciousness, or has a neurological deficit). The presence of a skull fracture also justifies the use of CT. NICE (National Institute for Health and Clinical Excellence) guidance has been issued on the use of imaging for head injuries for adults and children, specifically CT, listing the criteria for assessment based on best relevant data and consensus recommendations.

2. In suspected intracranial infection (the use of contrast enhancement is recommended).

3. For suspected intracranial haemorrhage and cases of ischaemic and haemorrhagic stroke.

4. In suspected raised intracranial pressure, and as a precaution before lumbar puncture once certain criteria are fulfilled. These would include reduced consciousness (a Glasgow coma score of less than 12), definite papilloedema, focal neurological deficit, immune suppression and bleeding dyscrasias.

5. In other situations, such as epilepsy, migraine, suspected tumour, demyelination, dementia and psychosis CT is a lesser quality tool. If imaging can be justified, MRI is greatly preferable and is recommended by NICE in these situations except for first episode of psychosis.

Technique

1. Most clinical indications are adequately covered by 3-mm sections parallel to the floor of the anterior cranial fossa, from the foramen magnum to the midbrain, with 7-mm sections to the vertex. In all trauma cases, window width and level should be adjusted to examine bone and any haemorrhagic, space-occupying lesions. Review of all trauma studies should be done on brain windows, bone and 'blood windows' (i.e. W175 L75).

2. In suspected infection, tumours, vascular malformations and subacute infarction, the sections should be repeated following intravenous (i.v.) contrast enhancement. Standard precautions with regard to possible adverse reactions to contrast medium should be taken.

3. Dynamic studies using iodinated contrast are increasingly being used as a routine in high-velocity head trauma, the assessment of intracerebral bleeding in young patients, aneurysmal SAH, ruptured arteriovenous shunts and dural venous sinus thrombosis. CT angiography (CTA) on a typical 4-slice multidetector scanner is performed using 120 ml of contrast injected at $3\,\mathrm{ml\,s}^{-1}$ with a delay of 20 s. Slices of 1.25 mm are reconstructed at increments of 0.8 mm. CT venography (CTV) involves a delay of 100 s. Images are usually reviewed both as three-dimensional rendered data and multiplanar reformats (MPRs).

Further reading

Bruening, R. & Flohr, T. (2003) *Protocols for Multislice CT 4- and 16-row Applications*. Berlin: Springer Verlag.

Yates, D., Aktar, R. & Hill, J. (2007) Assessment, investigation, and early management of head injury: summary of NICE guidance. *BMJ* **335**, 719–720.

MAGNETIC RESONANCE IMAGING OF THE BRAIN

13

Indications

MRI is indicated in all cases of suspected intracranial pathology. Techniques in use change with the development of new sequences and higher field strength magnets. The techniques described below are, therefore, only basic indications as to sequences in use.

The greatest advantages in the use of MRI are the improved contrast resolution between grey and white matter, brain and cerebrospinal fluid (CSF); the removal of artifact due to bone close to the skull base and in the posterior fossa; and in obtaining multiplanar images for lesion localization.

Technique

1. **Long TR sequences.** The whole brain can be examined with 5-mm sections with 1-mm interspaces using T2-weighted turbo spin echo imaging. Proton density sequences, long TR and short TE, are used mostly for the assessment of demyelination and intra-articular disc changes in the temporomandibular joints.

2. **Short TR sequences.** T1-weighted sequences are used for the demonstration of detailed anatomy but gadolinium chelate contrast agents are required to view pathology. Common practice is to obtain a sagittal or coronal T1-weighted sequence as part of a standard brain study. Volumetric sequences pre and post contrast are used for image guidance software interfaces for insertion of deep brain stimulators for movement disorders and the removal of intra- and extra-axial tumours.

3. **Gradient-echo T2-weighted sequences.** Although suffering from various artifacts, the sensitivity of these sequences to susceptibility effects makes them very sensitive to the presence of blood products, as in cases of previous head injury, SAH and cavernomas. Haemosiderin produces marked focal loss of signal in such cases, and all patients with a history of head injury or other causes of haemorrhage should be imaged with this sequence.

4. **FLAIR sequences (FLuid Attenuated Inversion Recovery)** provide very good contrast resolution in the detection of demyelinating plaques and infarcts, and have the advantage that juxta-ventricular pathology contrasts with dark CSF, and is not lost by proximity to the intense brightness of the ventricular CSF, as in spin-echo T2-weighted studies.

5. **Angiographic sequences.** There are many methods, of which 'time-of flight' is one of the more commonly used. This is a very short TR, T1-weighted gradient echo three-dimensional sequence, with sequential presaturation of each partition so that only non-presaturated inflowing blood gives a high signal. Image display is by so-called 'MIP' or maximum intensity projection, giving a three-dimensional model of the intracranial vessels. Contrast-enhanced MR angiography requires a pump injector and is less susceptible to flow artifacts.

6. **Echoplanar or diffusion weighted imaging (DWI).** This sequence is becoming widely available on scanners. Most units perform DWI on all patients with suspected stroke, vasculitis, encephalitis, abscesses and in the workup of intracranial tumours. DWI examines the free movement, or Brownian motion, of water molecules at a cellular level. In acute infarcts cytotoxic oedema prevents free movement of water whereas in tumours there is no restriction. All DWI should be reviewed together with conventional sequences and apparent diffusion coefficient (ADC) maps. Acute infarcts are hyperintense on DWI and hypointense on ADC.

IMAGING OF INTRACRANIAL HAEMORRHAGE

Imaging of suspected intracranial haemorrhage is one of the most common requests of clinicians, usually in the emergency setting. Follow-up of haematomas and formulating a differential diagnosis can sometimes be quite challenging. In the acute setting CT and the neurophysiological information available as a result of multidetector technology is often the first and only modality used to assess these patients. MRI is more often used in situations where the initial workup has been negative and a more sensitive modality is required.

COMPUTED TOMOGRAPHY

A conventional study consists of 3-mm sections through the brainstem and posterior fossa, and 7-mm sections through the cerebrum. This is the basic multi-detector CT protocol for brain imaging. This is done without contrast to avoid diagnostic difficulty in deciding whether a parenchymal lesion is due to enhancement or blood. Acute blood is typically hyperdense on CT. An exhaustive differential diagnosis for bleeding in different compartments of the brain can be sourced elsewhere but in general bleeding can be extra-axial (i.e. epidural, subdural, subarachnoid, intraventricular) or intra-axial. Intra-axial bleeding can be due to head trauma, ruptured aneurysms or arteriovenous malformations, bleeding tumours (either primary disease or secondaries), hypertensive haemorrhages (cortical or striatal) or haemorrhagic transformation of venous or arterial infarcts. In the assessment of subarachnoid haemorrhage and ischaemic stroke CTA is becoming increasingly used as the screening modality for deciding further intervention. Neurosurgeons are increasingly using CTA alone as the modality for planning microsurgical clipping, especially in the cases where a haematoma exerting mass effect needs to be evacuated immediately adjacent to a freshly ruptured intracranial

13

aneurysm. In ischaemic stroke CTA can localize an acute embolus and CT perfusion imaging can demonstrate the ischaemic core (irreversibly damaged brain) by calculating the relative cerebral blood volume and the ischaemic penumbra (recoverable brain parenchyma) by evaluating the relative cerebral blood flow (rCBF).

MAGNETIC RESONANCE IMAGING

MRI is used mostly to exclude the presence of an underlying tumour at an interval after the initial haemorrhage when there would be less perilesional brain swelling and obscuration of the anatomy due to blood degradation products. It is also used in the setting of subarachnoid bleeding where no aneurysm or arteriovenous malformation is found on CTA or catheter angiography. In these cases the entire neuraxis must be examined to exclude an 'occult' source of the haemorrhage. Diffuse axonal shear injuries, in patients with depressed coma scores post head injury, in light of a normal appearing CT scan, are best demonstrated on MRI with gradient echo imaging looking for susceptibility artifact due to 'microbleeds'. Where resources are optimal, and MRI is used as part of the initial imaging pathway in ischaemic stroke, MR will help to determine the volumes of brain that can be recovered as well as the presence of early haemorrhage that is not visible on CT which would contraindicate thrombolysis.

Further reading

Wada, R., Aviv R.I., Fox, A.J., et al. (2007) CT angiography 'spot sign' predicts hematoma expansion in acute intracerebral hemorrhage. *Stroke* **38(4)**, 1257–1262.

Westerlaan, H.E., Gravendeel, J., Fiore, D., et al. (2007) Multislice CT angiography in the selection of patients with ruptured intracranial aneurysms suitable for clipping or coiling. *Neuroradiology* **49(12)**, 997–1007.

IMAGING OF GLIOMAS

This is an all-encompassing term for a diverse group of primary brain tumours. This includes astrocytomas, oligodendrogliomas, choroid plexus tumours and ependymomas amongst others. The most commonly presenting tumour, however, is the WHO Grade IV astrocytoma or glioblastoma multiforme. Other brain tumours are derived from neuronal cell lines, mixed glial-neuronal cell lines, the pineal gland and embryonal cell lines, peripheral cranial nerves (such as the vestibular schwannoma), meningeal tumours and lymphoma. Appropriate differential diagnoses can be derived from noting the age of the patient, the tumour location (i.e. supra- or infratentorial, cortex or white matter, basal ganglia or brainstem, intra- or extra-axial), its consistency (i.e. cyst formation, mural nodule) and its enhancement characteristics.

COMPUTED TOMOGRAPHY

CT is often the first modality to demonstrate the presence of a brain tumour. The indications for scanning can include unrelenting morning headaches, drowsiness, stroke-like presentation and seizures. In addition to making the initial diagnosis, multidetector CT can be used for obtaining high-resolution datasets for image guidance for brain biopsies, with and without stereotactic frames. In the absence of advanced MR neuroimaging software and for patients who are unable to undergo MR, imaging multidetector CT can be used to obtain rCBF data for tumour matrix as well as the normal brain. Studies have been performed to correlate ratios of rCBF with tumour grade, assessment of radiation necrosis or dedifferentiation when following up tumours.

MAGNETIC RESONANCE IMAGING

MRI is the preferred modality for detailed assessment of brain tumours. In addition to using conventional imaging parameters to assess volume, location and tumour substance in multiple planes, advanced imaging techniques or 'multi-modality' imaging can reveal information about tumour grade and biology. Conventional T1 and T2 images are obtained. Diffusion-weighted imaging and diffusion tractography reveals information about tumour substance and effect on white matter tracts in the brainstem and the cerebrum. Multiple lesions, if present, can be better seen on post-contrast MRI, in which case metastatic disease becomes a consideration in the differential diagnosis. As grade IV gliomas can have a similar appearance, a search for a primary epithelial neoplasm elsewhere (for example breast and lung) would be indicated. MR spectroscopy is a technique whereby relative amounts of cell metabolites are detected to reflect the biochemical environment in a tumour. N-acetylaspartate, choline, creatine, lactate and myo-inositol are a few of the major metabolites assessed. Single voxel techniques are preferable using STEAM (stimulated echo acquisition mode) or point resolved spectroscopy (PRESS). Perfusion-weighted imaging can provide information about tumour grade and help to differentiate between tumour recurrence and radiation necrosis. Susceptibility perfusion imaging is most often used where gradient echo images are obtained of the entire brain during the first pass of gadolinium chelate and analysis of the collated data using small regions of interest is carried out looking at normal brain and the tumour. MPRAGE (magnetization-prepared rapid-acquisition gradient echo) volumetric data can also be used post contrast for image guidance for biopsy or tumour debulking.

13

Further reading

Al-Okaili, R.N., Krejza, J., Wang, S., et al. (2006) Advanced MR imaging techniques in the diagnosis of intra-axial brain tumors in adults. *RadioGraphics* **26**, S173–S189.

Stadlbauer, A., Gruber, S., Nimsky, C., et al. (2006) Preoperative grading of gliomas by using metabolite quantification with high-spatial-resolution proton MR spectroscopic imaging. *Radiology* **238**, 958–969.

IMAGING OF ACOUSTIC NEUROMAS

MRI is the definitive diagnostic method. The neurophysiological methods, although quite sensitive, produce a large number of false-positive studies.

COMPUTED TOMOGRAPHY

Some departments use 2-mm section i.v. contrast-enhanced CT with bone and soft-tissue windowed images for suspected acoustic neuroma to relieve pressure on their MRI services. This approach is usually reserved for elderly patients, mostly to exclude the presence of large lesions that may require debulking or excision. Intracanalicular tumours cannot be shown by this method but surgically these will not be addressed.

MAGNETIC RESONANCE IMAGING

Most imaging departments will have a 1.5-T scanner where MR cisternography sequences are available, nulling the CSF pulsation artifact and highlighting the appearances of cranial nerves, arteries and veins which may also be contributing to sensorineural deafness and tinnitus. Nulling the pulsation artifact from CSF provides the contrast required and images as thin as 0.8 mm, with no gap, can be obtained. From this kind of data multiplanar, reformatted images can be reviewed. Post-contrast studies are obtained when a change in the contour of the nerve is observed or a filling defect is seen in the labyrinthine structures.

Further reading

Rupa, V., Job, A., George, M., et al. (2003) Cost-effective initial screening for vestibular schwannoma: auditory brainstem response or magnetic resonance imaging? *Otolaryngol. Head Neck Surg.* **128(6)**, 823–828.

RADIONUCLIDE IMAGING OF THE BRAIN

There are currently two main modalities: regional cerebral blood flow imaging and PET imaging. Thallium imaging is also used in specialist centres for brain tumour assessment and there are niche agents in clinical practice used, for example in the diagnosis of Parkinson's disease. Conventional radionuclide brain scanning (blood–brain barrier imaging) is essentially never used in modern clinical practice.

Further reading
Freeman, L.M. & Blaufox, M.D. (eds) (2003) Functional brain imaging. *Sem. Nucl. Med.* **33**, (1 and 2)

CONVENTIONAL RADIONUCLIDE BRAIN SCANNING (BLOOD–BRAIN BARRIER IMAGING)

This technique is not indicated if CT and/or MRI are available. It was a technique that used i.v. injection of the radiopharmaceuticals ^{99m}Tc-DTPA and ^{99m}Tc-pertechnetate to detect areas of blood–brain barrier breakdown and demonstrate cerebral metastases, meningioma and high-grade glioma.

REGIONAL CEREBRAL BLOOD FLOW IMAGING

Indications
1. Localization of epileptic foci
2. Mapping of cerebrovascular disease
3. Investigation of dementias including Huntington's and Alzheimer's disease
4. Assessment of effects of treatment regimes
5. Confirmation of brain death.

Contraindications
None.

Radiopharmaceuticals
1. ^{99m}Tc-hexamethylpropyleneamineoxime (HMPAO or exametazime), 500 MBq (5 mSv ED).
   The most commonly used agent, HMPAO is a lipophilic complex that crosses the blood–brain barrier and localizes

13

roughly in proportion to cerebral blood flow. It is rapidly extracted by the brain, reaching a peak of 5–6% of injected activity within a minute or so, with minimal redistribution (about 86% remains in the brain at 24 h).

2. ^{99m}Tc-ethyl cysteinate dimer (ECD), 500 MBq (5 mSv ED). This localizes rapidly in proportion to cellular metabolism rather than blood flow, and the distribution has some differences to that of HMPAO, which may need to be taken into consideration for clinical diagnosis.[1,2] It currently has the advantage of greater stability than HMPAO and can be used for up to 6 h after reconstitution, which is of particular benefit for ictal epilepsy studies where an injection is only given once a seizure occurs.

Equipment

1. Single photon emission computed tomography (SPECT) gamma camera, preferably dual-headed
2. SPECT imaging couch with head extension
3. Low-energy high-resolution collimator (or more specialized slant-hole or fan-beam collimator).

Patient preparation

Since cerebral blood flow is continuously varying with motor activity, sensory stimulation, emotional arousal, etc., it is important to standardize the conditions under which the tracer is administered, especially if serial studies are to be undertaken in the same individual. Familiarization with the procedure to reduce anxiety and injection in a relaxing environment through a previously positioned i.v. cannula should be considered.

For localization of epileptic foci, ictal studies are much more sensitive than interictal, and if feasible the patient should be admitted under constant monitoring, with injection as soon as a seizure starts.

Technique

1. Administer 500 MBq of tracer
2. SPECT imaging is performed any time from 5 min to 2 h after injection with the patient supine.

Images

The acquisition protocol will depend upon the system available. Suitable parameters for a modern single-headed gamma-camera might be:

1. 360° circular orbit
2. 60–90° projections or continuous rotation over a 30-min acquisition

3. Combination of matrix size and zoom to give a pixel size of 3–4 mm.

Analysis

A cine film of the projections is looked at before the patient leaves to detect any movement. If significant movement has occurred and cannot be corrected by computer motion correction algorithms available, the patient must be re-scanned. SPECT reconstructions are made in three planes.

Additional techniques

1. If blood flow in the carotid and major cerebral arteries is of interest, a dynamic study during injection is performed.
2. Three-dimensional mapping of activity distributions onto standard brain atlases and image registration with MRI, CT and quantitative analysis are areas of increasing interest, particularly with the development of SPECT-CT scanners.

Aftercare

Radiation dose may be reduced by administration of a mild laxative on the day after the study and maintenance of good hydration to promote urine output.

Complications

None.

References
1. Asenbaum, S., Brücke, T., Pirker, W., et al. (1998) Imaging of cerebral blood flow with technetium-99m-HMPAO and technetium-99m-ECD: a comparison. *J. Nucl. Med.* **39(4)**, 613–618.
2. Koyama, M., Kawashima, R., Ito, H., et al. (1997) SPECT imaging of normal subjects with technetium-99m-HMPAO and technetium-99m-ECD. *J. Nucl. Med.* **38(4)**, 587–592.

Further reading
Murray, A. D. (2005) The brain, salivary and lacrimal glands. In: Sharp, P.F., Gemmell, H.G. & Murray, A.D. (eds) *Practical Nuclear Medicine*. 3rd edn. London: Springer-Verlag.

POSITRON EMISSION TOMOGRAPHY

Indications

1. Localization of epileptic foci
2. Investigation of dementias
3. Grading of brain tumours.

Contraindications

1. Recent chemotherapy – minimum interval of 2–3 weeks recommended
2. Recent radiotherapy – minimum interval of 8–12 weeks recommended
3. Poorly controlled diabetes, i.e. serum glucose >8.5 mmol l at time of scanning.

Radiopharmaceuticals

Fluorine-18 fluorodeoxyglucose (^{18}FDG) is a glucose analogue which is the most commonly used agent for oncological work and is also used for the investigation of dementias. There are other radio-pharmaceuticals, e.g. L-[methyl-^{11}C]methionine ([^{11}C] MET) or 3′-deoxy-3′-[^{18}F] fluorothymidine ([^{18}F] FLT) which have the advantage of little normal cerebral uptake.

Patient preparation

Fasting for 4–6 h, with plenty of non-sugary fluids.

Technique

1. ^{18}FDG -up to the UK limit of 400 MBq i.v. (10 mSv ED) is administered.
2. To reduce muscle uptake of ^{18}FDG, patients should remain in a relaxed environment such as lying in a darkened room, without talking if head and neck area are being imaged, between injection and scan.
3. Image at 1 h post injection. Later imaging has been reported to enhance tumour conspicuity due to a higher tumour to background ratio.
4. If combined with CT scanning:
   a. low-dose CT technique
   b. no i.v. contrast medium.
5. PET imaging of:
   a. brain
   b. whole body if indicated.

Alternative techniques

1. L-[methyl-^{11}C]methionine ([^{11}C] MET) or 3′-deoxy-3′-[^{18}F] fluorothymidine ([^{18}F] FLT) PET
2. ^{201}Thallium
3. MR spectroscopy.

^{201}THALLIUM BRAIN SCANNING

Indications

1. CNS (and other) tumours:
   a. grading
   b. differentiation of post surgical or radiotherapy change from residual or recurrent tumours.

   This radionuclide procedure has largely been superceded by PET.

Contraindications

None.

Radiopharmaceutical

^{201}Thallium 100 MBq (25 mSv ED).

Equipment

1. SPECT gamma camera
3. VerteX High Resolution (VXHR) gamma camera.

Technique

I.v. injection of radiopharmaceutical.

Analysis

SPECT.

Aftercare

None.

DOPAMINE TRANSPORTER LIGANDS

Indications

Ioflupane, 123-I FP-CIT (DatSCAN, GE Healthcare) contains a dopamine transporter radioligand and can be used to assess striatal uptake in possible Parkinson's disease, and differentiate from other movement disorders.

Contraindications

None.

Radiopharmaceuticals

^{123}I DatSCAN 185 MBq (4.5 mSv ED)

Equipment

1. SPECT gamma camera
2. VXHR.

Patient preparation

Thyroid blockade (400 mg potassium perchlorate orally 1 h before scan, 200 mg every 6 h for four doses).

Technique

I.v. injection of radiopharmaceutical.

Images

Image with SPECT at 3–6 h.

Analysis

Diagnosis depend on an assessment of relative uptake in the caudate and putamen.

Aftercare

None.

Further reading

Hammoud, D.A., Hoffman, J.M., Pomper, M.G., et al. (2007) Molecular neuroimaging: from conventional to emerging techniques. *Radiology* **245(1)**, 21–42.

ULTRASOUND OF THE INFANT BRAIN

Indications
Any suspected intracranial pathology, particularly suspected germinal matrix haemorrhage, extra-axial haematomas and hydrocephalus.

Equipment
4–7-MHz, sector transducer. A 7.5- or 10-MHz transducer to visualize superficial structures.

Patient preparation
None is required, though a recently fed infant is more likely to submit to examination without protest. An agitated child should be calmed by the mother or carer by any appropriate method.

Methods
1. Via the anterior fontanelle
2. Through the squamosal portion of the temporal bone to visualize extracerebral collections and the region of the circle of Willis
3. Via the posterior fontanelle, for the posterior fossa.

Technique
Six coronal and six sagittal images are obtained and supplemented with other images of specific areas of interest. The base of the skull must be perfectly symmetrical on coronal scans. The first image is obtained with the transducer angled forward and subsequent images obtained by angling progressively more posteriorly. The anatomical landmarks that define each view are given below.

Coronal
1. The orbital roofs and cribriform plate (these combine to produce a 'steer's head' appearance); anterior interhemispheric fissure; frontal lobes
2. Greater wings, lesser wings and body of sphenoid (these produce a 'mask' appearance); the cingulate sulcus; frontal horns of lateral ventricles
3. Pentagon view: five-sided star formed by the internal carotid, middle cerebral and anterior cerebral arteries
4. Frontal horns of lateral ventricles; cavum septum pellucidum; basal ganglia. Bilateral C-shaped echoes from the parahippocampal gyri; thalami
5. Trigones of lateral ventricles containing choroid plexus; echogenic inverted V from the tentorium cerebelli; cerebellum

13

6. Occipital horns of lateral ventricles; parietal and occipital cortex; cerebellum.

Sagittal

For the sagittal images, the reference plane should be a mid-line image with the third ventricle, septum pellucidum and fourth ventricle all on the same image. The more lateral parasagittal images are obtained with the transducer angled laterally and slightly oblique because the occipital horn of the lateral ventricle is more lateral than the frontal horn:

1. Two views of the mid-line
2. Parasagittal scans of the lateral ventricles. These are angled approximately 15° from the mid-line, to show the caudothalamic grooves
3. Steep parasagittal scans, approximately 30° from the mid-line, of the frontal, temporal and parietal cortices.

CEREBRAL ANGIOGRAPHY

Indications

1. Intracerebral and subarachnoid haemorrhage
2. Aneurysms presenting as space-occupying lesions
3. Brain arteriovenous shunts, carotico-cavernous fistulas (direct and indirect)
4. Cerebral ischaemia both of extracranial and intracranial origin
5. Pre-operative assessment of intracranial tumours.

Contraindications

1. Patients with unstable neurology (usually following subarachnoid haemorrhage or stroke)
2. Patients unsuitable for surgery
3. Patients in whom vascular access would be impossible or relatively risky
4. Iodine allergy. Relative contraindication as angiography could be performed with gadolinium chelates.

Equipment

A single or biplane digital subtraction angiography apparatus is required, with a C-arm allowing unlimited imaging planes, high-quality fluoroscopy, and road-mapping facility.

Three-dimensional rotational angiography is now increasingly available and forms an important part of the analysis of aneurysms during treatment. There should be access to the patient for both the radiologist and the anaesthetist, with appropriate head immobilization.

Preparation

When the patient is able to understand what is proposed, a clear explanation should be given, together with presentation of the risks and benefits. Most patients do not require sedation for diagnostic procedures and this would be contraindicated in acute neurological presentations. Children, patients who are excessively anxious, those who cannot cooperate because of confusion, or those who would be managed better during the procedure with full ventilation control are examined under general anaesthesia. Neurointerventional studies are done under general anaesthesia. Groin shaving is now regarded as unnecessary. Patients should not be starved unless general anaesthesia is to be used, but should, nevertheless, be restricted to fluid intake and only a light meal.

Technique

Catheter flushing solutions should consist of heparinized saline ($2500\,IU\,I^{-1}$ normal saline). Using standard percutaneous catheter introduction techniques, the femoral artery is catheterized. There is a wide range of catheters available and there are proponents of many types. In patients up to middle age without major hypertension, there will be little difficulty with any standard catheter and a simple 4F polythene catheter with a slightly curved tip or 45° bend will suffice in the majority. Older patients and those with atherosclerotic disease may need catheters offering greater torque control such as the JB2 or Simmons (Figs 13.1 & 13.2) as appropriate. Catheter control will be better if passed through an introducer set, and this is also indicated where it is anticipated that catheter exchange may be required. Selective studies of the common carotids and the vertebrals are preferable to super selective studies of the internal and external carotids unless absolutely necessary. The following points should be noted:

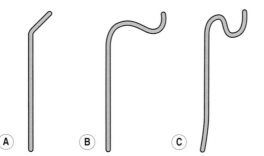

Ⓐ   Ⓑ   Ⓒ

13

Figure 13.1 (a) Vertebrale or Berenstein, (b) JB 2, (c) Mani. End holes: 1 Side holes: 0.

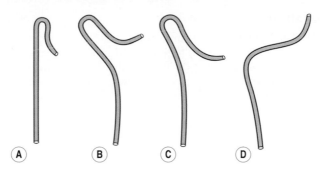

Figure 13.2 Simmons (sidewinder) catheters. (a) For narrow aorta. (b) For moderately narrow aorta. (c) For wide aorta. (d) For elongated aorta. End holes: 1 Side holes: 0.

1. The hazards of cerebral angiography are largely avoidable; they consist of the complications common to all forms of angiography (see Chapter 9) and those which are particularly related to cerebral angiography.
2. Any on-table ischaemic event has an explanation. Cerebral angiography does not possess an inherently unavoidable complication rate as has been suggested in the past. If an ischaemic event occurs there has been a complication, and its cause must be identified.
3. The most significant complications are embolic in origin, and the most important emboli are particulate. Air bubbles should be avoided as part of good angiographic practice, but are unlikely to cause a neurological complication.
4. Emboli may come from the injected solutions. Avoid contamination from glove powder, and dried blood or clot on gloves. Take care to avoid blood contamination of the saline or of the contrast medium, which is always dangerous. Avoid exposure of solutions to air. Contrast medium or heparin/saline in an open bowl is bad practice.
5. Emboli may arise from dislodgement of plaque or thrombus. Never pass a catheter or guidewire through a vessel that has not been visualized by preliminary injection of contrast medium. Use appropriate angled, hydrophilic guidewires. Do not try to negotiate excessively acute bends in vessels. The splinting effect of the catheter will cause spasm and arrest the flow in the artery. Dissections could occur which may lead to occlusion. Sharp curves can only be safely negotiated with microcatheters.
6. Emboli may arise from the formation of thrombus within a catheterized vessel. Always ensure that there is free blood flow past the catheter, and avoid forceful passage of a guidewire

or catheter in such a way as may damage the intima of the vessel and cause thrombus formation.

7. Emboli may arise within the catheter. Do not allow blood to flow back into the catheter, or if it does occur then flush regularly or by continuous infusion. Never allow a guidewire to remain within a catheter for more than 1 min without withdrawal and flushing, and never introduce a guidewire into a contrast filled catheter, but fill the catheter with heparinized saline first.

8. Keep study time to a minimum, but not at the expense of the diagnostic usefulness of the study.

Contrast medium

Non-ionic monomer, e.g. iohexol, iopamidol. The concentration required is equipment-dependent, but with modern DSA, $150\,g\,I\,ml^{-1}$ will be suitable.

Contrast medium volume

1. Common carotid –10 ml by hand in about 1.5–2 s
2. Internal carotid – 7 ml by hand in about 1.5 s
3. Vertebral artery – 7 ml by hand in about 1.5 s, but this volume can be diluted by 2 ml of saline to opacify the contralateral vertebral on the same injection.

Projections

As required, but basically 20° anterior-posterior (AP), Townes, lateral, occipitomental and oblique views as indicated. Multiple projections are especially needed for aneurysm studies to open loops and profile aneurysms; however, with three-dimensional rotational angiography, contrast runs can now be cut down to a minimum, and computer models of aneurysms and vessels can analysed instead.

Films

From early arterial to late venous, about 8 s in total in most cases, system acquisitions will be at 2–4 frames s^{-1} depending on the study. With digital fluoroscopy acquisitions typically will be 2 frames s^{-1} for 4 s, then 1 frame every 2 s for 4 s.

Aftercare

1. Standard nursing care for the arterial puncture site
2. Most departments adopt the practice of maintaining neurological observation for a period of 4 h or so after the procedure
3. Good hydration should be maintained.

13

Spine

Methods of imaging the spine

Many of the earlier imaging methods are now only of historical interest (e.g. conventional tomography, epidurography, epidural venography):

1. **Plain films.** These are widely available, but with low sensitivity. They are of questionable value in chronic back pain because of the prevalence of degenerative changes in both symptomatic and asymptomatic individuals of all ages beyond the second decade. They are, however, useful in suspected spinal injury, spinal deformity and post-operative assessment.

2. **Myelography/radiculography.** This is used when MRI is contraindicated or unacceptable to the patient. It is usually followed by CT for detailed assessment of abnormalities (CT myelography).

3. **Discography.** Advocates still regard it as the only technique able to verify the presence and source of discogenic pain.

4. **Facet joint arthrography.** Facet joint pain origin can be confirmed if it is abolished after diagnostic injection of local anaesthetic, and treated by steroid instillation. The radiological appearances of the arthrogram are not helpful for the most part except in showing a communication with a synovial cyst. Vertical and contralateral facet joint communications can arise in the presence of pars interarticularis defects.

5. **Arteriography.** This is used for further study of vascular malformations shown by other methods, usually MRI, and for assessment for potential embolotherapy. It is not appropriate for the primary diagnosis of spinal vascular malformations. It may be used for pre-operative embolization of vascular vertebral tumours (e.g. renal metastasis).

6. **Radionuclide imaging.** This is largely performed for suspected vertebral metastases and to exclude an occult painful bone lesion (e.g. osteoid osteoma) using a technetium scintigraphic agent, for which it is a sensitive and cost-effective technique.

7. **Computed tomography (CT).** CT provides optimal detail of vertebral structures and is particularly useful in spinal trauma, spondylolysis, vertebral tumours, spinal deformity and post-operative states, especially if multidetector CT (MDCT) is available.

8. **Magnetic resonance imaging (MRI).** This is the preferred technique for virtually all spinal pathology. It is the only technique that directly images the spinal cord and nerve roots. MRI with intravenous (i.v.) gadolinium-DTPA is indicated in spinal infection, tumours and post-operative assessment.

9. **Ultrasound (US).** Is of use as an intra-operative method, and has uses in the infant spine.

IMAGING APPROACH TO BACK PAIN AND SCIATICA

There are a variety of ways to image the spine, many of which are expensive. The role of the radiologist is to ensure that diagnostic algorithms are selected for diagnostic accuracy, clinical relevance and cost-effectiveness. Each diagnostic imaging procedure has a different degree of sensitivity and specificity when applied to a particular diagnostic problem. A combination of imaging techniques can be used in a complementary way to enhance diagnostic accuracy. The appropriate use of the available methods of investigating the spine is essential, requiring a sensible sequence and timing of the procedures to ensure cost-effectiveness, maximal diagnostic accuracy and clinical effectiveness with minimum discomfort to the patient.

The philosophy underlying the management of low back pain and sciatica encompasses the following fundamental points:

1. Radiological investigation is essential if surgery is proposed.
2. Radiological findings should be compatible with the clinical picture before surgery can be advised.
3. It is vital for the surgeon and radiologist to identify those patients who will and who will not benefit from surgery.
4. In those patients judged to be in need of surgical intervention, success is very dependent on precise identification of the site, nature and extent of disease by the radiologist.
5. The demonstration of degenerative disease of the spine by non-invasive methods cannot be assumed to be the cause of the patient's symptoms, as similar changes are often seen in asymptomatic individuals.

The need for radiological investigation of the lumbosacral spine is based on the results of a thorough clinical examination. A useful and basic preliminary step, which will avoid unnecessary investigations, is to determine whether the predominant symptom is back pain or leg pain. Leg pain extending to the foot is indicative of nerve root compression and imaging needs to be directed towards the demonstration of a compressive lesion, typically disc prolapse. This is most commonly seen at the L4/5 or L5/S1 levels (90–95%), and MRI should be employed as the primary mode of imaging. If the predominant symptom is back pain with or without proximal lower limb radiation, then invasive techniques may be required, including discography and facet joint arthrography. The presence of degenerative disc and facet disease demonstrated by plain films, CT or MRI has no direct correlation with the incidence of clinical symptomatology. The annulus fibrosus of the intervertebral disc and the facet joints are richly innervated, and only direct injection can assess them as a potential pain source. However, unless there are therapeutic implications there is no indication to go to these lengths, as many patients can be managed by physiotherapy and mild analgesics.

CONVENTIONAL RADIOGRAPHY

Routine radiographic evaluation at the initial assessment of a patient with acute low back pain does not usually provide clinically useful information. Eighty-five per cent of such patients will return to work within 2 months having received only conservative therapy, indicating the potential for non-contributory imaging. Despite the known limitations of radiographs, it is often helpful to obtain routine radiographs of the lumbar spine before another investigation is requested. The role of conventional radiographs can be summarized in the following points:

1. They assist in the diagnosis of conditions that can mimic mechanical or discogenic pain, e.g. infection, spondylolysis, ankylosing spondylitis and bone tumours, though in most circumstances ^{99m}Tc scintigraphy, CT and MRI are more sensitive.
2. They serve as a technical aid to survey the vertebral column and spinal canal prior to myelography, CT or MRI, particularly in the sense of providing basic anatomical data regarding segmentation. Failure to do this may lead to errors in interpreting correctly the vertebral level of abnormalities prior to surgery.
3. Correlation of CT or MRI data with radiographic appearances is often helpful in interpretation.

14

COMPUTED TOMOGRAPHY AND MAGNETIC RESONANCE IMAGING OF THE SPINE

CT and MRI have replaced myelography as the primary method for investigating suspected disc prolapse. High-quality axial imaging by CT is an accurate means of demonstrating disc herniation, but in practice many studies are less than optimal due to obesity, scoliosis and beam-hardening effects due to dense bone sclerosis. For these reasons, and because of better contrast resolution, MRI is the preferred technique and CT is only employed when MRI cannot be used. MRI alone has the capacity to show the morphology of the intervertebral disc, and can show ageing changes, typically dehydration, in the nucleus pulposus. It provides sagittal sections, which have major advantages for the demonstration of the spinal cord and cauda equina, vertebral alignment, stenosis of the spinal canal, and for showing the neural foramina. Far lateral disc herniation cannot be shown by myelography, but is readily demonstrated by CT or MRI. CT may be preferred to MRI where there is a suspected spinal injury, in the assessment of primary spinal tumours of bony origin, and in the study of spondylolysis and Paget's disease. MRI in spinal stenosis provides all the required information showing all the relevant levels on a single image, the degree of narrowing at each level and the secondary effects such as the distension of the vertebral venous plexus. The relative contributions of bone, osteophyte, ligament or disc, while better evaluated by CT, are relatively unimportant in the management decisions. Furthermore, MRI will show conditions which may mimic spinal stenosis such as prolapsed thoracic disc, ependymoma of the conus medullaris and dural arteriovenous fistula.

In addition to the diagnosis of prolapsed intervertebral disc, CT and MRI differentiate the contained disc, where the herniated portion remains in continuity with the main body of the disc, from the sequestrated disc where there is a free migratory disc fragment. This distinction may be crucial in the choice of conservative or surgical therapy, and of percutaneous rather than open surgical techniques. MRI studies have shown that even massive *extruded* disc lesions can resolve naturally with time, without intervention. Despite the presence of nerve root compression, a disc prolapse can be entirely asymptomatic. Gadolinium enhancement of compressed lumbar nerve roots is seen in *symptomatic* disc prolapse with a specificity of 95.9%.[1]

Finally, in the decision as to whether to choose CT or MRI it should be remembered that lumbar spine CT delivers a substantial radiation dose, which is important, particularly in younger patients.

The main remaining uses of myelography are in patients with claustrophobia or otherwise not suitable for MRI. There are advocates for the use of CT myelography in the investigation of MRI negative cervical radiculopathy. Myelography also allows a dynamic assessment of the spinal canal in instances of spinal stenosis and instability. The use of a special MR compatible spinal harness that provides axial loading, and the availability of open and upright MR scanners also provide non-invasive dynamic MR imaging capability.

The problems of the 'post-laminectomy' patient or 'failed back surgery syndrome' are well known. Accurate pre-operative assessment should limit the number of cases resulting from inappropriate surgery and surgery at the wrong level. The investigation of the post-operative lumbar spine is difficult, and re-operation has a poor outcome in many cases. Although the investigation of the post-operative lumbar spine is difficult, it is vital to make the distinction between residual or recurrent disc prolapse at the operated level and epidural fibrosis, in order to minimize the risk of a negative re-exploration. The best available technique is gadolinium-enhanced MRI.

Arachnoiditis is a cause of post-operative symptoms and its features are shown on myelography, CT myelography and MRI. In the past, many cases were caused by the use of myodil (Pantopaque) as a myelographic contrast medium. It is likely that the use of myodil as an intrathecal contrast agent caused arachnoiditis in most cases, but this became symptomatic in only a minority. The potentiating effects of blood in the CSF, particularly as a result of surgery, have been evident in many cases. New cases of arachnoiditis are now rarely seen, but there is residue of chronic disease still presenting from time to time.

Conclusions

MRI has revolutionized the imaging of spinal disease. Advantages include non-invasiveness, multiple imaging planes and lack of radiation exposure. Its superior soft tissue contrast enables the distinction of nucleus pulposus from annulus fibrosus of the healthy disc and enables the early diagnosis of degenerative changes. However, up to 35% of asymptomatic individuals less than 40 years of age have significant intervertebral disc disease at one or more levels on MRI images. Correlation with the clinical evidence is, therefore, essential before any relevance is attached to their presence and surgery is undertaken. As MRI is, at present, not as accurate as discography in the diagnosis and delineation of annular disease, and in diagnosing the pain source, there has been a resurgence of interest in discography. MRI should be used as a predictor of the causative levels contributing to the back pain with discography having a significant role in the investigation of discogenic pain prior to surgical fusion.[2]

References
1. Tyrrell, P.N., Cassar-Pullicino, V.N. & McCall, I.W. (1998) Gadolinium-DTPA enhancement of symptomatic nerve roots in MRI of the lumbar spine. *Eur. Radiol.* **8(1)**, 116–122.
2. Cassar-Pullicino, V.N. (1998) MRI of the ageing and herniating intervertebral disc. *Eur. J. Radiol.* **27(3)**, 214-228.

14

Further reading

Boden, S., Davis, D.O., Dina, T.S., et al. (1990) Abnormal magnetic resonance scans of the lumbar spine in asymptomatic subjects. *J. Bone Joint Surg. Am.* **72(3)**, 403–408.

Butt, W.P. (1989) Radiology for back pain. *Clin. Radiol.* **40(1)**, 6–10.

Cribb, G.L., Jaffray, D.C. & Cassar-Pullicino, V.N. (2007) Observations on the natural history of massive lumbar disc herniation. *J. Bone Joint Surg. Br.* **89(6)**, 782–784.

Du Boulay, G.H., Hawkes, S., Lee, C.C., et al. (1990) Comparing the cost of spinal MR with conventional myelography and radiculography. *Neuroradiology* **32(2)**, 124–136.

Horton, W.C. & Daftari, T.K. (1992) Which disc as visualized by magnetic resonance imaging is actually a source of pain? A correlation between magnetic resonance imaging and discography. *Spine* **17(6Suppl)**, S164–S171.

Hueftle, M.G., Modic, M.T., Ross, J.S., et al. (1988) Lumbar spine: post-operative MR imaging with gadolinium-DTPA. *Radiology* **167(3)**, 817–824.

MYELOGRAPHY AND RADICULOGRAPHY

CONTRAST MEDIA

Historically, the contrast media that have been used for myelography include gas (CO_2, air), lipiodol, abrodil, myodil, (Pantopaque, iodophenylate), meglumine iothalamate (Conray), meglumine iocarmate (Dimer X), metrizamide (Amipaque), iopamidol (Niopam), iohexol (Omnipaque) and iotrolan (Isovist). The early oil-based media were diagnostically poor and led to arachnoiditis. The early water-soluble media were very toxic and also led to arachnoiditis, and the first intrathecal contrast medium with acceptably low toxicity was metrizamide, a non-ionic dimer. Iohexol and iopamidol are non-ionic monomers licensed for intrathecal use and the ones most commonly used currently.

CERVICAL MYELOGRAPHY

This may be performed by introduction of contrast medium into the thecal sac by lumbar puncture and then run up to the cervical spine, or by direct cervical puncture at C1/2.

Indications

Suspected spinal cord pathology or root compression in patients unable or unwilling to undergo MRI imaging.

Lateral cervical or C1/2 puncture v lumbar injection

Cervical puncture is quick, safe and reliable but is contraindicated in patients with suspected high cervical or cranio-cervical pathology, and where the normal bony anatomy and landmarks are distorted or lost by anomalous development or rheumatoid disease. Complications are rare but include vertebral artery damage and inadvertent cord puncture. Cervical puncture is particularly indicated where there is severe lumbar disease, which may restrict the flow of contrast medium and may make lumbar puncture difficult, and when there is thoracic spinal canal stenosis. It is also required for the demonstration of the upper end of a spinal block. It is not a good technique for whole-spine myelography; after completion of a cervical myelogram, the contrast medium is too dilute for effective use in the remainder of the spinal canal. When lumbar injection is used, a good lumbar study is possible without dilution, following which a cervical and thoracic study is entirely feasible. Lumbar injection for cervical myelography is as effective as cervical injection when nothing restricts the upward flow of contrast medium. The post-procedural morbidity, mainly consisting of headache, is rather less after cervical puncture.

Contrast medium

Nonioic contrast medium is used (see above). The total dose should not exceed 3 g of iodine, i.e. 10 ml of contrast medium with a concentration of 300 mg ml^{-1}. Adequate filling for cervical myelography usually only requires 7–8 ml, or even less when the canal is narrow.

Equipment

Tilting X-ray table with a C-arm fluoroscopic facility for screening and radiography in multiple planes.

Patient preparation

Mild sedation with oral diazepam is appropriate in anxious patients, but is not essential. The skin puncture point is outside the hair line and no hair removal is generally needed, though the hair should be gathered into a paper cap.

Technique

1. The patient lies prone with arms at the sides and chin resting on a soft pad so that the neck is in a neutral position or in slight extension. Marked hyperextension is undesirable as it accentuates patient discomfort, particularly in those with spondylosis, who comprise the majority of patients referred for this procedure. In such cases it will further compromise a narrowed canal and may produce symptoms of cord compression. The patient must be comfortable and able to breathe easily.

2. Using lateral fluoroscopy the C1/2 space is identified. The beam should be centred at this level to minimize errors due to parallax. Head and neck adjustments may be needed to ensure a true lateral position. The aim is to puncture the subarachnoid space between the laminae of C1 and C2, at the junction of the middle and posterior thirds of the spinal canal, i.e. posterior to the spinal cord. A 20G spinal needle is used. There is better control with the relatively stiff 20G needle, and the requirement for a small needle size to minimize CSF loss does not apply in the cervical region, where CSF pressure is very low.

3. Using aseptic technique, the skin and subcutaneous tissues are anaesthetized with 1% lidocaine. The spinal needle is introduced with the stilette bevel parallel to the long axis of the spine, i.e. to split rather than cut the fibres of the interlaminar ligaments. Lateral fluoroscopy is used to adjust the direction of the needle, and ensure the maintenance of a perfect lateral position as the needle is advanced. It is very helpful if a nurse steadies the patient's head.

4. The sensation of the needle penetrating the dura is similar to that experienced during a lumbar puncture and the patient may experience slight discomfort at this stage. A feature that indicates that the needle tip is close to the dura is the appearance of venous blood at the needle hub as the epidural space is traversed. If the needle trajectory is too far posterior, tenting of the dura may occur, with failure to puncture the CSF space, even though anterior-posterior (AP) screening may show that the needle tip has crossed the midline. Repositioning may be needed in such cases. Severe acute neck or radicular pain indicates that the needle has been directed too far anteriorly and has come into contact with an exiting nerve root. Clumsy technique is known to have caused cord puncture, but permanent neurological damage as a result is unlikely.

5. Following removal of the stilette, CSF will drip from the end of the needle, and a sample may be collected if required.

6. Under fluoroscopy a small amount of contrast medium is injected to verify correct needle-tip placement. This will flow away from the needle tip and gravitate anteriorly to layer behind the vertebral bodies. Transient visualization of the dentate ligaments is obtained.

7. Injection is continued slowly until the required amount has been delivered. The cervical canal should be opacified anteriorly from the foramen magnum to C7/T1. If contrast tends to flow into the head before filling the lower cervical canal, tilt the table feet down slightly, and vice-versa if contrast is flowing into the thoracic region without filling the upper cervical canal.

Radiographic views

After needle withdrawal, two AP radiographs are obtained with the tube angulated cranially and caudally, in turn, along with both oblique views once again with cranial and caudal tube tilt. A soft and penetrated lateral views are needed to ensure full assessment of the cervico-thoracic junction. Lastly, a further lateral view of the craniocervical junction is taken with mild neck flexion because all too often the extended neck position prevents full visualization of the upper cervical cord up to the foramen magnum.

Aftercare

Although many centres request the patient to remain sitting or semi-recumbent for about 6 h, allowing the patient to remain ambulant does not increase the incidence of side-effects. A high fluid intake is generally encouraged; though evidence for its usefulness is lacking.

LUMBAR RADICULOGRAPHY

This may be performed by injection of contrast medium into the lumbar thecal sac. If for any reason lumbar puncture is not possible, e.g. because of lumbar spine deformity or arachnoiditis, it is possible to introduce the contrast medium from above by cervical injection. Dilution of the contrast as it passes downwards is a major disadvantage.

Indications

Suspected lumbar root or cauda equina compression, spinal stenosis and conus medullaris lesions in patients who are unable or unwilling to undergo MRI.

Contraindications

Lumbar puncture is potentially hazardous in the presence of raised intracranial pressure. It may be difficult to achieve satisfactory intrathecal injection in patients who have had a recent lumbar puncture, since subdural CSF accumulates temporarily, and this space may be entered rather than the subarachnoid space. Accordingly an interval of 1 week or so is advisable.

Contrast medium

The contrast medium is the same as that used for cervical myelography. The maximum dose is again the equivalent of 3 g of iodine, and may be given as 10 ml of contrast medium of 300 mg ml^{-1} concentration, or 12.5 ml of 240 mg ml^{-1}.

Equipment

Tilting fluoroscopic table.

Patient preparation

As for cervical myelography.

Preliminary radiographs

AP and lateral projections of the region under study are taken. Preliminary examination of radiographs is helpful to assess the anatomy of the spine, in order to facilitate the lumbar puncture, and to assist in interpretation of the images. It is important to draw the surgeon's attention to any question of ambiguous segmentation, either lumbarization or sacralization. There is a potential danger of operating at the wrong level if this is not made absolutely clear in the report. A clear description of any anomaly is required, together with a statement of how the vertebrae have been numbered in the report.

Technique

1. The lumbar thecal sac is punctured at L2/3, L3/4 or L4/5. The higher levels tend to be away from the most common sites of disc herniation and stenosis, and puncture may, therefore, be easier.
2. Lumbar puncture can technically be performed in the lateral decubitus position, in the sitting position, or even in the prone position. In the prone position the needle is guided under fluoroscopy, usually at the L2/L3 interspinous space with the patient lying on a folded pillow. This is important, because in the prone position the spinous processes are approximated due to lordosis, rendering puncture more difficult. In addition, spinal extension produces a relatively narrow thecal sac. The sitting position allows easy lumbar puncture, but is unsatisfactory for two reasons. First, the injected contrast medium drops through a large volume of CSF to accumulate in the sacral sac and becomes diluted as it descends. Second, patients may faint in this position, a complication that can be very dangerous, since the radiologist is on the wrong side of the table to help in preventing the patient from coming to any harm.
3. If lumbar puncture is carried out in the lateral decubitus position (described below) moderate spinal flexion is desirable, but there is no need for the extreme flexion sometimes demanded of the patient. A small pillow is placed under the dependent lumbar angle to keep the spine straight. The relevant interspace is one or two spinous processes above the plane of the iliac crest (L4/L5). If the spinous process cannot be felt, lateral fluoroscopy may help.
4. In obese patients the apparent soft-tissue midline gravitates below the spinal midline. The midline position may be verified while introducing local anaesthetic (1% lidocaine) into the skin

and subcutaneous tissue, though there is no need to infiltrate the interspinous ligament. A 22G spinal needle should be used. It should be introduced with only a 10–15° cranial angulation. The passage of the needle through the interspinous ligament has a very characteristic sensation of moderate smooth resistance. Lack of resistance implies passage in the fatty tissues lateral to the midline, and a gritty sensation means impingement on the bone of the spinous process.

5. There is a tendency in inexperienced operators to introduce the needle at too steep a cranial angle, which a casual inspection of the spinous process anatomy can show to be incorrect. While traversing the interspinous ligament, the bevel should be in the coronal plane to avoid deflection to one side or the other, but once well established in the ligament may be turned to penetrate the thecal sac parallel to its long axis.

6. There is a characteristic sudden loss of resistance as the needle enters the thecal sac, and at this time the stilette should be withdrawn to verify CSF flow out of the needle. In the prone position suction using a 2-ml syringe may be necessary to obtain CSF. It should then be reintroduced and the needle advanced about 2 mm to ensure that the whole of the bevel has entered the thecal sac. A flexible connector is attached, taking care not to disturb the needle position.

7. Most difficulties are technical, arising from non-midline positioning of the needle, but in the presence of canal stenosis it may be difficult to find a position among the crowded roots where good CSF flow will take place. In most cases, radiologists will prefer to observe the entry of contrast medium into the thecal sac on the fluoroscopic screen, and this is especially important if there has been any difficulty in achieving a good needle position.

8. After the contrast medium has been injected, the patient turns to lie prone, and a series of films is obtained. Before taking films ensure that the relevant segment of the spinal canal is adequately filled with contrast medium. This usually requires some degree of feet down tilt of the table, and a footrest should be in place to support the patient.

Radiographic views

1. AP and oblique views are obtained. (About 25° of obliquity is usual, but tailored in the individual case to profile the exit sleeves of the nerve roots of the cauda equina.)

2. A lateral view with a horizontal beam is useful, but further laterals in the erect or semi-erect position on flexion and extension are very useful, adding a dynamic dimension to the study.

3. Some radiologists advocate lateral decubitus frontal oblique views, to allow full entry of contrast medium into the dependent root sleeves of the whole lumbar and lower thoracic thecal sac. When turning patients from one side to the other ensure that they turn through the prone position, as turning supine will produce irretrievable contrast medium dilution.

At this stage the study will be complete as far as the question of root compression is concerned. The films should be carefully reviewed at this stage to ensure that all areas are fully covered, as the next manoeuvre will make any return to this area impossible. If the study is good, the patient should be screened in the lateral decubitus position, and tilted level or slightly head down until the contrast medium flows up to lie across the thoraco-lumbar junction. The patient may then be turned to lie supine and films of the conus and lower thoracic area obtained in the AP projection.

Additional technique

Post-myelographic MDCT is helpful for good visualization of the conus and cause of root compression and should routinely be done after myelography.

THORACIC MYELOGRAPHY

If the thoracic spine is the primary region of interest the lumbar puncture injection is made with the patient lying on one side, with the head of the table lowered and the patient's head supported on a bolster or pad to prevent contrast medium from running up into the head. If an obstruction to flow is anticipated, about half the volume of contrast medium may be injected and observed as it flows upwards. If an obstruction is encountered, the contrast medium is allowed to accumulate against it, and the remainder of the contrast medium is then injected slowly (this may cause some discomfort or pain and patience must be used). This manoeuvre will, in some cases, cause a little of the contrast medium to flow past the obstructing lesion and demonstrate its superior extent. If there is no obstruction, the full volume is injected. When the injection is complete, lateral radiographs may be taken and the patient then turned to lie supine. Further AP views are then taken.

CERVICAL MYELOGRAPHY BY LUMBAR INJECTION

The technique proceeds as for thoracic myelography, but the patient remains in the lateral decubitus position until the contrast medium has entered the neck. With the head raised on a pad or bolster contrast will not flow past the foramen magnum. When all the contrast has reached the neck the patient is turned to lie prone, and the study then completed as for a cervical injection study.

CT MYELOGRAPHY

CT myelography (CTM) should be delayed for up to 4 h after injection to allow dilution of the contrast medium. A very high concentration may cause difficulty in resolving the cervical nerve roots. Turning the patient a few times prior to CT ensures even distribution and reduces layering effects. In studying the spinal cord a delay is not required though, again, good mixing of the CSF with contrast medium is essential. The superior contrast resolution of CT allows the definition of very dilute contrast medium, e.g. beyond a spinal block, thus avoiding the need for a cervical puncture. Nerve root exit foramina may be studied by CTM in both the lumbar and cervical region, and it has been shown to be a sensitive technique, though it fails to demonstrate far lateral disc lesions. Delayed CTM is needed in suspected syringomyelia.

PAEDIATRIC MYELOGRAPHY

A few points need to be borne in mind when carrying out myelography in the paediatric age group:

1. General anaesthetic is essential for all children aged 6 years or younger, and for many children up to the age of 12 years.
2. Lumbar puncture in cases of spinal dysraphism carries the risk of damaging a low-lying cord due to tethering. The thecal sac is usually wide in these conditions and the needle should be placed laterally in the thecal sac. In addition, as low a puncture as possible will minimize the risk, though in practice spinal cord injury is very uncommon or masked by the neurologic deficit already present.
3. In dysraphism, the frequent association of cerebellar tonsillar herniation precludes lateral C1/2 puncture.

Aftercare

Most patients may be discharged home after being allowed to rest for a few hours after the study. The practice of automatic hospitalization for myelography can no longer be justified in the light of improved contrast media with very low rates of serious morbidity. The patient may remain ambulant. A good fluid intake is generally advised though its value is unproven.

Complications

1. Headache occurs in about 25% of cases, slightly more frequent in females
2. Nausea and vomiting in about 5%
3. Subdural injection of contrast medium. This occurs when only part of the needle bevel is within the subarachnoid space. Contrast medium initially remains loculated near the end of the needle, but can track freely in the subdural space to simulate

14

intrathecal flow. When in doubt, the injection should be stopped, and AP and lateral views obtained with the needle in situ. The temptation of interpreting such an examination should be resisted and the patient re-booked

4. Extradural injection of contrast medium outlines the nerve roots well beyond the exit foramina
5. Intramedullary injection of contrast medium. This is a complication of lateral cervical puncture or in a low-lying spinal cord, and is recognized as a slit-like collection of contrast medium in the spinal canal. Small collections are without clinical significance.

LUMBAR DISCOGRAPHY

Aims

There is strong evidence to support the role of discography in identifying patients with lumbar discogenic pain, but only moderate and limited supportive evidence in cervical and thoracic discogenic pain:

1. To opacify the disc with contrast medium injected into the nucleus pulposus in order to demonstrate degeneration and herniation.
2. To provoke and reproduce the pain for which the patient is being investigated and to assess its response to anaesthetic injection.

Indications

Given the present status of MRI, any request for discography must be considered with great care, as it is a painful procedure and not without risk. If infection occurs the disc will be permanently damaged. The indications are:

1. suspected discogenic pain without radicular signs
2. confirmation of normal discs above or below a proposed surgical fusion.

Contraindications

1. None absolute (except allergy to iodine)
2. Any local or distant sepsis will add to the risk of infective discitis
3. Patient not a surgical candidate due to comorbidity.

Contrast medium

Nonionic contrast media such as iopamidol or iohexol. A normal disc will usually allow up to 1.0 ml to be injected.

Equipment

1. Radiographic equipment as for myelography. Biplane screening is essential to ensure correct needle positioning.

2. Discography needles – a set of two needles are used for each level:
   a. Outer needle, 21G, 12.5 cm
   b. Inner needle, 26G, 15.8 cm.

Patient preparation

The procedure and its aim are explained to the patient. It is important (1) that patients are asked to describe what pain they experience and (2) that patients should not be told that they may get symptomatic pain. This precaution reduces the chance of obtaining a programmed response from the patient. No other preparation is needed. The procedure is done under local anaesthesia. Pre-medication and analgesia may alter the patient's subjective response to discography, diminishing its efficacy and usefulness. Diazepam may, however, be required in very anxious patients. Some authors recommend broad-spectrum antibiotic cover (e.g. cephalosporins) given immediately before the examination to minimize the risk of infection.

Preliminary radiographs

AP and lateral films should be available or obtained.

Technique

1. There are two possible needle approaches:
   a. The posterior approach, which traverses the spinal canal
   b. The lateral oblique extradural approach, which avoids puncture of the dura and the vulnerable part of the posterior annulus. This is the preferred approach and can be carried out with the patient in the prone or left lateral decubitus position. The left lateral decubitus position is preferred, with the patient's head resting on a pillow and a pad placed in the lumbar angle to maintain a straight spine. Moderate spinal flexion is useful, especially at L5/S1.
2. Full aseptic technique is mandatory; there should be no compromise on this point. The operator and any assistant should be gowned, masked, capped and gloved, and the patient should be draped. The level to be examined is determined by fluoroscopy, and the skin is anaesthetized, usually a hand's breadth from the spinous processes.
3. The outer 21G needle is then directed towards the posterior aspect of the disc under intermittent fluoroscopic control, at an angle of 45–60° to the vertical. An additional caudal tilt may be necessary for the L5/S1 level. This needle should reach but not traverse the annulus fibrosus. This point is recognized by a distinct feeling of resistance when the outer fibres are encountered. The 26G needle is then introduced through the 21G needle and the entry of its tip into the nucleus pulposus confirmed in two planes with the aid of the image intensifier prior to contrast medium injection.

4. Contrast medium is injected slowly using a 1-ml syringe. This is done under intermittent fluoroscopic control, while the pain response, the disc volume and its radiographic morphology are monitored. The resistance to flow will gradually increase in a normal disc during the 0.5–1.0-ml stage.

Radiographic views

1. AP and lateral films are obtained at each level examined.
2. At the end of the procedure after needle removal, AP and lateral films are taken in the standing position.
3. Films in flexion and extension may be useful.

Computed tomography post discogram

Thin-section CT slices aid in optimizing morphological grading of disc abnormalities, with particular reference to the status of the annulus and the degree and extent of annular tears.

Patient interrogation

Normal discs and some abnormal discs are asymptomatic. In the symptomatic abnormal discs, the pattern and distribution of pain are noted, together with any similarity to the usual symptomatology. At each symptomatic level local anaesthetic (bupivacaine hydrochloride 0.5%) may be injected to test its efficacy in producing symptomatic relief.

Aftercare

Simple analgesia may be required and overnight admission is usually advised to ensure adequate pain control.

Complications

1. Discitis is the most important complication. Pain with or without pyrexia after a few days indicates this development. Narrowing of the disc space with a variable degree of end-plate sclerosis is seen after a few weeks. Most cases are due to low-grade infection and require treatment with antibiotics.
2. With the transdural approach, post-lumbar puncture headache and/or vomiting may occur.

Further reading

Buenaventura, R.M., Shah, R.V., Patel, V., et al. (2007) Systematic review of discography as a diagnostic test for spinal pain: an update. *Pain Physician* **10(1)**, 147–164.

Colhoun, E., McCall, I.W., Williams, L., et al. (1988) Provocation discography as a guide to planning operations on the spine. *J. Bone. Joint. Surg. Br.* **70(2)**, 267–271.

McCulloch, J.A. & Waddell, G. (1978) Lateral lumbar discography. *Br. J. Radiol.* **51(607)**, 498–502.

Tehranzadeh, J. (1998) Discography 2000. *Radiol. Clin. North Am.* **36(3)**, 463–495.

INTRADISCAL THERAPY

The ability to carry out successful discography will enable the radiologist, with the cooperation of interested clinicians, to carry out therapeutic procedures such as mechanical percutaneous disc removal, laser therapy and intradiscal electrothermal therapy (IDET). While each has advocates, none is widely utilized, and the practice of such methods should be subject to very strict selection criteria and rigorous audit of the outcomes.

FACET JOINT ARTHROGRAPHY

Indications

This is performed for diagnostic and therapeutic purposes, primarily at the lumbar level. Intra-articular injection is the only effective means for assessing the facet joints as a source of back pain. The only indication, therefore, is suspected pain of facet joint origin. Such pain may strongly resemble radicular pain, and patients have often been managed on this basis over a long period of time without success.

Affected facets are usually degenerate as visualized on plain radiographs, CT or MRI. The facet joint capsule is richly innervated by the dorsal ramus of the lumbar spinal nerves. The procedure is valid in that many patients with degenerate facets do not have facet joint pain, and the role of the facet joint in the back pain of the individual patient cannot, therefore, be determined without facet joint injection. The arthrogram is not, therefore, a study of pathological anatomy; the visualization of the joint is important only to verify the needle position. Having visualized the joint, local anaesthetic can be injected to judge the patient's response. In cases obtaining good relief of symptoms, further management will then consist either of a programme of regular steroid injection therapy, cryolysis, radiofrequency or spinal fusion to prevent facet movement.

Equipment

1. As for myelography
2. A 22G spinal needle is appropriate for the study.

Contrast medium

Non-ionic contrast medium 0.1–0.2 ml should be used.

14

Technique

1. This is an outpatient procedure which involves the simultaneous injection of both joints at each level to be studied. More than one level should not be examined in each session to avoid diagnostic confusion. Needle placement can be done using fluoroscopy or CT guidance.
2. Using fluoroscopy the joint space is profiled by slowly rotating the patient from a prone position into a prone oblique orientation with the relevant side raised.
3. Sterile procedures are required.
4. The spinal needle is inserted and advanced perpendicularly to the facet joint, under fluoroscopic control. Caudal needle angulation is sometimes needed if the iliac crest overlies the L5/S1 facet joints. Alternatively the needles can be placed by simultaneous advancement into the joints using CT guidance.
5. In the majority of cases a noticeable 'give' indicates that the capsule is penetrated.
6. Contrast medium injection confirms correct needle placement by demonstrating immediate opacification of a superior and inferior recess.
7. Correct needle placement is documented showing intra-articular injection. The arthrographic appearances are not of any diagnostic consequence.
8. For diagnostic purposes up to 1 ml of 0.5% bupivacaine hydrochloride (Marcaine) is injected in the facet joint and the response over the ensuing 24-h period documented. For therapeutic injection, 0.5 ml of 0.5% Marcaine mixed with 0.5 ml of Depo-Medrone (methylprednisolone 40 mg ml^{-1}) is injected after arthrography.

Further reading

Fairbank, J.C., Park, W.M., McCall, I.W., et al. (1981) Apophyseal injection of local anaesthetic as a diagnostic aid in primary low back syndromes. *Spine* **6**, 598–605.

McCall, I.W., Park, W.M. & O'Brien, J.P. (1979) Induced pain referral from posterior lumbar elements in normal subjects. *Spine* **4(5)**, 441–446.

Maldague, B., Mathurin, P. & Malghem, J. (1981) Facet joint arthrography in lumbar spondylolysis. *Radiology* **140(1)**, 29–36.

Mooney, V. & Robertson, J. (1976) The facet syndrome. *Clin. Orthop. Relat. Res.* **115**, 149–156.

PERCUTANEOUS VERTEBRAL BIOPSY

The percutaneous approach to obtaining a representative sample of tissue for diagnosis prior to therapy is both easy and safe, avoiding the morbidity associated with open surgery. It has a success rate of around 90%. Accurate lesion localization prior to and during the procedure is required. Vertebral body lesions may be biopsied under either CT or fluoroscopic control. Small lesions, especially those located in the posterior neural arch, are best biopsied under CT control. A preliminary CT scan is helpful, whatever method is finally chosen to control the procedure.

Indications

Suspected vertebral or disc infection and vertebral neoplasia. Note that the presence of a more accessible lesion in the appendicular skeleton should be sought by radionuclide bone scanning, before vertebral biopsy is undertaken.

Contraindications

1. Biopsy should not be attempted under any circumstances in the presence of abnormal and uncorrected bleeding or clotting time or if there is a low platelet count.
2. Lesions suspected of being highly vascular, e.g. aneurysmal bone cyst or renal tumour metastasis are relatively dangerous, and a fine-needle aspiration should be used instead of a trephine needle for these cases.

Equipment

Numerous types of biopsy needle are available. The commonest type used is the Jamshidi set. A trephine needle with an internal diameter of 2 mm or more is required, minimizing histological distortion and reducing sampling error without increasing the complication rate. Specimen quality is higher with the Jamshidi type.

Patient preparation

Sedation/analgesia and, where necessary, general anaesthesia are required, preferably administered and monitored by an anaesthetist.

Technique

1. For a fluoroscopy-guided procedure the lateral decubitus position is used. For CT control the prone position is preferable.
2. The skin entry point distance from the mid-line is about 8 cm for the lumbar region and 5 cm in the thoracic region.
3. The aim of the procedure is to enter the vertebral body at about 4 o'clock or 8 o'clock (visualizing the body with the spinous process at 6 o'clock). Local anaesthetic may be

injected via a 21G spinal needle to allow deep infiltration of the soft tissues into close proximity to the periosteum.

4. The biopsy needle is advanced at between 30 and 45° to the sagittal plane in the thoracic and lumbar spine, respectively.

5. When the biopsy needle impinges on the cortex of the vertebral body its position is confirmed fluoroscopically in both AP and lateral planes, or on a single CT section. The trocar and cannula are then advanced through the cortex and the trocar is then withdrawn.

6. Using alternate clockwise and anticlockwise rotation the biopsy cannula is advanced approximately 1 cm.

7. By twisting the needle firmly several times in the same direction the specimen is severed.

8. At least two cores of bone may be obtained by withdrawing the needle back to the cortex, angulating and re-entering the vertebral body.

9. The needle is then withdrawn while simultaneous suction is applied by a syringe attached to the hub.

10. To remove the specimen, the plunger is inserted at the sharp end of the needle and the tissue is pushed out. Any blood clot should be included as part of the specimen.

11. In suspected infection the end-plate rather than the disc is biopsied. Most cases are due to osteomyelitis extending to the disc space. If there is a para-vertebral abscess, aspiration and culture of its contents is preferable to vertebral biopsy.

Aftercare

1. Overnight stay with routine nursing observation and analgesia if needed.

2. The approach to a thoracic lesion should be extra-pleural, but if any doubt exists, a chest X-ray should be obtained after the procedure, as there is a small risk of pneumothorax or haemothorax.

Complications

These are rare, but there are potential risks to nearby structures in poorly controlled procedures, including the lung and pleura, aorta, nerve roots and spinal cord. Local bleeding is an occasional problem.

Further reading

Babu, N.V., Titus, V.T., Chittaranjan, S., et al. (1994) Computed tomographically guided biopsy of the spine. *Spine* **19(21)**, 2436–2442.

Shaltot, A., Michell, P.A., Betts, J.A., et al. (1982) Jamshidi needle biopsy of bone lesions. *Clin. Radiol.* **33**, 193–196.

Stoker, D.J. & Kissin, C.M. (1985) Percutaneous vertebral biopsy: a review of 135 cases. *Clin. Radiol.* **36**, 569–577.

Tehranzadeh, J., Tao, C. & Browning, C.A. (2007) Percutaneous needle biopsy of the spine. *Acta Radiol.* **48(8)**, 860–868.

BONE AUGMENTATION TECHNIQUES

The vertebral bodies can collapse in osteoporosis and metastatic disease. The injection of small amounts of bone cement directly into the vertebral body (vertebroplasty) strengthens the vertebral body and is successful in control of spinal pain. Pre-procedure radiographs and an MRI scan are obtained, while a spinal surgeon is on standby should any complications require surgical intervention. Multiple levels can be treated in this manner with placement of the needle in the vertebral body using either a transpedicular approach or a posterolateral approach. Careful aseptic technique and fluoroscopic/CT guidance during cement injection is essential to avoid cement migration into the canal and/or veins. An allied technique (kyphoplasty) in addition partially restores vertebral body height in osteoporotic vertebral fractures.

Further reading

Burton, A.W., Rhines, L.D. & E. Mendel, E. (2005) Vertebroplasty and kyphoplasty: a comprehensive review. *Neurosurg. Focus* **18(3)**, e1.

Hide, I.G. & Gangi, A. (2004) Percutaneous vertebroplasty: history, technique and current perspectives. *Clin. Radiol.* **59(6)**, 461–467.

NERVE ROOT BLOCKS

LUMBAR SPINE

This is undertaken in difficult diagnostic cases, usually in the presence of multilevel pathology, especially in post-operative situations. If the injected local anaesthetic in the perineural space abolishes the patient's symptoms it is concluded that pain is originating from the injected nerve root. Therapeutic instillation of local anaesthetic with steroid (e.g. triamcinolone, betamethasone [Celestone Soluspan]) has proved successful as a means of treating sciatica in patients with disc prolapse, especially in a foraminal location. It is crucial that a review of the MRI images takes place before the procedure is carried out to ensure that the correct level and side are in accordance with the patient's symptoms. The objective is to place the needle *outside* the nerve root sleeve so that the injected substances diffuse between the disc prolapse and the compressed nerve. Reduction of the inflammatory response induced by the herniated disc can be slow and improvement of symptoms can take up to 8–12 weeks.

The accurate placement of the tip of a spinal needle is confirmed by the injection of a small amount of contrast medium. This is important to avoid injection in one of the lumbar vessels as, rarely, paraplegia presumed to be due to inadvertent intra-arterial injection has been reported. This risk needs to be communicated in the informed consent with the patient prior to the procedure.

Under local anaesthetic control, the needle is advanced using fluoroscopic or CT guidance, to a point inferior and lateral to the ipsilateral pedicle. The extra-foraminal nerve roots are outlined by contrast medium and for diagnostic purposes a small amount of 0.5% bupivacaine is instilled as a means of assessing the correct level responsible for the patient's sciatica.

CERVICAL SPINE

Perineural root sleeve therapy can also be used in cervical radiculopathy. Correct needle placement using CT and fluoroscopy is very important, utilizing contrast medium injection for confirmation prior to the therapeutic injection of lidocaine (bupivacaine is not used in the cervical spine) and steroid. There is a real risk of inadvertent vascular injection, particularly in the vertebral artery. CT fluoroscopic guidance at the required foraminal level is used to ensure the needle traverses in a horizontal or slightly downward course posterior to the carotid and jugular vessels. The needle tip is aimed towards the outer rim of the posterior bone outline of the foramen so as to avoid the vertebral vessels and the nerve root.

Further reading

Blankenbaker, D.G., De Smet, A.A., Stanczak, J.D., et al. (2005) Lumbar radiculopathy: treatment with selective lumbar nerve blocks. Comparison of effectiveness of triamcinolone and betamethasone injectable suspensions. *Radiology* **237(2)**, 738–741.

Herron, L.D. (1989) Selective nerve root block in patient selection for lumbar surgery: surgical results. *J. Spinal Disord.* **2(2)**, 75–79.

Schellhas, K.P., Pollei, S.R., Johnson, B.A., et al. (2007) Selective cervical nerve root blockade: experience with a safe and reliable technique using an anterolateral approach for needle placement. *Am. J. Neuroradiol.* **28(10)**, 1909–1914.

Wagner, A.L. (2004) Selective lumbar nerve root blocks with CT fluoroscopic guidance: technique, results, procedure time, and radiation dose. *Am. J. Neuroradiol.* **25(9)**, 1592–1594.

Wagner, A.L. (2005) CT fluoroscopic-guided cervical nerve root blocks. *Am. J. Neuroradiol.* **26(1)**, 43–44.

Weiner, B.K, & Fraser, R.D. (1997) Foraminal injection for lateral lumbar disc herniation. *J. Bone Joint Surg. Br.* **79(5)**, 804–807.

Lacrimal system and salivary glands

Methods of imaging the lacrimal system

1. Conventional/digital subtraction dacryocystography.
2. Conventional/digital subtraction dacryocystography + computed tomography (CT) dacryocystography
3. Magnetic resonance imaging.

Further reading

Ansari, S.A., Pak, J. & Shields, M. (2005) Pathology and imaging of the lacrimal drainage system. *Neuroimaging Clin. N. Am.* **15(1)**, 221–237.

DIGITAL SUBTRACTION AND CT DACRYOCYSTOGRAPHY

Dacryocystography allows visualization of the lacrimal system by direct injection of contrast into the cannalicus of the eyelid. It may be combined with CT imaging performed immediately after lacrimal system contrast injection. CT imaging gives additional diagnostic information, particularly about adjacent structures.[1]

Indications

Epiphora – to demonstrate the site and degree of obstruction.

Contraindications

None.

Contrast medium

Low osmolar contrast material (LOCM) 300, 0.5–2.0 ml per side.
The use of lipiodol is to be discouraged.

Equipment

1. Digital subtraction radiography unit
2. Silver dilator and lacrimal cannula, or 18G blunt needle with polythene catheter (the catheter technique has the advantage that the examination can be performed on both sides simultaneously).

Patient preparation

0.5 % bupivacaine eye drops.

Technique

1. The lacrimal sac is massaged to express its contents prior to injection of the contrast medium. The lower eyelid is everted to locate the lower canaliculus at the medial end of the lid. The lower canaliculus is dilated and the cannula or catheter is inserted. The lower lid should be drawn laterally during insertion to straighten the bend in the canaliculus, and so avoid perforation by the cannula.
The upper canaliculus may also be cannulated if there is difficulty with the lower canaliculus.
2. The contrast medium is injected and a digital subtraction run at one image per second is obtained. This allows for a dynamic study in real time.

Images

Appropriate images are filmed /digitally stored.

Aftercare

A protective eye patch for 30–60 min may be necessary in view of the local anaesthetic used.

Complications

Perforation of the canaliculus.

Reference

1. Freitag, S.K., Woog, J.J., Kousoubris, P.D., et al. (2002) Helical computed tomographic dacryocystography with three dimensional reconstruction: a new view of the lacrimal drainage system. *Opthal. Plast. Reconstr. Surg.* **18(2)**, 121–132.

MRI OF LACRIMAL SYSTEM

The lacrimal system can be assessed with MRI (MR dacryocystography) either following topical administration of eye drops containing a dilute gadolinium solution (sterile 0.9% NaCl solution containing 1:100 diluted gadolinium chelate) or by direct injection of a dilute gadolinium solution into the lacrimal canaliculus.[1] The less invasive, topical administration technique is more widely used. MR is useful in the diagnosis of obstruction level in the lacrimal system for patients with epiphora and in assessment of surrounding soft tissues.

Reference

Manfrè, L., de Maria, M., Todaro, E., et al. (2000) MR dacryocystography: comparison with dacryocystography and CT dacryocystography. *Am. J. Neuroradiol.* **21(6)**, 1145–1150.

Methods of imaging the salivary glands

1. **Plain films:** for calculus disease (sialithiasis)
2. **Conventional sialography:** less commonly performed than in the past; many indications replaced by non-invasive cross-sectional imaging
3. **CT:** thin-section unenhanced CT for diagnosis of sialithiasis ± intravenous (i.v.) contrast medium, e.g. in suspected tumour or abscess
4. **Ultrasound (US):** ideal investigation for superficial salivary gland disease and a sensitive test for sialithiasis
5. **MRI:** ± i.v. contrast medium for assessment of inflammatory or malignant disease, may include MR spectroscopy for characterization of focal mass and MR sialography
6. **Radionuclide imaging (sialoscintigraphy).**

Further reading

Bialek, E.J., Jakubowski, W., Zajkowski, P., et al. (2006) US of the major salivary glands: anatomy and spatial relatinships, pathological conditions and pitfalls. *Radiographics* **26(3)**, 745–763.

Freling, N.J. (2000) Imaging of salivary gland disease. *Semin. Roentgenol.* **35(1)**, 12–20.

15

Rabinov, J.D. (2000) Imaging of salivary gland pathology. *Radiol. Clin. North Am.* **38(5)**, 1047–1057.

Yousem, D.M., Kraut, M.A. & Chalian, A.A. (2000) Major salivary gland imaging. *Radiology* **216(1)**, 19–29.

CONVENTIONAL AND CT SIALOGRAPHY

Indications

1. Pain
2. Swelling
3. Sicca syndrome.

Contraindications

Acute infection or inflammation.

Contrast medium

1. LOCM 240–300
2. Lipiodol Ultra Fluid.

   Neither contrast medium has a clear advantage over the other.

Equipment

1. Skull unit (using macroradiography technique)
2. Silver lachrymal dilator
3. Silver cannula or 18G blunt needle and polythene catheter.

Patient preparation

Any radio-opaque artifacts are removed (e.g. false teeth).

Preliminary film

Parotid gland

1. Antero-posterior (AP) with the head rotated 5° away from the side under investigation. Centre to the mid-line of the lower lip
2. Lateral, centred to the angle of the mandible
3. Lateral oblique, centred to the angle of the mandible, and with the tube angled 20° cephalad.

Submandibular gland

1. Inferosuperior using an occlusal film. This is a useful view to show calculi
2. Lateral, with the floor of the mouth depressed by a wooden spatula
3. Lateral oblique, centred 1 cm anterior to the angle of the mandible, and with the tube angled 20° cephalad.

Technique

1. The orifice of the parotid duct is adjacent to the crown of the second upper molar, and that of the submandibular duct is at the base of the frenulum of the tongue. If they are not visible, a sialogogue (e.g. citric acid) is placed in the mouth to promote secretion from the gland, and so render the orifice visible.
2. The orifice of the duct is dilated with the silver wire probe and the cannula or polythene catheter is introduced into the duct. The catheter can be held in place by the patient gently biting on it.
3. Up to 2 ml of contrast medium are injected. The injection is terminated immediately if any pain is experienced. The duct must not be overfilled
4. If the cannula method is used, films are taken immediately after the injection. The catheter method has the advantage that films can be taken during the injection, with the catheter in situ, and that both sides can be examined simultaneously.

Films

1. *Immediate* – the same views as for the preliminary films are repeated. The occlusal film for the submandibular gland may be omitted, as this is only to demonstrate calculi.
2. *Post-secretory* – the same views are repeated 5 min after the administration of a sialogogue. The purpose of this is to demonstrate sialectasis.

Aftercare

None.

Complications

1. Pain
2. Damage to the duct orifice
3. Rupture of the ducts
4. Infection.

ULTRASOUND AND MRI OF SALIVARY GLANDS

MR is very useful in the diagnosis of lesions of the salivary glands.

A heavily T2-weighted sequence can image the ductal system of the major salivary glands in the diagnosis of sialolithiasis and sialadenitis (MR sialography). Non-contrast studies can be useful in differentiating benign or low-grade malignant from high-grade malignant tumours. Contrast enhancement is useful in the differential diagnosis

15

of cystic from solid lesions, and when determining the degree of perineural spread of malignant disease.[1] Diffusion weighted imaging and MR spectroscopy are increasingly used for the characterization of salivary gland masses.[2]

Pulse sequences

Thin, T1-weighted and T2-weighted unenhanced images are taken. Fast spin-echo T2-weighted images may require fat suppression. Gadolinium-enhanced scans with T1 weighting and fat suppression are obtained in the axial plane; sagittal and coronal images may be obtained at the radiologist's discretion.

References

1. Yousem, D.M., Kraut, M.A. & Chalian, A.A. (2000) Major salivary gland imaging. *Radiology* **216(1)**, 19–29.
2. Lee, Y.Y., Wong, K.T., King, A.D., et al. (2008) Imaging of salivary gland tumours. *Eur. J. Radiol.* **66(3)**, 419–436.

Further reading

Shah, G.V. (2004) MR imaging of salivary glands. *Neuroimaging Clin. N. Am.* **14(4)**, 777–808.

16

Thyroid and parathyroids

Methods of imaging the thyroid and parathyroid glands

1. Plain film
2. Ultrasound (US)
3. Computed tomography (CT)
4. Magnetic resonance imaging (MRI)
5. Radionuclide imaging.

ULTRASOUND OF THYROID

Indications

1. Palpable thyroid mass
2. Suspected thyroid tumour
3. 'Cold spot' on radionuclide imaging
4. Suspected retrosternal extension of thyroid
5. Guided aspiration or biopsy.

Contraindications

None.

Patient preparation

None.

Equipment

5–10-MHz transducer. Linear array for optimum imaging.

Technique

The patient is supine with the neck extended. Longitudinal and transverse scans are taken of both lobes of the thyroid. The isthmus is imaged in a transverse scan as it crosses anterior to the trachea. If there is retrosternal extension, angling downwards and scanning during swallowing may enable the lowest extent of the thyroid to be visualized.

ULTRASOUND OF PARATHYROID

The normal parathyroid glands are not visualized at US because of their small size and similar texture to surrounding tissue. US is performed with a 5–10 MHz transducer for the detection of parathyroid adenoma, hyperplasia and carcinoma and to guide aspiration or biopsy.

Further reading

American Institute of Ultrasound in Medicine (2003) AIUM guideline for the performance of thyroid and parathyroid ultrasound examination. *J. Ultrasound Med.* **22(10)**, 1126–1130.

Gritzmann, N., Koischwitz, D. & Rettenbacher, T. (2000) Sonography of the thyroid and parathyroid glands. *Radiol. Clin. North Am.* **38(5)**, 1131–1145.

Solbiati, L., Osti, V., Cova, L., et al. (2001) Ultrasound of thyroid, parathyroid glands and neck lymph nodes. *Eur. Radiol.* **11(12)**, 2411–2424.

CT AND MRI OF THYROID AND PARATHYROID

In thyroid disease CT or MRI are indicated:

1. for assessment of a thyroid mass over 3 cm in size
2. for differentiation of thyroid tissue from adjoining neck mass
3. in staging of known thyroid malignancy
4. to assess extension of substernal goitre.

As a result of its iodine content, normal thyroid is hyperdense relative to adjacent soft-tissue structures on non-contrast enhanced CT. Unless otherwise contraindicated, CT of thyroid is routinely performed with intravenous (i.v.) contrast. Particular care must be taken in the administration of iodinated i.v. contrast to hyperthyroid patients (see Chapter 2) and in the timing of any subsequent radionuclide thyroid imaging.

In parathyroid disease, CT and MRI are used:

1. to detect parathyroid adenoma in primary hyperparathyroidism
2. in patients with persistent or recurrent hyperparathyroidism following neck exploration.

Further reading

Gotway, M.B. & Higgins, C.B. (2000) MR imaging of the thyroid and parathyroid glands. *Magn. Reson. Imaging Clin. N. Am.* **8(1)**, 163–182.

Weber, A.L., Randolph, G. & Aksoy, F.G. (2000) The thyroid and parathyroid glands. CT and MR imaging and correlation with pathology and clinical findings. *Radiol. Clin. North Am.* **38(5)**, 1105–1129.

RADIONUCLIDE THYROID IMAGING

Indications

1. Evaluation of likely malignancy of thyroid nodules
2. Assessment of goitre including retrosternal extension
3. Assessment of thyroid uptake prior to radio-iodine therapy
4. Assessment of neonatal hypothyroidism[1]
5. To locate ectopic thyroid tissue, e.g. lingual or in a thyroglossal cyst
6. Evaluation of thyroiditis.

Contraindications

None.

Radiopharmaceuticals

1. ^{99m}*Tc-pertechnetate*, 80 MBq max (1 mSv ED). Pertechnetate ions are trapped in the thyroid by an active transport mechanism, but are not organified. Cheap and readily available, it is an acceptable alternative to ^{123}I.
2. ^{123}*I-sodium iodide*, 20 MBq max (4 mSv ED). Iodide ions are trapped by the thyroid in the same way as pertechnetate, but are also organified, allowing overall assessment of thyroid function. The agent of choice, but ^{123}I is a cyclotron product and is, therefore, relatively expensive with limited availability. ^{131}*I-sodium iodide* can also be used for imaging but is associated with a significantly higher radiation dose, so is generally used in the context of whole-body imaging post ^{131}I ablation.

Equipment

1. Gamma-camera
2. Pinhole, converging or high-resolution parallel hole collimator.

Patient preparation

None, but uptake may be reduced by antithyroid drugs, iodine-based preparations and radiographic iodinated contrast media.

Technique

^{99m}Tc-pertechnetate

1. I.v. injection of pertechnetate
2. After 15 min, immediately before imaging, the patient is given a drink of water to wash away pertechnetate secreted into saliva
3. Start imaging 20 min post injection when the target-to-background ratio is maximum
4. The patient lies supine with the neck slightly extended and the camera anterior. For a pinhole collimator, the pinhole should be positioned to give the maximum magnification for the camera field of view (usually 7–10 cm from the neck)
5. The patient should be asked not to swallow or talk during imaging. An image is acquired with markers on the suprasternal notch, clavicles, edges of neck and any palpable nodules.

^{123}I-sodium iodide

The technique is similar to that for pertechnetate except:

1. sodium iodide may be given i.v. or orally
2. imaging is performed 3–4 h after i.v. administration or 24 h after an oral dose
3. a drink of water is not necessary, since ^{123}I is not secreted into saliva in any significant quantity.

Films

200 kilocounts or 15 min maximum:

1. Anterior
2. LAO and RAO views as required, especially for assessment of multinodular disease
3. Large field of view image if retrosternal extension or ectopic thyroid tissue is suspected.

Analysis

The percentage thyroid uptake may be estimated by comparing the background-subtracted attenuation-corrected organ counts with the full syringe counts measured under standard conditions before injection.

Additional techniques

1. Whole-body ^{131}I imaging is often performed after thyroidectomy and ^{131}I ablation for thyroid cancer to locate sites of metastasis

2. Perchlorate discharge tests can be performed to assess possible organification defects, particularly in congenital hypothyroidism.[1]

Aftercare

None.

Complications

None.

Other techniques

Metastatic thyroid cancer can be evaluated using diagnostic ^{123}I or therapeutic ^{131}I whole body scans as above. When these scans are negative, but serum thyroglobulin is raised FDG PET is often positive.[2]

Metastatic medullary carcinoma of the thyroid can be imaged with either pentavalent DMSA, indium-labelled octreotide, MIBG or, more recently, FDG PET. These techniques are discussed in Chapter 11.

References

1. El-Desouki, M., Al-Jurayyan, N., Al-Nuaim, A., et al. (1995) Thyroid scintigraphy and perchlorate discharge test in the diagnosis of congenital hypothyroidism. *Eur. J. Nucl. Med.* **22**, 1005–1008.
2. Intenzo, C.M., Jabbour, S., Dam, H.Q., et al. (2005) Changing concepts in the management of differentiated thyroid cancer. *Semin. Nucl. Med.* **35**, 257–265.

Further reading

Martin, W.H., Sandler, M.P. & Gross, M.D. (2005) Thyroid, parathyroid, and adrenal gland imaging. In: Sharp, P.F., Gemmell, H.G. & Murray, A.D. (eds) *Practical Nuclear Medicine.* 3rd edn. London: Springer-Verlag; 247–272.
Sarkar, S.D. (2006) Benign thyroid disease: what is the role of nuclear medicine? *Semin. Nucl. Med.* **36(3)**, 185–193.

RADIONUCLIDE PARATHYROID IMAGING

Indications

Pre-operative localization of parathyroid adenomas and hyperplastic glands, usually before second-look surgery.

Contraindications

None.

Radiopharmaceuticals

1. ^{99m}Tc-*methoxyisobutylisonitrile (MIBI or sestamibi)*, 500 MBq typical, 900 MBq max (11 mSv ED) and ^{99m}Tc-*pertechnetate*, 80 MBq max (1 mSv ED). Both MIBI and pertechnetate are trapped by the thyroid, but only MIBI accumulates in hyperactive parathyroid tissue. With computer subtraction of pertechnetate from MIBI images, abnormal accumulation of MIBI may be seen. MIBI also washes out of normal thyroid tissue faster than parathyroid, so delayed images (1–4 h) can highlight abnormal parathyroid activity.

2. ^{99m}Tc-*tetrofosmin (Myoview)* can be used as an alternative to MIBI, and is as effective if the subtraction technique is used, but not as good for delayed imaging since differential washout is not as great as for MIBI.

3. ^{201}Tl-*thallous chloride* (80 MBq max, 18 mSv ED) was previously used in conjunction with ^{99m}Tc-pertechnetate, but is increasingly being replaced by the technetium agents due to their superior imaging quality and lower radiation dose.

Equipment

1. Gamma-camera (small field of view preferable for thyroid images, large field of view for chest images)
2. High-resolution parallel hole collimator. A pinhole collimator can also be used, but may result in repositioning magnification errors that compromise subtraction techniques
3. Imaging computer capable of image registration and subtraction.

Patient preparation

None, but uptake may be modified by antithyroid drugs and iodine-based medications, skin preparations and contrast media.

Technique

A variety of imaging protocols have been used, with either pertechnetate or MIBI administered first, with subtraction and possibly additional delayed imaging, and using MIBI alone with early and delayed imaging. Subtraction techniques are most sensitive, but additional delayed imaging may increase sensitivity slightly and improve confidence in the result. The advantage of administering pertechnetate first is that MIBI injection can follow within 30 min with the patient still in position to minimize movement, and if subtraction shows a clearly positive result, the patient does not need to stay for delayed imaging. With MIBI injected first, pertechnetate can only be administered after several hours when washout has occurred:

1. 80 MBq ^{99m}Tc-pertechnetate is administered i.v. through a cannula which is left in place for the second injection.

2. After 15 min the patient is given a drink of water immediately before imaging, to wash away pertechnetate secreted into saliva.
3. The patient lies supine with the neck slightly extended and the camera is positioned anteriorly over the thyroid.
4. The patient should be asked not to move during imaging. Head immobilizing devices may be useful, and marker sources may aid repositioning.
5. 20 min post injection, a 10-min 128×128 image is acquired.
6. Without moving the patient, 500 MBq ^{99m}Tc-MIBI is injected i.v. through the previously positioned cannula (to avoid a second venepuncture which might cause patient movement).
7. 10 min post injection, a further 10-min 128×128 image is acquired.
8. A chest and neck image should then be acquired on a large field of view camera to detect ectopic parathyroid tissue.
9. Computer image registration and normalization is performed and the pertechnetate image subtracted from the 10-min MIBI image.
10. If a lesion is clearly visible in the subtracted image, the patient can leave.
11. If the lesion is not obvious, late MIBI imaging can be performed at hourly intervals up to 4 h if necessary to look for differential washout.

Additional techniques

1. In patients in whom pertechnetate thyroid uptake is suppressed, e.g. with use of iodine-containing contrast media or skin preparations, oral ^{123}I (20 MBq) administered several hours before MIBI may be considered.
2. SPECT may be used to improve localization and small lesion detection.
3. Dynamic imaging with motion correction may reduce motion artifact.

Aftercare

None.

Complications

None.

Further reading

Kettle, A.G. & O'Doherty, M.J. (2006) Parathyroid imaging: how good is it and how should it be done? *Semin. Nucl. Med.* **36(3)**, 206–211.
Palestro, C.J., Tomas, M.B. & Tronco, G.G. (2005) Radionuclide imaging of the parathyroid glands. *Semin. Nucl. Med.* **35(4)**, 266–276.

Breast

Methods of imaging the breast

1. Mammography
2. Ultrasound (US)
3. Magnetic resonance imaging (MRI)
4. Radionuclide imaging
5. Imaging guided biopsy/pre-operative localization.

MAMMOGRAPHY

Indications

1. Focal signs in women aged >35 years in the context of triple (i.e. clinical, radiological and pathological) assessment at a specialist, multi-disciplinary diagnostic breast clinic.
2. Following diagnosis of breast cancer, to exclude multi-focal/multi-centric/bilateral disease.
3. Breast cancer follow-up, no more frequently than annually or less frequently than biennially.
4. Population screening of asymptomatic women with screening interval of 3 years, in accordance with NHS Breast Screening Programme policy:
   a. By invitation, women aged 47–73 years in England, Northern Ireland and Wales and 50–70 years elsewhere in UK.
   b. Women >73 years, by self referral (there is no upper age limit).
5. Screening of women with a moderate/high risk of familial breast cancer who have undergone genetic risk assessment in accordance with National Institute of Clinical Excellence (NICE) guidance.
6. Screening of a cohort of women who underwent the historical practice of mantle radiotherapy for treatment of Hodgkin's

disease when aged <30 years. These women have a breast cancer risk status comparable to the high-risk familial history group.[1]

7. Investigation of metastatic malignancy of unknown origin.

Not indicated

1. Asymptomatic women without familial history of breast cancer, aged <35 years
2. Investigation of generalized signs/symptoms, e.g. cyclical mastalgia or non-focal pain/lumpiness
3. Prior to commencement of hormone replacement therapy
4. To assess the integrity of silicone implants
5. Individuals affected by ataxia-telangiectasia mutated (ATM) gene mutation with resultant high sensitivity to radiation exposure, including medical X-rays
6. Routine investigation of gynaecomastia.

Equipment

Conventional film-screen mammographic imaging must be carried out on a dedicated unit which includes in its specification:

1. dual-focus X-ray tube: 0.1/0.3 focal spot size
2. dual filtration: molybdenum/rhodium
3. choice of rotating target material: molybdenum/rhodium/tungsten
4. 18×24 cm and 24×30 cm interchangeable buckys
5. automatic/semi-automatic and manual exposure control
6. carbon fibre table top assembly with reciprocating or oscillating grid, average grid ratio 5:1
7. magnification assembly; magnification factors 1.8/2.0
8. contact spot compression.

Technique

Standard mammographic examination comprises imaging of both breasts in two views, namely the mediolateral oblique (MLO) and craniocaudal (CC) positions. Screening methodology is bilateral, two-view (MLO and CC) mammography at all screening rounds.

Additional views may be required to provide adequate visualization of specific anatomical sites:

1. Lateral/medial extended CC
2. Axillary tail
3. Mediolateral/lateromedial.

Compression of the breast is an integral part of mammographic imaging resulting in:

1. reduction in radiation dose
2. immobilization of the breast, thus reducing blurring
3. uniformity of breast thickness allowing even penetration
4. reduction in breast thickness thus reducing scatter/noise achieving higher resolution.

Adaptation of the technique can provide additional information:

1. Spot compression, to remove overlapping composite tissue
2. Magnification (smaller focal spot combined with air-gap), to provide morphological analysis.

In the presence of subpectoral implants, the push back technique of Ecklund[2] can aid visualization of breast tissue.

Digital mammography

Conventional film-screen technology has largely been superseded by full-field digital mammography (FFDM) which has a higher sensitivity in:

1. women aged <50 years
2. pre/peri-menopausal women
3. dense fibroglandular breast tissue.[3]

Ongoing developments of FFDM include:

1. *tomosynthesis* which creates a single three-dimensional image of the breast by combining data from a series of two-dimensional radiographs acquired during a single sweep of the X-ray tube. This technique may improve diagnostic accuracy in screening, reduce recall by an estimated 40% and has a radiation dose of approximately 50% of that of a single mammographic exposure
2. *contrast-enhanced digital mammography,* i.e. angiomammography. Two approaches are being developed: temporal sequencing (in which images pre and post contrast are subtracted with a resultant angiomammogram) and dual energy imaging (in which imaging at low and high energies detailing, respectively, parenchyma and fat with and without iodine are obtained. The subsequent views can then be subtracted
3. *computer-aided detection (CAD)* software can assist film reading by placing prompts over areas of potential mammographic concern. Evidence is emerging that, even in the screening setting, single reading in association with CAD may offer sensitivities and specifities comparable to that of double reading.[4]

References
1. Hancock, S.L., Tucker, M.A. & Hoppe, R.T. (1993) Breast cancer after treatment of Hodgkin's disease. *J. Natl. Cancer Inst.* **85**, 25–31.
2. Eklund, G.W., Busby, R.C., Miller, S.H., et al. (1988) Improved imaging of the augmented breast. *Am. J. Roentgenol.* **151**, 469–473.

3. Pisano, E.D., Gatsonis, C., Hendrick, E., et al. (2005) Diagnostic performance of digital versus film mammography for breast cancer screening. *N. Engl. J. Med.* **353**, 1773–1783.
4. Gilbert, F.J., Astley, S.M., McGee, M.A., et al. (2006) Single reading with computer-aided detection and double reading of screening mammograms in the United Kingdom National Breast Screening Program. *Radiology* **241**, 47–53.

Further reading
James, J.J. (2004) The current status of digital mammography. *Clin. Radiol.* **59**, 1–10.
NHS Breast Screening Programme on website www.cancerscreening.nhs.uk
NICE Clinical Guidelines (CG 41 October 2006) Classification and Care of Women at Risk of Familial Breast Cancer in Primary, Secondary and Tertiary Care on website www.nice.org.uk
Tucker, A.K. & Yin Yuen Ng (eds) (2000) *Textbook of Mammography.* 2nd edn. Edinburgh: Churchill Livingstone; 18–64.
Royal College of Radiologists, UK (1995) *The Use of Imaging in the Follow-up of Patients with Breast Cancer.* Royal College of Radiologists **(95)3**.

ULTRASOUND

Indications
1. Focal signs in women aged <35 years in the context of triple (i.e. clinical, radiological and pathological) assessment at a specialist, multi-disciplinary diagnostic breast clinic.
2. As an adjunctive method to improve diagnostic sensitivity and specificity in women aged >35 years with a mammographic and/or clinical abnormality.
3. Following diagnosis of breast cancer to assess initial tumour size or response to neo-adjuvant therapy.
4. Assessment of implant integrity.
5. Diagnosis, drainage guidance and follow-up of breast abscess.
6. Targeting diagnostic biopsy/pre-operative localization of both palpable and impalpable breast lesions.
7. To guide axillary lymph node biopsy, thus informing choice of surgical management.[1]

Not indicated
1. For screening in any age group
2. In the investigation of generalized signs/symptoms, e.g. cyclical mastalgia or non-focal pain/lumpiness
3. In the routine investigation of gynaecomastia.

Equipment

Hand-held, high-frequency (8–18 MHz) contact US is widely used in breast imaging, with concomitant advantages of cost, accessibility and safety. Proprietary stand off gels can be useful when assessing superficial lesions and the nipple-areolar complex.

Technique

1. The patient's arm on the side to be examined should be placed behind the head.
2. The patient lies supine for examination of the medial aspect of the breast.
3. The patient lies in the lateral, oblique position for examination of the lateral and axillary aspects of the breast and axilla.

Additional technique

Elastography[2] is a non-invasive US technique, which provides a visual representation of the stiffness (elasticity) of both normal and abnormal tissue. US imaging is used to examine tissue, both before and after minimal compression. A colour coded image is generated with dark tissue representing least compressible tissue, i.e. with a higher index of suspicion of malignancy.

References

1. Damera, A., Evans, A.J., Cornford, E.J., et al. (2003) Diagnosis of axillary nodal metastases by ultrasound guided core biopsy in primary operable breast cancer. *Br. J. Cancer.* **89**, 1310–1313.
2. Zhi, H., Ou, B., Luo, B.-M., et al. (2007) Comparison of ultrasound elastography, mammography and sonography in the diagnosis of solid breast lesions. *J. Ultrasound. Med.* **26**, 807–815.

Further reading

Stavros, A.T. (2004) *Breast Ultrasound.* Philadelphia: Lippincott, Williams & Wilkins.

MAGNETIC RESONANCE IMAGING

Indications

1. Detection/exclusion of recurrent malignant disease in the conserved breast $\geq$ 6 months following surgery. Mature scar tissue, which may mimic malignancy morphologically, does not enhance with resultant high negative predictive value.

2. Assessment of implant integrity.
3. Monitoring response to neo-adjuvant therapy.
4. Combined with mammography, as a screening tool[1] in women deemed to be at high risk of developing breast cancer (see above, mammography section).
5. In carefully selected cases, to clarify equivocal or suspicious mammographic and US findings.
6. Investigation of occult breast cancer. 0.3% of patients present with malignant axillary lymphadenopathy but normal breast triple assessment.[2]

Indications under evaluation

1. Detection of unsuspected multi-focal/multi-centric/contralateral disease. This may be of particular value in the pre-operative staging of invasive lobular disease. A high proportion of lesions identified on MRI can be located on second look US and are, therefore, amenable to conventional biopsy. All biopsy techniques can be adapted for use with MRI guidance.
2. MRI may have a role in the pre-operative evaluation of the extent of high grade (Grade 3) ductal carcinoma in situ (DCIS).

Technique

1. Contraindications as for standard MRI examinations.
2. Lying prone, with breasts placed in a dedicated surface coil, images are obtained pre and post contrast (0.1–0.2 mmol kg gadolinium chelate contrast, given i.v. via pump injector) in either axial fat suppression or coronal subtraction sequences. The presence, amount, speed and morphology of the pattern of enhancement are analysed.
3. For implant integrity non-enhanced scanning is adequate.

References
1. Leach, M.O., Boggis, C.R., Dixon, A.K., et al. (2005) Screening with magnetic resonance imaging of a UK population at high familial risk of breast cancer: a prospective multi-centre cohort study (MARIBS). *Lancet* **365**, 1769–1778.
2. Porter, B.A. (2005) Current best clinical indications for breast MRI. *Summary Proceedings: 29th Annual Symposium of American Society of Breast Disease.* http://asbd.org/images/Porter_1.pdf

Further reading
Morris, E.A. (2007) Diagnostic breast MR imaging: current status and future directions. *Radiol. Clin. North Am.* **45**, 863–880.

RADIONUCLIDE IMAGING

Intra-operative sentinel node identification (see p. 256)

A sentinel lymph node is the first node to which malignant cells are likely to spread from the primary tumour. The lower axillary sentinel lymph node(s) can be identified at operation following injection of a combination of radioisotope (^{99m}Tc colloidal albumin, particle size 3–80 nm) and blue dye. The subareolar route allows rapid (i.e. within minutes) uptake to lymph nodes via the plexus of Sappey.

Positron emission tomography scanning (see Chapter 11)

Hybrid positron emission tomography (PET)-CT scanning with ^{18}F-fluorodeoxyglucose (FDG) may provide additional information in carefully selected cases where re-staging of disease, monitoring response to treatment or the detection of distant metastases is required.

Further reading

Clarke, D., Khonji, N.I. & Mansel, R.E. (2001) Sentinel node biopsy in breast cancer: ALMANAC trial. *World J. Surg.* **25**, 819–822.

Lim, H.S., Yoon, W., Chung, T.W., et al. (2007) FDG PET/CT for the detection and evaluation of breast diseases: usefulness and limitations. *Radiographics* **27(Suppl 1)**, S197–213.

IMAGE-GUIDED BREAST BIOPSY

Indications

1. Diagnostic biopsy: to obtain specimen of tissue for histological analysis. Comprise the majority of biopsy procedures.
2. Therapeutic biopsy: US guided, large volume (up to 7G needle), vacuum-assisted techniques can be used to excise:
   a. small (<2 cm) fibroadenomata
   b. parenchymal distortion (with no evidence of atypia on diagnostic core)
   c. impalpable papillary lesions
   d. complex cysts.

Equipment

1. Require either:
   a. US guidance; using hand held, high frequency (8–18 MHz) probe. The avoidance of radiation combined with accessibility of the technique results in this approach being used wherever possible

   OR

   b. X-ray guidance; applying the principle of stereotaxis whereby imaging a static object from two known angles from a known zero point can provide data from which the X, Y and Z co-ordinates can be calculated. Small field digital stereotactic equipment can be purchased as an add-on to conventional mammography machines, thus providing the most common approach to X-ray-guided biopsy, namely with the patient in the seated, upright position. Less commonly, the small field digital stereotactic system is attached to a prone table (dedicated to biopsy use) with resultant increased accessibility for posteriorly sited lesions and reduction in syncopal episodes – advantages which can be reproduced by the use of an appropriate biopsy chair allowing the adoption of the lateral decubitus position in conjunction with an upright imaging system.

2. Automated biopsy gun. Choice of needle depends on the nature of the mammographic abnormality. For US-guided biopsy of masses, 14 gauge biopsy needle delivered by automated (not disposable) biopsy gun is adequate. For biopsy of clustered microcalcifications and parenchymal distortions, large volume (up to 7 gauge) needles in conjunction with vacuum assisted techniques increase diagnostic accuracy.

Patient preparation

1. Consent
2. For patients receiving anticoagulant treatment:
   a. Aspirin – no contraindication
   b. Warfarin – if decision taken to proceed to biopsy the INR must be <1.5
   c. Clopidogrel – cessation for no less than 7 days prior to biopsy.

Technique

1. Standard skin cleansing and local anaesthetic infiltration
2. Biopsy needle introduced via automated biopsy gun
3. At the time of biopsy, when the mammographic target *may* be completely removed by diagnostic biopsy or to confirm concordance of the target site with other imaging modalities,

a titanium marker can be deployed either via an introducer or the large volume biopsy needle. Some tissue markers comprise not only a radio-opaque clip but a series of collagen pellets rendering the marker ultrasonically visible for up to 6 weeks

4. Confirmatory imaging should accompany all cases:
   a. non-calcified lesion – US (orthogonal views) of needle position during procedure
   b. calcified lesion – X-ray of microcalcification in cores obtained by US or X-ray guidance.

Complications

1. Bleeding
2. Infection
3. Milk fistula (in the lactating breast)
4. Damage to adjacent tissue, e.g. pneumothorax. Careful technique, with needle alignment parallel to chest wall should avoid this.

PRE-OPERATIVE LOCALIZATION

Pivotal to the success of this technique is close multidisciplinary team working at pre-operative discussion/planning, accurate communication between the imaging department and theatre, and post-operative confirmation of adequacy of surgery at the multidisciplinary team (MDT) meeting.

The technique involves the insertion of a thin metal wire (or several wires) through the skin with the wire tip positioned within the lesion itself. The position of the wire is secured and the wire is then used by the surgeon to guide excision of the lesion.

Equipment

1. Localizing wire
2. Non-allergenic adhesive to fix the wire to adjacent skin
3. Swabs – coloured to be easily identifiable as separate from those used in theatre
4. Image guidance:
   a. The avoidance of radiation and accessibility of the technique results in US being the method of image guidance of choice, particularly if the original pre-operative biopsy was achieved via US guidance. Lesions which on US are visible <4 cm from skin can be amenable to the technique of skin marking, avoiding the requirement of a localizing wire. Following discussion with the surgeon, the operative position of the

17

patient should be reproduced. With the US probe immediately overlying the lesion, the skin is marked and the depth to target is measured. At operation, the site of the skin mark is incised and dissection through the relevant distance is undertaken

b. X-ray guidance using fenestrated grid or stereotactic devices can be used for the placement of the localizing wire.

Patient preparation

As for image-guided biopsy.

Technique

1. Standard skin cleansing and local anaesthetic infiltration
2. In cases of extensive (i.e. >2 cm) microcalcification, the placement of multiple wires may aid adequacy of excision
3. After wire placement, mammograms (orthogonal views) indicating the precise position of the tip of the localizing wire are taken. These must be available to the surgeon at the time of operation
4. Using magnification technique (see Mammography section), X-ray of the surgical specimen is undertaken to confirm excision of the mammographic lesion both at the time of operation (allowing further sampling) and at the post-operative MDT.

Further reading

Liberman, L. (2002) Percutaneous image-guided core breast biopsy. *Radiol. Clin. North Am.* **40**, 483–500.

NHSBSP Publication No 20 (2003) *Quality Assurance Guidelines for Surgeons in Breast Cancer Screening.* 3rd edn. Sheffield: NHSBSP.

Sedation and monitoring

SEDATION

Sedation is the use of a drug or drugs to produce a state of depression of the central nervous system that enables interventional procedures or treatment to be carried out. Over recent years the complexity and number of interventional procedures in radiology departments has increased; often these patients are frail or medically unfit for surgery. Sedation is only part of a 'package' of care comprising pre-assessment, properly informed consent, adequate facilities, good techniques and risk avoidance.[1]

Sedative drugs may be combined with drugs used for pain relief (analgesia). Some drugs, such as benzodiazepines, have purely sedative effects but others, such as opioids, have combined sedative and analgesic effects. Although sedative and analgesic agents are generally safe, catastrophic complications related to their use can occur, often as a result of incorrect drug administration or inadequate patient monitoring.[2] The incidence of adverse outcomes is reduced by improved understanding of the pharmacology of drugs used, appropriate monitoring of sedated patients and by recognizing those at increased risk of adverse event.

There is a continuum between the main types of sedation (see Fig. 18.1) defined as:

1. **anxiolysis**: the patient is alert and calm
2. **conscious sedation**: a state of depression of the central nervous system that enables diagnostic and therapeutic procedures to be carried out, but during which the patient remains conscious, retains protective reflexes and is able to understand and respond to verbal commands
3. **deep sedation**: in which these criteria are not fulfilled and airway or ventilation intervention may be required. Deep sedation requires the presence of an anaesthetist
4. **general anaesthesia.**

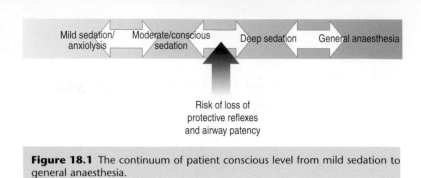

Figure 18.1 The continuum of patient conscious level from mild sedation to general anaesthesia.

The joint Royal College of Radiologists/Royal College of Anaesthetists Working Party on Sedation and Anaesthesia in Radiology[3] recommended establishment of local guidelines for sedation in radiology. These should include:

1. each patient must have a pre-procedure evaluation to assess their suitability for sedation
2. the operator must not supervise the sedation
3. nurses and technicians should not administer drugs without medical supervision
4. all staff carrying out sedation should have undertaken training in sedation and resuscitation, and should have knowledge and experience of the sedative drugs, monitoring and resuscitation equipment
5. there should be periodic retraining and assessment of staff
6. there should be an appropriate recovery area
7. resuscitation equipment and appropriate reversal drugs must be immediately available.

Preparation

Sympathetic patient management with an explanation of the procedure may reduce anxiety and remove the need for any medication. Sedation should be explained and consent obtained. Patients who are to be given intravenous (i.v.) sedation should undergo a period of fasting before the procedure; 6 h fasting for solid food and 2 h for clear liquids.

Resuscitation and monitoring equipment and oxygen delivery devices should be checked and venous access established.

Equipment

1. Appropriate drugs, including reversal agents
2. Monitoring equipment – see page 360
3. Resuscitation equipment – see page 363.

Pre-assessment

It is essential to anticipate and reduce the risk of potential problems before the procedure. Pre-assessment must include:

1. evaluation of the patient's airway
2. full assessment of the patient's medical, drug and allergy history
3. cardio-respiratory reserve assessment.

18

DRUGS

As part of a sedation protocol the following may be used:

1. Combination of a sedative drug and an analgesic drug (e.g. i.v. midazolam and i.v. opiate). Intravenous analgesic and sedative drugs have a synergistic sedative effect and the dose of each drug must be reduced by up to 70% when administered together. It is best to give the i.v. analgesic first then titrate the dose of i.v. sedative
2. Analgesic drug alone (e.g. i.v. opiate)
3. Sedative drug alone (e.g. i.v. midazolam).

Analgesic drugs

Analgesic drugs are used for pain control and improve patient comfort. For some procedures local anaesthesia or oral analgesia (using paracetamol 1 g or ibuprofen 400 mg taken 1–2 h before the procedure) will be appropriate. For more invasive interventional radiology procedures the use of intravenous analgesia may be required.

LOCAL ANAESTHESIA

For recommended doses see Table 18.1.

Table 18.1 Recommended doses of local anaesthetic drugs

Drug	Onset of effect	Duration of effect	Maximum total recommended dose	Route of administration
Lidocaine 1% (1% = 10 mg ml^{-1})	10–15 min	1–2 h	3 mg kg^{-1} (max 200 mg) without adrenaline 7 mg kg^{-1} (max 500 mg) with adrenaline	Subcutaneous injection
Bupivacaine 0.25% (0.25% = 2.5 mg ml^{-1})	15–30 min	2–3 h	2 mg kg^{-1} (max 150 mg)	Subcutaneous injection

Commonly used local anaesthetics for subcutaneous infiltration are:

1. *Lidocaine 1%.* Lidocaine may be used in combination with adrenaline and is supplied in pre-mixed ampoules for this purpose. Adrenaline causes local vasoconstriction, decreases drug absorption and will increase the intensity and duration of action of lidocaine. Lidocaine is also available as a 2% solution.
2. *Bupivacaine 0.25%.* Has slower onset but longer duration of action than lidocaine. The effect of adrenaline is much less pronounced in combination with bupivacaine. Bupivacaine is also available as a 0.5% solution.

INHALATIONAL ANALGESIA

A mixture of 50% nitrous oxide and 50% oxygen (Entonox®) may be used. This has both analgesic and sedative properties.

INTRAVENOUS ANALGESIA

These drugs are used for pain control but also have a dose-dependant sedative effect. Most commonly used are the opioid drugs morphine, pethidine and fentanyl. These drugs must be given in small, divided doses and dose titrated to the patient's need. It is extremely important to titrate the dosage to effect rather than assume a fixed dose based on body weight. The maximum recommended dose must not be exceeded because of the risk of adverse events, particularly respiratory depression. For recommended dosage see Table 18.2.

The opioid drugs can cause:

1. nausea and vomiting
2. hypotension
3. respiratory depression
4. bradycardia.

Table 18.2 Recommended doses of intravenous analgesic drugs

Drug	Maximum total recommended dose	Onset of effect	Duration of effect	Route of administration
Morphine	$100 \, \mu g \, kg^{-1}$ body weight	5–10 min	4–5 h	Intravenous injection
Pethidine	$1 \, mg \, kg^{-1}$ body weight	5 min	1–2 h	Intravenous injection
Fentanyl	$1 \, \mu g \, kg^{-1}$ body weight	1 min	0.5–1 h	Intravenous injection

These drugs should be used in divided doses and the maximum total dose must not be exceeded. It is always important to titrate the dosage of medication to effect rather than assume a fixed dose based on body weight.

Effects of opioids can be reversed by the competitive antagonist naloxone (dose 0.4–2 mg). Naloxone should be administered intravenously in a solution containing 0.4 mg in 10 ml and given in 1 ml increments. It has peak effect at 1–2 min with duration of 20–60 min. As a result of the relatively short duration of action, repeated doses of naloxone may be necessary.

SEDATIVE DRUGS

18

For conscious sedation in the radiology department, the water-soluble benzodiazepine midazolam is the drug of choice. Midazolam has superseded diazepam because the latter has active metabolites and longer duration of effect. Midazolam produces:

1. dose-dependant anxiolysis
2. intense amnesia (for 20–30 min)
3. sedation
4. muscle relaxation.

Midazolam is given i.v. It has a rapid onset of effect, within 1–5 min, and duration of less than 6 h. The sedative dose is 70 μg kg^{-1} body weight (for average adult approx. 4–5 mg) and the sleep dose is 100–200 μg kg^{-1} (>7 mg). Typically, 2–2.5 mg is administered i.v. over 30–120 s with further 0.5 mg doses titrated as required. Rarely are total doses of more than 5 mg required. Smaller doses of 1–3 mg must be used in the elderly.

The effects of midazolam can be reversed by the competitive antagonist flumazenil; onset of flumazenil is within 1–3 min with a half-life of 7–15 min. The dose of flumazenil should be titrated every 1–2 min starting with 200 μg and giving a maximum of 1 mg. The clinical effect depends on the dose of flumazenil and sedative given. The half-life of flumazenil is shorter than that of midazolam, therefore, re-sedation effects can occur.

The use of i.v. anaesthetic agents, such as ketamine and propofol, can result in the patient moving quickly from a state of sedation to anaesthesia with concomitant risks. These drugs should only be used by those who have undergone appropriate specialist training.

Sedation of children

Each child should be individually assessed. In most circumstances parents should stay with the child, and with patience and encouragement the need for sedation may be avoided in some cases. Short procedures such as CT can often be achieved in neonates by keeping them awake and then feeding the child and swaddling just prior to the procedure. Often, children over the age of 4–5 years will not need sedation and will cooperate. Local anaesthetic cream, e.g. Ametop, can be applied to a suitable vein prior to insertion of a venous cannula if venous access is required. Oral sedation does not work well in children over the age of 4 and older children who are unable to co-operate will usually require general anaesthetic.

It is important to ensure that all monitoring and resuscitation equipment is suitable for paediatric use. A nurse, experienced in the care of sedated children, should be present throughout. When drugs are given which are likely to result in loss of consciousness, the primary care of the patient should be under the direct supervision of an anaesthetist.

For many years chloral hydrate has been the mainstay for sedation of young children for a variety of procedures. Triclofos is an active metabolite of chloral hydrate which causes less gastric irritation and vomiting. Alimemazine (Vallergan) is a sedating antihistamine, with anticholinergic effects. The recommendations in Table 18.3 are made as being suitable for the majority of patients, in respect of both safety and efficacy. It is recognized that, for certain patients, deviation from these guidelines will be appropriate on clinical or weight grounds (Table 18.3).

Vomiting is not uncommon after oral sedation is given. If the child vomits within 10 min the dose can be repeated. After 10 min a reduced dose of 50–70% of the Triclofos + Alimemazine dose can be repeated. The dose should not be repeated after 20 min as significant absorption may have occurred.

On the night before the procedure or scan parents should be asked to try to keep the child awake for as long as possible. The child should be woken early on the relevant day and no 'naps' allowed on the journey to the hospital. This will ensure that the child is already tired prior to administration of the sedation. The sedative medication usually takes about 45 min to take effect.

Table 18.3 Sedation recommendations made as being suitable for the majority of child patients. These doses are used to acheive deep sedation: a nurse should be present throughout.

Age/weight	Sedation	Dose
<1 month old	Feed only or Triclofos	$30\,\text{mg}\,\text{kg}^{-1}$
>1 month old but <5 kg	Triclofos	50–$70\,\text{mg}\,\text{kg}^{-1}$
5–10 kg	Triclofos	$100\,\text{mg}\,\text{kg}^{-1}$
>10 kg–4 years	Triclofos + Alimemazine	$100\,\text{mg}\,\text{kg}^{-1}$ (maximum 2 g) $1\,\text{mg}\,\text{kg}^{-1}$ (maximum 30 mg)
Over 4 years	Consider oral sedation as above or general anaesthetic	

Children should have nothing to eat or drink prior to sedation as follows:

1. *Breast fed only*: Last feed 2 hours before sedation
2. *Under 1 year or on formula, or weaning onto a soft diet*: Last feed/ milk 4 h before sedation, but can have clear fluids up to 2 h before
3. *Over 1 year*: Light meal, such as fruit juice, milk, toast or cereal 4 h before sedation, clear fluids up to 2 h before sedation.

Complications

Early recognition and treatment of complications is essential to reduce morbidity and mortality from sedation in all patients.

Minor complications include:

1. syncope
2. phlebitis
3. emesis
4. agitation
5. rash.

Major complications are rare, but include:

1. bradycardia
2. hypotension
3. hypoxia
4. death.

Sedation causes a reduction in muscle tone of the oropharynx and at deeper levels of sedation the glottic reflexes may fail. Major complications of sedation are most often due to airway obstruction and respiratory depression. The following patient groups are at high risk:

1. *Elderly patients*. Old age is an independent risk factor for sedation. The effects of sedative drugs are more pronounced and prolonged in the elderly. Small incremental doses of sedatives are required.
2. *Chronic obstructive pulmonary disease*. These patients have a blunted ventilator drive. Supine position impairs chest wall function and oxygenation. Patients may need supplemental oxygen and bronchodilators. Local anaesthesia should be used for pain whenever possible and sedative drugs should be used sparingly.
3. *Coronary artery disease*. Under-sedation will increase cardiac oxygen demand but over-sedation can cause hypotension, hypoxaemia and decrease myocardial oxygen delivery leading to myocardial ischaemia. Patients should be given supplemental oxygen.
4. *Hepatic dysfunction or renal failure*. Altered drug metabolism in renal and liver disease increases the risk of overdose when

using opioids and benzodiazepines. These drugs should be used in reduced doses.

In children, similarly, Triclofos should be avoided in those with end-stage liver failure and used with caution in cholestasis. In renal impairment dose reduction should be considered.

5. *Drug addicts*. These patients may exhibit unpredictable requirements and drug-seeking behaviour. Local anaesthetics and short-acting benzodiazepines are preferred, reversal agents should be avoided.

References

1. Royal College of Radiologists (2003) *Safe Sedation, Analgesia and Anaesthesia within the Radiology Department*. London: The Royal College of Radiologists.
2. Martin, M.L. & Lennox, P.H. (2003) Sedation and analgesia in the interventional radiology department. *J. Vasc. Interv. Radiol.* **14(9 Pt 1)**, 1119–1128.
3. Royal College of Radiologists/Royal College of Anaesthetists joint publication (1992) *Sedation and Anaesthesia in Radiology*. London: The Royal College of Radiologists.

Further reading

Shabanie, A. (2006) Conscious sedation for interventional radiology procedures: a practical guide. *Tech. Vasc. Interv. Radiol.* **9(2)**, 84–88.
Sury, M.R., Harker, H., Begent, J., et al. (2005) The management of infants and children for painless imaging. *Clin. Radiol.* **60(7)**, 731–741.

MONITORING

Monitoring should be used:

1. in all patients receiving any form of sedation
2. for those at risk of haemorrhage
3. in any prolonged or complicated procedure.

The purpose is to observe and assess response of the patient to any psychological or physiological stress imposed by the procedure or sedative agents administered and allow appropriate therapeutic action to be taken.

Equipment

1. *Pulse oximetry*. Pulse oximetry is the most sensitive monitoring method to detect hypoxaemia. It is the minimum requirement for safe monitoring and may suffice as the sole monitoring

device in the young and fit. It accurately measures the oxygen saturation of blood and provides information on pulse rate and adequacy of the circulation. The oxygen saturation should be maintained at or above 95%. Most pulse oximeters have a short lag time in demonstrating desaturation. Due to the nature of the oxygen dissociation curve, patients may rapidly desaturate from 90% to 70%. Oxygen saturation of 90% is an emergency and corrective action should be taken immediately. The pulse oximeter signal may be affected by interference from nail polish, light, movement and cold extremities.

2. *Electrocardiograph.* A continuous electrocardiography monitor will provide information on pulse rate and rhythm, presence of arrhythmia and signs of ischaemia, but does not monitor circulation or cardiac output.

3. *Automated blood pressure monitor.* Minimum acceptable mean arterial pressure is 60 mmHg, but patients with cardiac disease or hypertension require higher pressures. False high arterial pressure readings are obtained with cuffs which are too small. Manual blood pressure measurements are inconvenient and inconsistent. The blood pressure monitor may impede function of the pulse oximeter so should not be on the same arm. The monitor should be set to 5 min recording intervals; nerve damage has been reported with prolonged use.

Monitor alarms may be the first signal of an adverse event and should not be silenced. If there is any doubt repeat measurement should be performed.

Technique

Monitoring should include assessment of:

1. the patient's level of consciousness
2. ability to maintain airway
3. adequacy of respiratory function – respiratory rate and pattern
4. adequacy of cardiac function – pulse and skin colour
5. pain level
6. side-effects or complications of any drugs administered
7. hydration and urine output during prolonged procedures.

The patient should be monitored by a trained professional who should have no other role at the time of the procedure than to continuously monitor these parameters. The radiologist performing the procedure should not monitor the patient.

Vital signs (pulse, blood pressure and respiratory rate) should be regularly measured. Any adverse events must be fully recorded in the patient's notes. Monitoring should continue into the recovery period.

18

SEDATION AND MONITORING FOR MAGNETIC RESONANCE IMAGING

Sedation should be given in a quiet area close to the scanner and there should be an appropriate recovery area available.

The MRI scan room is a challenging environment in which to monitor the patient. The scanner is noisy, potentially claustrophobic and any patient inside the scanner is relatively inaccessible.

All equipment used for monitoring and all anaesthetic equipment must be MR compatible, e.g. MR compatible pulse oximeters with fibre-optic cabling. Potential problems include effects from the gradient field and radiofrequency fields. Heat induction in conducting loops formed by ECG leads can cause superficial burns and induced current in monitoring equipment may produce unreliable readings or malfunction of syringe drivers resulting in incorrect drug-dose delivery (see Chapter 1). Responsibility for safe use of MRI monitoring equipment should be allocated to a small number of experienced and appropriately trained staff.

Further reading
Berlin, L. (2001) Sedation and analgesia in MR imaging. *Am. J. Roentgenol.* **177(2)**, 293–296.

RECOVERY AND DISCHARGE CRITERIA

The effects of most agents used for sedation and analgesia last longer than the duration of the procedure; therefore, monitoring of the patient must continue into the recovery period. Once the patient is alert and orientated and vital signs have returned to their baseline values or acceptable levels, the patient can be considered fit to be moved from the radiology department. The overall responsibility for the patient's care until discharge is with the consultant radiologist or main operator and every unit should have written guidelines for discharge criteria.

Medical emergencies

Medical emergencies occurring in the radiology department may be due to:

1. medication or radiographic contrast given
2. procedure-related complications
3. deterioration of pre-existing morbidities.

Patients may develop cardiac arrhythmias, hypotension, inadequate ventilation or adverse drug/radiographic contrast reactions. Complications arise from sedative drug administration, invasive procedures and human error; poor monitoring and organizational failings may contribute.

If a complication occurs, rapid recognition of the problem and effective management are essential. A call must be made to summon the hospital medical emergency or cardiac arrest team for any medical emergency event that is not immediately reversed or if ongoing care will be required.

The basic principles are summarized in the ABC of resuscitating the acutely ill patient:

A. Airway – ensuring a patent airway
B. Breathing – providing supplemental oxygen and adequate ventilation
C. Circulation – restoration of circulating volume.

These early interventions should proceed in parallel with diagnosis and definitive treatment of the underlying cause. If cardiac arrest is suspected, the adult advanced life support algorithm in Figure 19.1 should be followed.

EQUIPMENT

A resuscitation trolley, which is regularly checked, should be kept in the radiology department and contain:

1. a defibrillator
2. a positive pressure breathing device (Ambu bag) and mask
3. supplemental oxygen and oxygen delivery devices
4. suction equipment

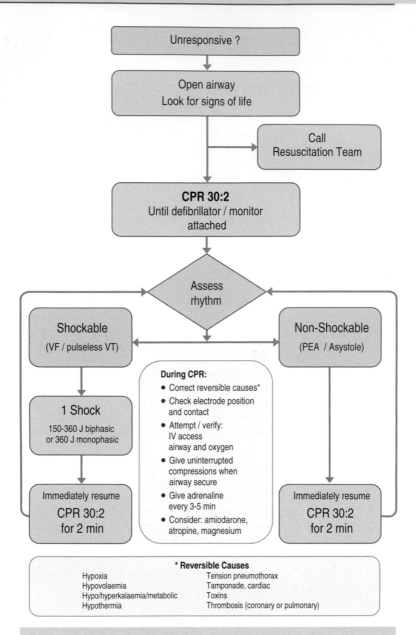

Figure 19.1 Adult Advanced Life Support Algorithm. Reproduced by kind permission of the Resuscitation Council (UK).

5. an intubation tray with airways, laryngoscopes and endotracheal tubes
6. intravenous (i.v.) cannulas and i.v. fluids
7. drugs:
   a. sedative reversal drugs including naloxone and flumazenil
   b. resuscitation drugs including adrenaline, atropine and hydrocortisone
8. pulse oximeter
9. non-invasive blood pressure device and appropriately sized cuffs
10. an electrocardiograph.

19

RESPIRATORY EMERGENCIES

In all cases it is essential to call for urgent anaesthetic assistance if the medical emergency event is not immediately reversed.

RESPIRATORY DEPRESSION

Sedative and analgesic drugs can cause depression of respiratory drive and compromise of the airway leading to hypoxia and hypercapnia. The clinical signs are:

1. decreased, shallow, laboured breathing
2. decreased oxygen saturations
3. in partial airway obstruction, snoring and paradoxical chest wall movement.

The patient should immediately be placed in the supine position. If the airway is compromised it should be maintained by opening the mouth, tilting and extending the head, and lifting the chin. Supplemental oxygen must be provided. If respiratory depression is due to sedative drugs then reversal agents should be considered.

LARYNGOSPASM

This is airway obstruction due to tonic contractions of laryngeal and pharyngeal muscles. Risk factors include excessive secretions and mechanical irritation:

1. In partial obstruction stridor will be present. Partial airway obstruction can be treated with oxygen, coughing and calming measures.
2. In complete obstruction there will be chest wall but no air movement. Immediate anaesthetic assistance is required.

BRONCHOSPASM

This is constriction of bronchial airways by increased smooth muscle tone leading to small-airway obstruction. Risk factors are preexisting asthma, airway irritation, histamine release and smoking. The signs include:

1. wheeze
2. tachypnoea and dyspnoea
3. decreased oxygen saturations
4. use of accessory respiratory muscles
5. tachycardia
6. silent chest.

Treatment includes high flow oxygen, nebulized salbutamol 2.5–5 mg, nebulized ipratropium bromide 0.25–0.5 mg and i.v. hydrocortisone 100–200 mg.

ASPIRATION OF BLOOD OR GASTRIC CONTENTS INTO THE LUNGS

This occurs when protective reflexes are lost and, if severe, can cause hypoxia, requiring mechanical ventilation. Risk factors are:

1. post-procedure nausea and vomiting
2. obesity
3. hiatus hernia
4. non-adherence to fasting guidelines.

The patient should be placed on their side in the head down position, high-flow oxygen should be administered, airway adjuncts should be removed and the airway suctioned.

PNEUMOTHORAX

This is likely to be related to a procedure such as lung biopsy. Presentation is with unilateral pleuritic chest pain and dyspnoea:

1. For asymptomatic small pneumothorax the patient should be observed.
2. For symptomatic small pneumothorax simple aspiration should be performed and the patient subsequently observed.
3. If the pneumothorax is >2 cm in depth (which is equivalent to 49% of the volume of the hemithorax) an intercostal chest drain should be inserted.
4. If the dyspnoea increases rapidly and the patient becomes cyanosed, tension pneumothorax should be suspected and air should be aspirated immediately by insertion of a 16G cannula through the second intercostal space in the mid-clavicular line.

CARDIOVASCULAR EMERGENCIES

In all cases it is essential to call for urgent anaesthetic assistance if the medical emergency event is not immediately reversed.

HYPOTENSION

This is defined as a fall of greater than 25% from the patient's pre-procedure systolic blood pressure. Hypotension may be a manifestation of shock, which is a state of circulatory failure resulting in inadequate tissue perfusion to vital organs. The signs of hypotension are pallor, faints, tachycardia, a reduction in capillary refill and oliguria. The common causes are:

1. pharmacological vasodilatation
2. myocardial depression
3. hypovolaemia due to procedure-related haemorrhage or haematoma
4. sepsis
5. vasovagal event.

The treatment depends on cause; pressure should be applied to any developing haematoma, the patient placed in the Trendelenburg position and oxygen administered. In the case of haemorrhage or haematoma, normal blood pressure will not be achievable until bleeding is controlled. For treatment of hypotension, i.v. fluid such as Hartmann's solution should initially be given as a 500 ml bolus and the patient immediately re-assessed.

TACHYCARDIA

This is classified as a heart rate greater than 100 beats per min and is associated with stimulation of the sympathetic nervous system due to:

1. under-sedation
2. pain
3. hypotension
4. hypoxia.

Heart rates of up to 160 beats per min are generally well tolerated, but tachycardia-induced hypotension or myocardial ischaemia require urgent treatment.

BRADYCARDIA

This is classified as a heart rate less than 60 beats per min and may be due to sedative depressant effect, vasovagal or secondary to hypoxia or pain. Management is as follows:

19

1. If the patient is non-symptomatic, monitor closely.
2. If hypotension or bradycardia <40 beats per min is present an anticholinergic drug such as atropine 0.3–0.6 mg may be given i.v.
3. If the patient develops asystole or ventricular fibrillation then confirm diagnosis – unconscious, apnoeic, absent carotid pulse. Call for help, defibrillator and cardiac arrest team, and follow the advanced life support algorithm outlined in Figure 19.1.

ADVERSE DRUG REACTIONS

CONTRAST MEDIA REACTION

This is also discussed in detail in Chapter 2. Suggested management is as follows:

1. Nausea/vomiting – patient reassurance. Retain i.v. access and observe
2. Urticaria – retain i.v. access and observe. If troublesome give an antihistamine by slow i.v. injection, e.g. chlorphenamine maleate 10–20 mg. If severe urticaria add i.v. hydrocortisone 100 mg
3. Hypotension with bradycardia (vasovagal reaction)
4. Mild wheeze (see above)
5. Anaphylaxis – rare, most often mild, but may be life threatening. Iodinated i.v. contrast media are the commonest cause of anaphylaxis in the radiology department; however, other possible causes include gadolinium agents, opioid drugs, antibiotics, aspirin, latex and local anaesthetics. Anaphylaxis is a hypersensitivity reaction which causes a range of symptoms and signs including: oedema of face and airway, wheeze, cyanosis, tachycardia, hypotension, erythema and urticaria. Anaphylaxis is likely when all of the following three criteria are met:
   a. Sudden onset and rapid progression of symptoms
   b. Life-threatening Airway ± Breathing ± Circulation problems
   c. Skin or mucosal changes (flushing, urticaria, angio-oedema)
   However, it should be noted that skin or mucosal changes alone do not indicate anaphylactic reaction and that these changes are subtle or absent in up to 20% of anaphylactic reactions. The recommended management plan for anaphylaxis is the UK Resuscitation Council algorithm in Figure 19.2
5. Unconscious/unresponsive/pulseless/collapse – see Figure 19.1.

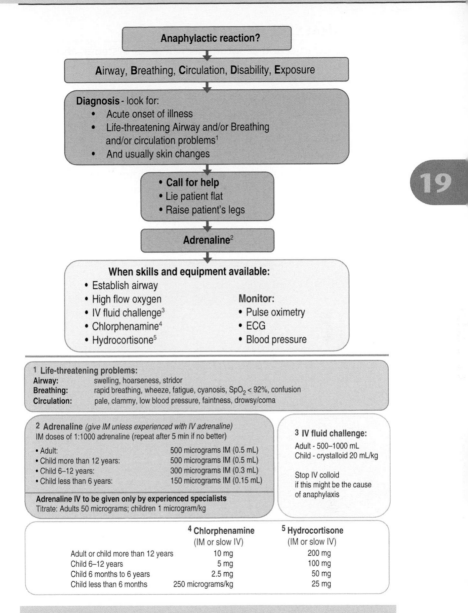

Anaphylactic reaction?

↓

Airway, **B**reathing, **C**irculation, **D**isability, **E**xposure

↓

Diagnosis - look for:
- Acute onset of illness
- Life-threatening Airway and/or Breathing and/or circulation problems[1]
- And usually skin changes

↓

- **Call for help**
- Lie patient flat
- Raise patient's legs

↓

Adrenaline[2]

↓

When skills and equipment available:
- Establish airway
- High flow oxygen
- IV fluid challenge[3]
- Chlorphenamine[4]
- Hydrocortisone[5]

Monitor:
- Pulse oximetry
- ECG
- Blood pressure

---

1 Life-threatening problems:

Airway:	swelling, hoarseness, stridor
Breathing:	rapid breathing, wheeze, fatigue, cyanosis, $SpO_2 < 92\%$, confusion
Circulation:	pale, clammy, low blood pressure, faintness, drowsy/coma

2 Adrenaline *(give IM unless experienced with IV adrenaline)*
IM doses of 1:1000 adrenaline (repeat after 5 min if no better)

- Adult: 500 micrograms IM (0.5 mL)
- Child more than 12 years: 500 micrograms IM (0.5 mL)
- Child 6–12 years: 300 micrograms IM (0.3 mL)
- Child less than 6 years: 150 micrograms IM (0.15 mL)

Adrenaline IV to be given only by experienced specialists
Titrate: Adults 50 micrograms; children 1 microgram/kg

3 IV fluid challenge:
Adult - 500–1000 mL
Child - crystalloid 20 mL/kg

Stop IV colloid
if this might be the cause
of anaphylaxis

	4 Chlorphenamine (IM or slow IV)	**5 Hydrocortisone** (IM or slow IV)
Adult or child more than 12 years	10 mg	200 mg
Child 6–12 years	5 mg	100 mg
Child 6 months to 6 years	2.5 mg	50 mg
Child less than 6 months	250 micrograms/kg	25 mg

Figure 19.2 Anaphylaxis Algorithm. Reproduced by kind permission of the Resuscitation Council (UK).

LOCAL ANAESTHETIC TOXICITY

Accidental i.v. injection of local anaesthetic or systemic absorption can result in toxicity due to membrane effects on the heart and central nervous system:

1. Early signs of toxicity are tingling around mouth and tongue, light headedness, agitation and tremor.
2. More severe reactions include sudden loss of consciousness, with or without tonic-clonic convulsions and cardiovascular collapse.

The immediate management includes stopping injection, calling for help, maintaining airway (including securing the airway with intubation if required), 100% oxygen, ensuring adequate i.v. access, ventilator and cardiovascular support, and control of seizures. In the event of a cardiac arrest, resuscitation should be prolonged.

Appendix I

Dose limits – the Ionising Radiation Regulations 1999[1]

Body part etc	Dose limit (mSv)			
	Employees 18 years or over	Special circumstances[#]	Trainees aged under 18 years	Other persons (including any person below 16 years)
Effective dose in any calendar year	20	50 (not more than 100 mSv averaged over 5 years)	6	1 (5*)
Equivalent dose for the skin in a calendar year as applied to the dose averaged over any area of 1 cm^2, regardless of the area exposed. Equivalent dose for hands, forearms, feet and ankles in a calendar year	500	500	150	50
Equivalent dose for the lens of the eye in a calendar year	150	150	50	15
Equivalent dose for the abdomen of a woman of	13	13	n/a	n/a

Continued

Body part etc	Dose limit (mSv)			
	Employees 18 years or over	Special circumstances[#]	Trainees aged under 18 years	Other persons (including any person below 16 years)
reproductive capacity at work, being the equivalent dose from exposure to ionizing radiation averaged throughout the abdomen in any consecutive 3-monthly period				

[#]If an employer demonstrates to the Health and Safety Executive (HSE) that it cannot meet the 20 mSv/calendar year limit. It may apply this limit after notifying HSE, the employees concerned and the approved dosimetry service.

*The dose limit for persons who are exposed to ionizing radiation from a medical exposure of another person but are not 'comforters or carers'[2] is 5 mSv in any period of 5 consecutive calendar years.

References
1. Crown copyright 1999 with the permission of the Controller of Her Majesty's Stationery Office.
2. A 'comforter and carer' is defined in IRR 99 as an individual who (other than as part of his occupation) knowingly and willingly incurs an exposure to ionizing radiation resulting from the support and comfort of another person who is undergoing or who has undergone any medical exposure.

Appendix II

Average effective dose equivalents for some common examinations

Examination	Effective dose equivalent (mSv)	Miles travelled by car*	Equivalent period of natural background radiation	Probability of radiation effect occurring ($\times 10^{-6}$) (fatal somatic)	
				Male	Female
Chest (PA)	0.02	50	3 days	0.27	0.47
Skull	0.1	250	2 weeks	1.7	1.7
Cervical spine	0.1	250	2 weeks		
Thoracic spine	1.0	2500	6 months	7.0	11
Lumbar spine	2.4	5000	14 months	25	26
Hip (1 only)	0.3	750	2 months		
Pelvis	1.0	2500	6 months	3.9	3.9
Abdomen	1.5	3750	9 months	9.4	9.5
Extremity (e.g. hand, foot)	<0.01	<25	<1.5 days		

Barium
  Meal
  Small bowel
  Large bowel
	
	5.0
	6.0
	9.0
		
		12500
		15000
		22500
			
			2.5 years
			3 years
			4.5 years
				
				26
				
				37
					
					31
					
					38

i.v. urography	4.6	11500	2.5 years	26	37

Continued

Examination	Effective dose equivalent (mSv)	Miles travelled by car*	Equivalent period of natural background radiation	Probability of radiation effect occurring ($\times 10^{-6}$) (fatal somatic)	
				Male	Female
Computed tomography					
Head	2.0	5000	1 year	62	69
Chest	8.0	20000	4 years	330	370
Abdomen	8.0	20000	4 years	330	370

*ICRP 60.

Appendix III

The Ionising Radiation (Medical Exposure) Regulations 2000[1]

These Regulations, together with the Ionising Radiations Regulations 1999 (S.I. 1999/3232) partially implement, as respects Great Britain, Council Directive 97/43/Euratom (OJ No. L180, 9.7.97, p. 22) laying down basic measures for the health protection of individuals against dangers of ionizing radiation in relation to medical exposure. The regulations impose duties on those responsible for administering ionizing radiation to protect persons undergoing medical exposure whether as part of their own medical diagnosis or treatment or as part of occupational health surveillance, health screening, voluntary participation in research or medico-legal procedures.

They replaced The Ionising Radiation (Protection of Persons Undergoing Medical Examination or Treatment) Regulations 1988.

1. Commencement

These regulations came into force:

a. except for regulation 4(1) and 4(2) on 13 May 2000;
b. as regards regulation 4(1) and 4(2) on 1 January 2001.

2. Glossary of [some of the] terms

adequate training means training which satisfies the requirements of Schedule 2; and the expression *adequately trained* shall be similarly construed;

appropriate authority means the Secretary of State as regards England, the National Assembly for Wales as regards Wales, or the Scottish Ministers as regards Scotland;

child means a person under the age of 18 in England and Wales or a person under the age of 16 in Scotland;

clinical audit means a systematic examination or review of medical radiological procedures which seeks to improve the quality and the outcome of patient care through structured review whereby radiological practices, procedures and results are examined against agreed standards for good medical radiological procedures, intended to lead to modification of practices where indicated and the application of new standards if necessary;

diagnostic reference levels means dose levels in medical radiodiagnostic practices or, in the case of radioactive medicinal products, levels of activity, for typical examinations for groups of standard-sized patients or standard phantoms for broadly defined types of equipment;

dose constraint means a restriction on the prospective doses to individuals which may result from a defined source;

the Directive means Council Directive 97/43/Euratom laying down measures on health protection of individuals against the dangers of ionizing radiation in relation to medical exposure;

employer means any natural or legal person who, in the course of a trade, business or other undertaking, carries out (other than as an employee), or engages others to carry out, medical exposures or practical aspects, at a given radiological installation;

employer's procedures means the procedures established by an employer pursuant to regulation 4(1);

equipment means equipment which delivers ionizing radiation to a person undergoing a medical exposure and equipment which directly controls or influences the extent of such exposure;

individual detriment means clinically observable deleterious effects that are expressed in individuals or their descendants the appearance of which is either immediate or delayed and, in the latter case, implies a probability rather than a certainty of appearance;

ionizing radiation means the transfer of energy in the form of particles or electromagnetic waves of a wavelength of 100 nanometres or less or a frequency of 3×10^{15} hertz or more capable of producing ions directly or indirectly;

medical exposure means any exposure to which regulation 3 applies and which involves an individual being exposed to ionizing radiation;

medical physics expert means a person who holds a science degree or its equivalent and who is experienced in the application of physics to the diagnostic and therapeutic uses of ionizing radiation;

medico-legal procedure means a procedure performed for insurance or legal purposes without a medical indication;

operator means any person who is entitled, in accordance with the employer's procedures, to carry out practical aspects including those to whom practical aspects have been allocated pursuant to regulation 5(3), medical physics experts as referred to in regulation 9 and, except where they do so under the direct supervision of a person who is adequately trained, persons participating in practical aspects as part of practical training as referred to in regulation 11(3);

patient dose means the dose concerning patients or other individuals undergoing medical exposure;

practical aspect means the physical conduct of any of the exposures referred to in regulation 3 and any supporting aspects including handling and use of radiological equipment, and the assessment of technical and physical parameters including radiation doses, calibration and maintenance of equipment, preparation and administration of radioactive medicinal products and the development of films;

practitioner means a registered medical practitioner, dental practitioner or other health professional who is entitled in accordance with the employer's procedures to take responsibility for an individual medical exposure;

quality assurance means any planned and systematic action necessary to provide adequate confidence that a structure, system, component or procedure will perform satisfactorily and safely complying with agreed standards and includes quality control;

quality control means the set of operations (programming, coordinating, implementing) intended to maintain or to improve quality and includes monitoring, evaluation and maintenance at required levels of performance;

radioactive medicinal product has the meaning given in the Medicines (Administration of Radioactive Substances) Regulations 1978;

referrer means a registered medical practitioner, dental practitioner or other health professional who is entitled in accordance with the employer's procedures to refer individuals for medical exposure to a practitioner.

3. These Regulations apply to the following medical exposures:

a. the exposure of patients as part of their own medical diagnosis or treatment;

b. the exposure of individuals as part of occupational health surveillance;

c. the exposure of individuals as part of health screening programmes;

d. the exposure of patients or other persons voluntarily participating in medical or biomedical, diagnostic or therapeutic, research programmes;

e. the exposure of individuals as part of medico-legal procedures.

4. Duties of the Employer

1. The employer shall ensure that written procedures for medical exposures including the procedures set out in Schedule 1 are in place and:

a. shall take steps to ensure that they are complied with by the practitioner and operator; or

b. where the employer is concurrently practitioner or operator, he shall comply with these procedures himself.

2. The employer shall ensure that written protocols are in place for every type of standard radiological practice for each equipment.

3. The employer shall establish:

   a. recommendations concerning referral criteria for medical exposures, including radiation doses, and shall ensure that these are available to the referrer;

   b. quality assurance programmes for standard operating procedures;

   c. diagnostic reference levels for radiodiagnostic examinations falling within regulation 3(a), (b), (c) and (e) having regard to European diagnostic reference levels where available;

   d. dose constraints for biomedical and medical research programmes falling within regulation 3(d) where no direct medical benefit for the individual is expected from the exposure.

4. The employer shall take steps to ensure that every practitioner or operator engaged by the employer to carry out medical exposures or any practical aspect of such exposures:

   a. complies with the provisions of regulation 11(1); and

   b. undertakes continuing education and training after qualification including, in the case of clinical use of new techniques, training related to these techniques and the relevant radiation protection requirements; or

   c. where the employer is concurrently practitioner or operator, he shall himself ensure that he undertakes such continuing education and training as may be appropriate.

5. Where the employer knows or has reason to believe that an incident has or may have occurred in which a person, while undergoing a medical exposure was, otherwise than as a result of a malfunction or defect in equipment, exposed to ionizing radiation to an extent much greater than intended, he shall make an immediate preliminary investigation of the incident and, unless that investigation shows beyond a reasonable doubt that no such overexposure has occurred, he shall forthwith notify the appropriate authority and make or arrange for a detailed investigation of the circumstances of the exposure and an assessment of the dose received.

6. The employer shall undertake appropriate reviews whenever diagnostic reference levels are consistently exceeded and ensure that corrective action is taken where appropriate.

5. Duties of the Practitioner, Operator and Referrer

1. The practitioner and the operator shall comply with the employer's procedures.
2. The practitioner shall be responsible for the justification of a medical exposure and such other aspects of a medical exposure as is provided for in these Regulations.
3. Practical aspects of a medical exposure or part of it may be allocated in accordance with the employer's procedures by the employer or the practitioner, as appropriate, to one or more individuals entitled to act in this respect in a recognized field of specialization.
4. The operator shall be responsible for each and every practical aspect which he carries out as well as for any authorization given pursuant to regulation 6(5) where such authorization is not made in accordance with the guidelines referred to in regulation 6(5).
5. The referrer shall supply the practitioner with sufficient medical data (such as previous diagnostic information or medical records) relevant to the medical exposure requested by the referrer to enable the practitioner to decide on whether there is a sufficient net benefit as required by regulation 6(1)(a).
6. The practitioner and the operator shall cooperate, regarding practical aspects, with other specialists and staff involved in a medical exposure, as appropriate.
7. For the avoidance of doubt, where a person acts as employer, referrer, practitioner and operator concurrently (or in any combination of these roles) he shall comply with all the duties placed on employers, referrers, practitioners or operators under these Regulations accordingly.

6 Justification of Individual Medical Exposures

1. No person shall carry out a medical exposure unless:
   a. it has been justified by the practitioner as showing a sufficient net benefit giving appropriate weight to the matters set out in paragraph (2); and
   b. it has been authorized by the practitioner or, where paragraph (5) applies, the operator; and
   c. in the case of a medical or biomedical exposure as referred to in regulation 3(d), it has been approved by a Local Research Ethics Committee; and
   d. in the case of an exposure falling within regulation 3(e), it complies with the employer's procedures for such exposures; and
   e. in the case of a female of child-bearing age, he has enquired whether she is pregnant or breast feeding, if relevant.

2. The matters referred to in paragraph (1)(a) are:
   a. the specific objectives of the exposure and the characteristics of the individual involved;
   b. the total potential diagnostic or therapeutic benefits, including the direct health benefits to the individual and the benefits to society, of the exposure;
   c. the individual detriment that the exposure may cause; and
   d. the efficacy, benefits and risk of available alternative techniques having the same objective but involving no or less exposure to ionizing radiation.
3. In considering the weight to be given to the matters referred to in paragraph (2), the practitioner justifying an exposure pursuant to paragraph (1)(a) shall pay special attention to:
   a. exposures on medico-legal grounds;
   b. exposures that have no direct health benefit for the individuals undergoing the exposure; and
   c. the urgency of the exposure, where appropriate, in cases involving:
      i. a female where pregnancy cannot be excluded, in particular if abdominal and pelvic regions are involved, taking into account the exposure of both the expectant mother and the unborn child; and
      ii. a female who is breast feeding and who undergoes a nuclear medicine exposure, taking into account the exposure of both the female and the child.
4. In deciding whether to justify an exposure under paragraph (1)(a) the practitioner shall take account of any data supplied by the referrer pursuant to regulation 5(5) and shall consider such data in order to avoid unnecessary exposure.
5. Where it is not practicable for the practitioner to authorize an exposure as required by paragraph (1)(b), the operator shall do so in accordance with guidelines issued by the practitioner.

7. Optimization

1. In relation to all medical exposures to which these Regulations apply except radiotherapeutic procedures, the practitioner and the operator, to the extent of their respective involvement in a medical exposure, shall ensure that doses arising from the exposure are kept as low as reasonably practicable consistent with the intended purpose.
2. In relation to all medical exposures for radiotherapeutic purposes the practitioner shall ensure that exposures of target volumes are individually planned, taking into account that doses of non-target volumes and tissues shall be as low as reasonably practicable and consistent with the intended radiotherapeutic purpose of the exposure.

3. Without prejudice to paragraphs (1) and (2), the operator shall select equipment and methods to ensure that for each medical exposure the dose of ionizing radiation to the individual undergoing the exposure is as low as reasonably practicable and consistent with the intended diagnostic or therapeutic purpose and in doing so shall pay special attention to:
   a. quality assurance;
   b. assessment of patient dose or administered activity; and
   c. adherence to diagnostic reference levels for radiodiagnostic examinations falling within regulation 3(a), (b), (c) and (e) as set out in the employer's procedures.
4. For each medical or biomedical research programme falling within regulation 3(d), the employer's procedures shall provide that:
   a. the individuals concerned participate voluntarily in the research programme;
   b. the individuals concerned are informed in advance about the risks of the exposure;
   c. the dose constraint set down in the employer's procedures for individuals for whom no direct medical benefit is expected from the exposure is adhered to; and
   d. individual target levels of doses are planned by the practitioner for patients who voluntarily undergo an experimental diagnostic or therapeutic practice from which the patients are expected to receive a diagnostic or therapeutic benefit.
5. In the case of patients undergoing treatment or diagnosis with radioactive medicinal products, the employer's procedures shall provide that, where appropriate, written instructions and information are provided to:
   a. the patient, where he has capacity to consent to the treatment or diagnostic procedure; or
   b. where the patient is a child who lacks capacity so to consent, the person with parental responsibility for the child; or
   c. where the patient is an adult who lacks capacity so to consent, the person who appears to the practitioner to be the most appropriate person.
6. The instructions and information referred to in paragraph (5) shall:
   a. specify how doses resulting from the patient's exposure can be restricted as far as reasonably possible so as to protect persons in contact with the patient;
   b. set out the risks associated with ionizing radiation; and
   c. be provided to the patient or other person specified in paragraph (5) as appropriate prior to the patient leaving the hospital or other place where the medical exposure was carried out.

III

7. In complying with the obligations under this regulation, the practitioner and the operator shall pay special attention to:
   a. the need to keep doses arising from medico-legal exposures as low as reasonably practicable;
   b. medical exposures of children;
   c. medical exposures as part of a health screening programme;
   d. medical exposures involving high doses to the patient;
   e. where appropriate, females in whom pregnancy cannot be excluded and who are undergoing a medical exposure, in particular if abdominal and pelvic regions are involved, taking into account the exposure of both the expectant mother and the unborn child; and
   f. where appropriate, females who are breast feeding and who are undergoing exposures in nuclear medicine, taking into account the exposure of both the female and the child.
8. The employer shall take steps to ensure that a clinical evaluation of the outcome of each medical exposure, is recorded in accordance with the employer's procedures or, where the employer is concurrently practitioner or operator, shall so record a clinical evaluation, including, where appropriate, factors relevant to patient dose.
9. In the case of fluoroscopy:
   a. the operator shall ensure that examinations without devices to control the dose rate are limited to justified circumstances; and
   b. no person shall carry out an examination without an image intensification or equivalent technique.

8. Clinical Audit

The employer's procedures shall include provision for the carrying out of clinical audit as appropriate.

9. Expert advice

1. The employer shall ensure that a medical physics expert shall be involved in every medical exposure to which these Regulations apply in accordance with paragraph (2).
2. A medical physics expert shall be:
   a. closely involved in every radiotherapeutic practice other than standardized therapeutic nuclear medicine practices;
   b. available in standardized therapeutic nuclear medicine practices and in diagnostic nuclear medicine practices;
   c. involved as appropriate for consultation on optimization, including patient dosimetry and quality assurance, and to give advice on matters relating to radiation protection concerning medical exposure, as required, in all other radiological practices.

10. Equipment

1. The employer shall draw up, keep up-to-date and preserve at each radiological installation an inventory of equipment at that installation and, when so requested, shall furnish it to the appropriate authority.
2. The inventory referred to in paragraph (1) shall contain the following information:
   a. name of manufacturer,
   b. model number,
   c. serial number or other unique identifier,
   d. year of manufacture, and
   e. year of installation.
3. The employer shall ensure that equipment at each radiological installation is limited to the amount necessary for the proper carrying out of medical exposures at that installation.

11. Training

1. Subject to the following provisions of this regulation no practitioner or operator shall carry out a medical exposure or any practical aspect without having been adequately trained.
2. A certificate issued by an institute or person competent to award degrees or diplomas or to provide other evidence of training shall, if such certificate so attests, be sufficient proof that the person to whom it has been issued has been adequately trained.
3. Nothing in paragraph (1) above shall prevent a person from participating in practical aspects of the procedure as part of practical training if this is done under the supervision of a person who himself is adequately trained.
4. The employer shall keep and have available for inspection by the appropriate authority an up-to-date record of all practitioners and operators engaged by him to carry out medical exposures or any practical aspect of such exposures or, where the employer is concurrently practitioner or operator, of his own training, showing the date or dates on which training qualifying as adequate training was completed and the nature of the training.
5. Where the employer enters into a contract with another to engage a practitioner or operator otherwise employed by that other, the latter shall be responsible for keeping the records required by paragraph (4) and shall supply such records to the employer forthwith upon request.

12. Enforcement

1. The provisions of these Regulations shall be enforced as if they were health and safety regulations made under section 15 of the Health and Safety at Work etc. Act 1974 and, except as provided in paragraph (2), the provisions of that Act, as regards

enforcement and offences, shall apply for the purposes of these Regulations.

2. The enforcing authority for the purposes of these Regulations shall be the appropriate authority.

13. Defence of due diligence

In any proceedings against any person for an offence consisting of the contravention of these Regulations it shall be a defence for that person to show that he took all reasonable steps and exercised all due diligence to avoid committing the offence.

SCHEDULE 1

Regulation 4(1)

Employer's Procedures

The written procedures for medical exposures shall include:

a. procedures to identify correctly the individual to be exposed to ionizing radiation;

b. procedures to identify individuals entitled to act as referrer or practitioner or operator;

c. procedures to be observed in the case of medico-legal exposures;

d. procedures for making enquiries of females of child-bearing age to establish whether the individual is or may be pregnant or breast feeding;

e. procedures to ensure that quality assurance programmes are followed;

f. procedures for the assessment of patient dose and administered activity;

g. procedures for the use of diagnostic reference levels established by the employer for radiodiagnostic examinations falling within regulation 3(a), (b), (c) and (e), specifying that these are expected not to be exceeded for standard procedures when good and normal practice regarding diagnostic and technical performance is applied;

h. procedures for determining whether the practitioner or operator is required to effect one or more of the matters set out in regulation 7(4) including criteria on how to effect those matters and in particular procedures for the use of dose constraints established by the employer for biomedical and medical research programmes falling within regulation 3(d) where no direct medical benefit for the individual is expected from the exposure;

i. procedures for the giving of information and written instructions as referred to in regulation 7(5);

j. procedures for the carrying out and recording of an evaluation for each medical exposure including, where appropriate, factors relevant to patient dose;

k. procedures to ensure that the probability and magnitude of accidental or unintended doses to patients from radiological practices are reduced so far as reasonably practicable.

SCHEDULE 2
Regulation 2(1)
Adequate Training

Practitioners and operators shall have successfully completed training, including theoretical knowledge and practical experience, in:

i. such of the subjects detailed in section A as are relevant to their functions as practitioner or operator; and

ii. such of the subjects detailed in section B as are relevant to their specific area of practice.

A. Radiation production, radiation protection and statutory obligations relating to ionizing radiations

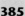

1. Fundamental Physics of Radiation
    1.1. Properties of radiation
        Attenuation of ionizing radiation
        Scattering and absorption
    1.2. Radiation hazards and dosimetry
        Biological effects of radiation
        Risks/benefits of radiation
        Dose optimization
        Absorbed dose, dose equivalent, effective dose and their units
    1.3. Special attention areas
        Pregnancy and potential pregnancy
        Infants and children
        Medical and biomedical research
        Health screening
        High dose techniques
2. Management and Radiation Protection of the Patient
    2.1. Patient selection
        Justification of the individual exposure
        Patient identification and consent
        Use of existing appropriate radiological information
        Alternative techniques
        Clinical evaluation of outcome
        Medico-legal issues
    2.2. Radiation protection
        General radiation protection
        Use of radiation protection devices

- patient
- personal
Procedures for untoward incidents involving
overexposure to ionizing radiation
3. Statutory Requirements and Advisory Aspects
   3.1. Statutory requirements and non-statutory
recommendations
Regulations
Local rules and procedures
Individual responsibilities relating to medical
exposures
Responsibility for radiation safety
Routine inspection and testing of equipment
Notification of faults and Health Department hazard
warnings
Clinical audit
B. Diagnostic radiology, radiotherapy and nuclear medicine
4. Diagnostic Radiology
   4.1. General
Fundamentals of radiological anatomy
Fundamentals of radiological techniques
Production of X-rays
Equipment selection and use
Factors affecting radiation dose
Dosimetry
Quality assurance and quality control
   4.2. Specialized techniques
Image intensification/fluoroscopy
Digital fluoroscopy
Computed tomography scanning
Interventional procedures
Vascular imaging
   4.3. Fundamentals of image acquisition etc.
Image quality vs. radiation dose
Conventional film processing
Additional image formats, acquisition, storage and
display
   4.4. Contrast media
Non-ionic and ionic
Use and preparation
Contra-indications to the use of contrast media
Use of automatic injection devices
5. Radiotherapy
   5.1. General
Production of ionizing radiations
Use of radiotherapy

    – benign disease
    – malignant disease
    – external beam
    – brachytherapy

  5.2. Radiobiological aspects for radiotherapy
    Fractionation
    Dose rate
    Radiosensitization
    Target volumes

  5.3. Practical aspects for radiotherapy
    Equipment
    Treatment planning

  5.4. Radiation protection specific to radiotherapy
    Side-effects – early and late
    Toxicity
    Assessment of efficacy

6. Nuclear Medicine

  6.1. General
    Atomic structure and radioactivity
    Radioactive decay
    The tracer principle
    Fundamentals of diagnostic use
    Fundamentals of therapeutic use
    – dose rate
    – fractionation
    – radiobiology aspects

  6.2. Principles of radiation detection, instrumentation and equipment
    Types of systems
    Image acquisition, storage and display
    Quality assurance and quality control

  6.3. Radiopharmaceuticals
    Calibration
    Working practices in the radiopharmacy
    Preparation of individual doses
    Documentation

  6.4. Radiation protection specific to nuclear medicine
    Conception, pregnancy and breast feeding
    Arrangements for radioactive patients
    Disposal procedures for radioactive waste

Reference

1. Crown copyright 2000. With the permission of the Controller of Her Majesty's Stationery Office.

Artifacts in Magnetic Resonance Imaging

Chemical shift

This is the most noticeable of the artifacts.

Protons in fat and water have different resonant frequencies. Signal arising from protons in fat will be interpreted as arriving from a different point along the frequency encoded read-out axis relative to signal from water. This difference will depend on the strength of the main magnetic field and will be more apparent at higher field strengths. Shift artifact will also be greater when the field gradient is less. Chemical shift artifact is most noticeable around the bladder, kidneys and vertebral endplates (regions with fat/water interfaces).

Motion

All motion – cardiac, CSF pulsation, gastrointestinal, respiratory and that due to blood vessel pulsation – causes artifact. This increases noise, edge blurring and streaking. Respiratory and cardiac artifact can be minimized by gating or compensation, but this adds significantly to the scan time. Peristalsis can be minimized by using relaxants such as glucagon. Blood flow produces signal loss as protons in arterial blood are moving rapidly and phase mismatches occur. Ghosting can occur, particularly noticeable in axial sections, in which faint images of blood vessels are seen at points distant from their true location in the phase encoded readout axis. Saturation radiofrequency (RF) pulses applied to tissue outside the region of interest can help reduce motion artifact.

Ferromagnetic

Ferromagnetic objects alter the T1 and T2 decay characteristics of the local magnetic environment and usually result in a signal void around the object. Non-ferromagnetic metals can induce similar though less marked artifact due to induced eddy currents.

Radiofrequency

Radiofrequency (RF) noise degrades MR images. Patient generated noise can occur due to eddy currents from thermal movement of ions. System-generated noise from coils or amplifiers may produce specific patterns such as herringbone artifact. Extrinsic RF may produce linear streaking and can arise from any malfunctioning electrical device, e.g. light bulb or leaking RF door seals.

Aliasing

If the field of view is smaller than the area of tissue excited, structures that are peripheral to the field of view will wrap around the image and be seen on the opposite edge.

Partial volume averaging

This is analogous to similar artifact occurring in CT. The signal intensity of any particular voxel is determined by the average signal intensity within it. Artifact due to partial volume averaging increases with the section thickness.

Further reading

Bernstein, M.A., Huston, J 3rd & Ward, H.A (2006) Imaging artifacts at 3.0 T. *J. Magn. Reson. Imaging* **24(4)**, 735–746.

McRobbie, D.W., Moore, E.A., Graves, M.J., et al. (2007) *MRI from Picture to Proton.* 2nd edn. Cambridge: Cambridge University Press; 79–107.

Mirowitz, S.A. (1999) MR imaging artifacts. Challenges and solutions. *Magn. Reson. Imaging Clin. N. Am.* **7(4)**, 717–732.

Index

Index

Index

Index